TAXI
CDG
JFK
PEK
LHR
I ♥ NY
Virginia Slims 120's
Charcoal

BIPOLAR BLONDE

A True Story of Suicide, Soulmates, and Starting Again

MORGAN HUTCHINSON

83 press

COVER ART BY DONALD ROBERTSON

83 Press
2323 2nd Avenue North
Birmingham, Alabama 35203
83press.com

ISBN 978-1-971708-00-3
Printed in China

DEDICATION

To my mom—who is my forever cheerleader, equal parts laughter and lifeline. You're always ready with a hug, a call, and, when truly necessary, Virginia Slims.

To my mother-in-law—who we miss every day, you welcomed me, a bipolar divorcée, with open arms and zero hesitation. Your kindness changed everything.

To my three incredible children—who inspire me every day to become the very best version of myself and who remind me, in a thousand quiet and beautiful ways, that my life matters. Mommy loves you one zillion times infinity.

And to Brett—who fell in love with me, manic and all, on the other end of a 10-inch pay phone cord in a place most people try to forget. I will love you forever.

A VERY IMPORTANT AUTHOR'S NOTE

This memoir, for lack of a better word, is 19 years in the making. A few more, if you count the years spent misdiagnosed, living it without a name. It's a window into my soul. The true story of a finite period, a mere six months, that changed everything. The months that almost ended my life, and somehow, in the end, saved it.

I was 27 years old when I received my official bipolar diagnosis. I'm 46 now. I've wanted to tell this story for a long time. But stories like this don't just ask to be told—they demand something of you. Strength. Distance. A willingness to return to places you barely survived the first time.

I'm not entirely sure I'm ready, even now. I'm not sure anyone ever is. Bipolar disorder is not a chapter you close. It's a day-by-day negotiation. But the subject of mental health is too important to keep hidden, too urgent to wait for perfect readiness. I'm sharing now because my story is not unique. It's one of thousands. The failures. The shame. The highs. The lows. The humiliation. The elation.

Too many people are still living in silence. Still carrying the weight of stigma. Still not getting the help they need because they don't feel safe enough to speak—and because too few are speaking for them. So, I thought, why not start with my own messy story? My uncomfortable truth. Maybe, it will open a door. Maybe, it will start a conversation. Better yet, maybe I can tell it in a way people will actually read.

A nonfiction book that moves like a novel. Because, if we're being honest, the clinical reads aren't cutting it. The stack of books I handed Brett, my husband, trying to explain what was happening to me in 2009, were not exactly compelling. Informative, yes. Human, not always.

For the last nine years, I've called myself an accidental designer as cofounder of Buru, a clothing brand Brett and I started together and continue to run as a family business in Los Angeles, California. I suppose, now, I can add accidental author to the list.

But this book, it's entirely me.

My perspective. My voice. Around 120,000 words, hand-typed from dozens of seats: bleachers at my kids' games, Comfort+ on Delta flights, the corner of my sofa, club chairs in hotel lobbies, and loungers by the pool. Written in the margins of a full life—running a business, raising three children, and loving Brett.

It's too important not to share. I'm over the stigma. Aren't you?

But here's the thing—I'm over the tiptoeing, too.

To live with the darkness, I've had to learn how to make light. And sometimes, that means making light of my situation, not of bipolar disorder itself, and never of mental illness as a whole, but of the edges that might otherwise swallow me.

You'll see terms like crazy, cuckoo's nest, manic, looney bin. They come easily to me now. Sometimes, the softer words are the harder ones to say. Even the title leans in—not just bipolar, but blonde. I'm Southern. I love hairspray. And in the summer of 2009, I really loved hair bleach.

Who am I kidding? I still do.

But truly, there are moments in this book that may be difficult for some readers. The subtitle hints at it, but it's not just the suicide attempts. There are threads of self-harm, eating disorders, religious tension, psychiatric wards, infidelity, even the indignities of institutional life.

If those feel too close, too heavy, you may want to move gently through certain pages.

But if you love New York City, friendships with history, first kisses, and high-velocity romance, then there's plenty here for you, too. Because this story, like most, isn't just one thing. It's the darkest chapter of my life. And also, unexpectedly, the beginning of everything, wrapped up in an unshakeable love story.

Threaded throughout this story are the friends who held me up, girls who knew me as a child or met me in college, walked beside me into adulthood, and never let go, even when I made it difficult. The kind of friends who protect you, tell you the truth, and stay anyway.

And alongside them, my family—supportive, complicated, and deeply human. The ones who loved me through it and still carry me in ways big and small.

Some of these moments are remembered through the lens of my 17-year-old self. They're earnest, reactive, and still forming. I felt everything as it happened, without the space that time eventually provides, and my voice carries that immediacy.

But time does what it does best. It heals. It teaches. It softens. It adds dimension where there was once only feeling, and it offers understanding where there was once confusion.

What may read as sharp in these pages was never meant to wound. It was simply honest, at the time. With distance, those same moments now live differently in me, held with more grace, more empathy, and a fuller appreciation for the people who were doing the best they could, just as I was.

I love my family, immediate and extended, deeply, broadly, and without reservation. That has never been the question. If anything, time has only expanded that love, giving it more room to hold both memory and understanding at once.

This is a story about growth as much as it is about truth, about how I saw things then, and how I come to see them later. From the outside, my life now looks . . . steady and whole, like it all worked out. A happy marriage. Three beautiful, healthy children. A business my husband and I built from the ground up that continues to grow in ways I once only imagined. But that is only the polished version of it.

This book is the behind-the-scenes glimpse of how messy it all started. And how that undercurrent, the one I once tried so hard to outrun, is still part of our everyday lives.

Bipolar doesn't end. It's managed. It's supported. And, if you're lucky, it's embraced.

I'm one of the lucky ones.

Brett knew it the night we met.

A VERY IMPORTANT NOTE FOR READERS

This book contains personal accounts and scenes that may be difficult for some readers. Care has been taken to tell this story honestly, but with that honesty comes subject matter that may be sensitive.

Please be aware that this book includes references to:

- Suicide and suicide attempts
- Self-harm
- Depression and mental illness
- Psychiatric hospitals and treatment settings
- Divorce and the impact of family separation

Reader discretion is encouraged. You are invited to move through these pages in whatever way feels right for you—pausing, skipping, or returning when you're ready.

This story is told from my perspective, shaped by my memory, time, and experience. Many, though not all, names, places, and identifying details have been changed to protect the privacy of those who appear in this book.

IF YOU'RE STRUGGLING

If anything written in this book feels close to home—you're not alone. I know how isolating it can feel to sit with thoughts you don't quite understand, or don't feel safe saying out loud. But there are people who will listen. People who want to help you carry it, even if just for a moment.

Reaching out can feel like the hardest step. It's also the most important one. If you're in immediate distress or thinking about harming yourself, please call or text 988 (Suicide & Crisis Lifeline in the US).

If you are elsewhere, you can find local helplines at *findahelpline.com.*

If calling feels like too much, consider reaching out to someone you trust: a friend, a family member, or a therapist. You don't have to explain everything. You just have to start.

There is support. There is care. And even when it doesn't feel like it, there is a way through.

If you're interested in joining others to END THE STIGMA, contact Bring Change to Mind at *bringchange2mind.org* to discover opportunities to help.

Chapter 1

THE MEET-CUTE

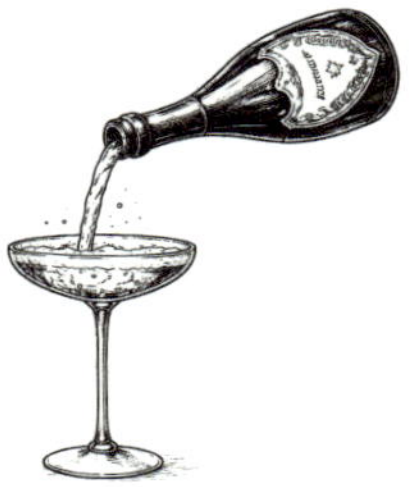

JUNE 18, 2009
9:30 p.m.—Bemelmans Bar at The Carlyle
Upper East Side, New York City

Behind an antiqued gold-framed door with a single gilded "B" pressed into the blackened glass, Bemelmans is abuzz. Inside, Ray Gilbert's "Zip-A-Dee-Doo-Dah" floats above the champagne-laced chatter. The air is sweet with the scent of citrus peels, gin, and something faintly nostalgic.

Gold leaf accents reflect flickering light across the ceiling, casting a forgiving glow that makes everyone look and feel luminous. Not that this crowd needs much help. There probably isn't a blonde in the room who doesn't have her color done by Frédéric Fekkai himself, stylist to the elite and inventor of laid-back-luxe hair care, or at the very least, someone trained in the Fekkai lineage. Everyone, that is, except me.

At first glance, every woman appears ageless and stunningly natural, but I've lived in this neighborhood long enough to know better. Any Southern girl, like me, knows that looking this unadorned takes serious work. Good genes and moisturizer don't get you here. This is curated elegance: subtle mink lash extensions; bimonthly facials with renowned celebrity esthetician Joanna Vargas; a discreet 50 units of Botox, placed with surgical restraint; daily SoulCycle fitness classes to keep everything lifted and taut; and, likely, a personal chef somewhere in the background, ensuring the calories behave.

Still, there's an unspoken rule: you can't look like you're trying. This isn't Beverly Hills. No one announces their maintenance schedule. No one brags about injectables. On the Upper East Side, refinement whispers. It never shouts. My budget doesn't exactly allow for this level of upkeep, but at 28, with perky tatas, freshly touched-up blonde roots, and glowing skin courtesy of the humid night air, I can fake it. Yet, somehow, sitting in a sea of curated perfection doesn't faze me tonight.

As I blend into the crowd, less curated than the glossy regulars, I'm oblivious to my lack of belonging. Tonight happens to be one of those nights when unwavering confidence shows up uninvited. Maybe, it's the adrenaline of my recent escape from a town I hate and the box I allow people to put me in. Maybe, it's the innocence of the song hovering above the room. Maybe, it's the jolly wall paintings by Ludwig Bemelman himself, scenes filled with puppies on park benches, clowns holding handfuls of balloons, bunny rabbits dressed as bartenders, and sweet Madeleine with eleven little girls in two straight lines. Whatever the reason is, my confidence is soaring. Tonight, I'm not trying to measure up to anyone's expectations. I'm not softening my opinions or editing my history. I'm just me. Though, I suppose it's easier to make bold proclamations when you're completely alone.

I didn't plan to be here alone, but I know it's a safe place to land. The crowd skews older. Most of the men have graduated from middle-aged silver fox to full grandfather territory. They are content to observe not pursue. If they speak to a young woman at all, it's only to note how much she resembles a granddaughter.

They're all wearing some version of the same uniform: a summer blazer, a crisp blue or white button-down, and pleated trousers. Nothing flashy. Nothing loud. Perfectly tailored. Quietly expensive. The kind of precision you only notice if you're looking for it. It's subtle, much like the cosmetic work of the women in the room, but it speaks volumes if you pay proper attention.

The view from the bar poses a much different perspective than in the booths or at the tables. From up here, I have a bird's-eye view of waiters dancing through crowded shiny black tables, shuffling cocktails on red linen napkins to make room for a silver-plated caddy overflowing with cheese straws, potato chips, and mixed nuts. There isn't a bar in Manhattan that does snack service better than Bemelmans. I could eat my weight in their cheese straws. It's been my dinner too many times to admit. At the bar, however, the snack service is underwhelming, but that's not an issue tonight. I haven't been hungry lately anyways—a side effect from life moving so fast.

I stay perched at the bar, collecting little snippets of conversation, a quick exchange with a passerby and a longer chat with two bankers at the far end. And then . . . In walks tall, dark, and handsome.

His white button-down isn't as crisp as the others in the room. It's softened, slightly rumpled, and unbuttoned one notch lower than Upper East Side protocol would typically allow. In this sea of navy suits and disciplined tailoring, he is perfectly undone yet still polished.

He's clearly come in from the rain. No umbrella. His dark waves are pushed back from his forehead as the gold-framed door swings shut behind him. He combs his fingers through his hair once, casually, as if he's unaware that half the room just shifted a degree warmer.

I glance toward the piano player, pretending interest in the melody. But I feel him with my whole body, as if there's an invisible string pulling us together, drawing him closer with each step. The murmur of the room dulls.

In seconds, he's beside me. I look up and lock onto his hazel eyes. They're kind and framed with faint, charming lines that suggest laughter comes easily to him. And then he smiles, wide and unguarded; it's the happiest smile I've ever seen. Suddenly, the night rearranges itself.

He extends his hand towards me and with a refreshing blend of confidence and vulnerability, loud enough to overshadow the crowd—he says, "Hi, I'm Brett. I'm unemployed."

Same night, 6:30 p.m.—Bvlgari, Fifth Avenue

Bvlgari is celebrating its 125th anniversary with the launch of a new watch collection benefiting Save the Children. The flagship store is packed wall-to-wall, the rain outside pressing everyone inward. No one wants to venture back into the damp, so they linger. Champagne refills, strategic networking, and air kisses take place under glittering lights.

Lydia asks if I'm ready to leave. I glance at the time. It's earlier than I thought. We definitely haven't overstayed our welcome. She has an early flight, so no late-night antics for her. No pushback from me. My small-talk game is unraveling by the minute. I'm scattered and frenzied—talking too quickly and laughing a beat too loud. I need an exit. Placing our empty flutes on the nearest caterer's tray, Lydia and I head toward the door.

We hug goodbye at the corner of 57th and Fifth, the mist strengthening as we part ways. Lydia disappears into a waiting black town car. I linger for a moment, letting the drizzle kiss my bare shoulders before putting on my black trench coat. The fuchsia duchess satin of my skirt gathers spots from the rain.

I consider heading home. But "home" is a temporary, sparsely furnished apartment. The thought of slipping out of this vintage Dolce & Gabbana number to sit alone in my nightgown feels deflating. My outfit deserves better.

The Four Seasons is an obvious and convenient choice, a catty-corner block away, but the moment I walk through the revolving doors, I remember why a girl can't come here alone. The crowd is more high-end prostitutes, partnered with predatory bankers visiting from sister cities, than small-town girls turned Manhattanites.

While briefly observing the bar scene drenched in a sea of white table linens set aglow with monochrome table lamps, I overhear just enough lame pickup lines, each one more grotesque than the next. My favorite is: "Do you like to party?" It's made complete with a less-than-subtle hand brush against the nose, suggesting the man's love for the smell of a certain white powder.

Time to leave. Drugs have always made me nervous. Over the years, I've seen more neat little white lines on palm-tree-protected tables downtown at Bungalow 8 than I care to count. I never quite numbed to it, never found it glamorous. I suppose the Southern prude in me surfaces more often than I admit. Though she's not around as much lately, just at moments like these.

I shake my head "no" to the hostess when she signals an open seat at the bar, turning to make my way back through the marble lobby, heels clicking against the hushed grandeur as I head out. On instinct, I swipe one of the oversized umbrellas stationed near the exit. I round the corner up Madison Avenue.

Concrete glistens on the quiet street. The only noise comes from the soft hush of rain puddles splashing under taxi tires. Without the sea of mismatched moving blankets, covered in terribly fake Louis Vuitton and Gucci bags, prepared to be pulled up in a moment's notice, the sidewalks at 59th Street feel double in size. The speed in which counterfeit vendors can pack up and escape has always felt like more of a luxury to me than the real designer goods themselves.

It's pitch dark now, but the store windows light up my walk like tiny runways, showcasing every luxury brand imaginable. Summer tweeds from Chanel. Bold colors from Valentino. Enticing prints from ETRO. Moody silhouettes from Prada.

This is my favorite time of day to walk Madison. With the stores closed, I can ogle the collections freely, sans concern of the "always be selling" shop girls who mistakenly assume my own designer wares mean that I can afford their goods. Yet, it's not in their hallowed halls I buy my threads. Mine, hunted expertly at thrift stores, help me look more Manhattan than Murray (Murray, Kentucky, that is).

Shielded from the drizzling summer rain by my giant, stolen umbrella, I feel no rush to be anywhere, though my feet carry me, as if on autopilot, to where I always end up—on the Upper East Side at Bemelmans.

As I cross over 61st Street, a wave of nostalgia overtakes me . . .

My first NYC apartment is just two blocks to my right, between Park and Lex. It's a spot where so much life happened in such a short period. When I moved in, back in 2004, I began lovingly referring to the apartment as "she/her." She was a fourth-floor walk-up. My mother insisted, correctly, that she was, in fact, on the fifth floor.

By the time you reached the top of the stairs, breathless and a little triumphant, the space felt like such a reward that I shaved off an entire flight in her honor. She deserved the simple courtesy. A true floor-through in a prewar townhome, she donned high plaster ceilings, crown molding with stories embedded in, and sunlight that moved slowly from front to back as the day unfolded. Most impressive of all was an in-unit washer and dryer, which in Manhattan, felt nothing short of divine intervention.

She wasn't just an apartment. She was proof. Proof that I had made it to The City and carved out something that felt entirely my own. Every creak in her floorboards sounded familiar. Every window draft felt earned. That walk-up was mine. Even if she was technically on the fifth floor.

Inside her walls, I transformed from a small-time country girl into someone who belonged. That walk-up housed the early days of my company Jet Set Lingerie, when sketches were drawn on any scrap of paper I could find and packaging prototypes were spread out on every surface. Those were long days with my business partners, Greer and Addy, a.k.a. the Twins, as we convinced ourselves this wild idea might work. A lingerie company born in that walk-up sells products in over 500 specialty stores across the country. It still feels improbable.

That walk-up was where I sat after my first diagnosis, made too quickly, too confidently. I remember popping my first Celexa with a glass of red wine. It was a miscalculation, a detour, but I didn't know that yet.

I remember packing boxes too soon, leaving before I was ready. Though, if I'm honest, I don't know that I ever would have been.

Some places hold your becoming. That apartment did. Standing here now, rain tapping softly against the umbrella, I feel it settle into my bones. I'm meant to be here. Back in the "New York Groove."

I make it to 76th Street just as the rain subsides. Through the revolving doors and down the hall, I carefully take each step, doing my best not to wipe out on the rainwater tracked in by other guests. I pass through The Carlyle's Gallery, the zigzag carpet drying the soles of my shoes. Then, through the side door, I slip into the bar.

Goodness, it's loud tonight. A good loud—festive and buoyant. Far more crowded than typical weeknights at Bemelmans, which are usually reserved for regulars and neighborhood fixtures who know the bartenders by name.

Typically, the Twins and I would nestle into our favorite corner booth by the piano. More intimate than the bar, and decidedly less social, it offered us a reprieve to drink, snack, and unwind from our busy days as burgeoning business owners. At the bar, I am in the middle of the social movement. While attempting to order a second glass of house bubbly, which in Bemelmans' case is Moët, I am intercepted by two young bankers with strong opinions about my drink of choice.

"Sorry to interrupt," Suit Number One says, leaning in just enough to be polite but not presumptuous. "Any chance you're in the mood to try something a little bolder?"

He gestures toward Suit Number Two and says, "He's a banker, like me, but also a stellar sommelier. He might have a better suggestion."

My eyes flash to the bottom of my empty glass. Nothing better than cold champagne served in a classic coupe over the more predictable flute. There's something deliciously nostalgic about drinking from the shallow bowl with a delicate stem. It feels like stepping into another decade.

Maybe the Suits are right. Perhaps I've reached my bubbles quota for the night. Time to try something else, something bold. The two of them seem sweet. Harmless. Crisp in that freshly pressed finance way.

Still, I wish Lydia, my "queen of the social circuit" friend, who scooped me under her wing any chance she got this summer, could have joined me tonight. She would love this—a proper post-party recap, dissecting outfits and overheard conversations, rating charm levels on a ten-point scale. Lydia is a force—a powerhouse auctioneer at the most famous auction house in the world. She raises millions in a single evening with nothing more than a gavel, her quick wit, and razor-sharp emotional intelligence. She reads a room the way other people read a menu, with instinct and strategy. Her statuesque presence doesn't hurt. At nearly 6 feet tall, with glossy black hair and legs for days, Lydia commands attention before she ever opens her mouth.

The Twins and I may not share Lydia's impressive height, but put the three of us together, and we still manage to make a splash with the same shade of blonde, similar builds, and a shared love of eclectic, colorful style that refuses to play it safe. We gravitate toward loud prints, unexpected silhouettes, and anything that suggests we didn't come to blend in.

Individually, we're noticeable. Together, we're a moment. And none of us has ever minded making an entrance. After 24 years of friendship, we're not just separate individuals; we're a shared language.

We're lucky Lydia lets us tag along for the ride. Parties here, there, everywhere! She pulls me and the Twins into her orbit. Over the years, she's introduced us to oodles of chic city dwellers. Lydia doesn't just enter a room; she expands it.

There's a common thread between the four of us, something stitched together by our Southern roots. Our shared hunger for big-city life, something beyond the easy comforts of middle-class America, runs deep. It's not just ambition; it's also understanding. We know what it means to leave, to want more, and to build something different than what is familiar.

Other than consistently seeing Lydia over the past month, my summer back in the city has been a bit solitary and delightfully freeing. I'm like a bird out of its cage. For the first time in my life, no one knows where I am. Better yet, no one is asking. My BlackBerry sits silently on the bar, resting near my empty champagne glass. The device's lack of notifications feels almost suspicious. I check it anyway, out of habit more than expectation.

Nothing. No missed calls. No urgent texts. No "Where are you?" or "Call me." Just stillness. I'm as free as a bird—a blue bird on my shoulder . . . After a slightly uncomfortable silence, I turn to the Suits.

"Well, something bold it is," I respond to Suit Number One. I punctuate it with a wink. Unfortunately, my face interprets "wink" as "minor eye spasm." God didn't grant me that skill.

I can hear their words floating around in the air, the mentions of "full body" this or "region" that, but none of it sticks. Though, I do catch their names, Josh and Oliver, and a mention of Shana, the girlfriend, who is on the way to join them.

"You'll love her," the Suits say in unison.

Funny how I selected this spot initially, with open stools on either side to provide a buffer to banker types, chatting about mergers over martinis, but their company is fun and light, and now, I have this "bold" glass of red wine in front of me that I would have likely never tried otherwise.

When Shana, Josh's girlfriend, arrives, I feel another burst of energy. I should be tired after a long day, but I haven't needed more than three hours of sleep all summer. I feel great, almost electric.

Shana glides into the room like she belongs in it. She's willowy and dressed head to toe in black, a fitted silk camisole tucked into a high-waisted pencil skirt, with sharp heels that add height to her petite frame. It's minimal but far sexier than anything I ever wear. Her big, dark curls spill over her shoulders in a way that feels effortless and dramatic all at once. She doesn't need color; she is the contrast.

A shift change catches my eye. The addition of a double bass and guitar round out the jazz trio, signaling that I've been here well over an hour—and that my tab just went up $40 thanks to the cover charge. The hum from tucked-away booths, each packed tightly with guests, continues to rise. They engage only with each other, operating like tiny islands, completely unaware of the others around them.

It's nearly impossible to feel sad in this dreamy room.

I feel almost untethered, as if I'm floating just slightly above myself. Observing it all from a softened distance. Watching my own movements unfold—the tilt of my head, the curve of my smile, the way my hand reaches for the stem of my glass. It's like I'm both participant and audience at once. Hyperaware. Absorbing every detail. Even the ones that belong to me.

To think that just a month earlier, I was in Dallas, Texas, endlessly in and out of my car, circling strip malls in the thick heat and driving from one beige building to the next. I was either alone or with Greer, working on our business or hunting for the perfect diner for lunch to break up the day. The time with her was joyful, but outside of that, I was miserable.

Not that I could say it out loud, and certainly not to Greer. I wore the optimism required of a company founder. I kept the tone light, forward-looking, and productive. But when a short-term, furnished apartment near Bryant Park in New York City fell into my lap almost casually, I took it as a sign. A door had cracked open, and I walked through. Then, with surprising confidence, I persuaded my entire circle to follow my lead, or, at least, to trust the move. The crazy part was that I barely had to sell it. Moving back to New York required far less convincing than I'd braced myself for. It was as if some part of all of us already knew it was where I should be.

Greer didn't want me to leave. She had only just returned to Texas after a year of living in London with her husband, Rhett, for his job. Her absence had made Dallas feel even flatter, colorless, and lonely.

I visited her in London, and she'd come back to Texas. And, in between, we met in Paris, in New York, and wherever else we could justify. We had a ball every time. With Addy often in tow, the three of us would slip easily into our old rhythm in foreign cities, laughing too loudly at dinners that ran too long. Ordering second helpings of dessert and cheese and more wine. We were indulgent in every way, but mostly in our friendship.

But it wasn't the same without the day-in, day-out grind of building our business, Jet Set Lingerie, side by side. It wasn't the comfort of our 50-shades-of-pink office, with colorful samples spilling off desks, Diet Coke cans multiplying by noon, and the three of us solving problems in real time.

Life was shifting. I felt it in my bones. In some ways, I was guiding the shift, but it was coming whether I wanted it to or not. Addy was pregnant. She was living in Knoxville, Tennessee, now with her happy husband and darling dog in their grown-up house. Our days of disco naps were behind us. Painting the town pink as vintage-inspired Jet Set Lingerie flight attendants in perfectly pressed skirt suits with little red pillbox hats perched just so was part costume, part concept. A wink to the golden age of travel, when everything felt more polished, more playful.

It captured exactly what we were building—lingerie designed for women in motion. Pieces you could tuck into a carry-on and throw on between destinations to feel put-together, no matter where you landed.

There was a whimsy to it that we loved. Not taking ourselves too seriously, but knowing what we were doing. Even if the Twins weren't quite ready to admit it was the end of an era, I knew it was the truth.

The day I left Dallas, Greer cried. Only two weeks before, we had made the tough decision to pack up the Jet Set Lingerie office and move most things into a storage unit. Our office lease was ending, and the economy was not in a good place. The housing crash was affecting us all. It was the bottom line for most but the top drawer for us.

Our wholesale orders were shrinking, and our new direct-toconsumer website wasn't exactly breaking the Internet. Although it did have the cutest cartoon intro video featuring a pink plane, branded as "Airforce Blonde," landing on a pink runway with Jet Set Lingerie flight attendants filing out, train cases full of panties in hand. An intro video didn't sell products if no one was going to the website.

The day we moved, we carted bins of overstock inventory, racks of samples, our matching desks, and framed artwork out onto the sidewalk and into a rented U-Haul truck. Greer stood still for a moment, watching it all disappear into the back of the truck. Then, she looked at me, eyes glossy.

"Pippy," she said softly, "I don't think you're going to come back."

There have been a dozen nicknames over our 24 years of friendship, but "Pippy" is the one that stuck—as in Pippi Longstocking, freckled, wild, inexplicably strong. I don't have any freckles, but strength, I've got in spades.

It started our sophomore year of high school. Greer, Addy, and I pulled over to the side of the road to cut down our annual "Charlie Brown Christmas tree." It was a silly tradition we began as a prank on my mom the year before. She secretly loved it. We decorated the ugliest cedar tree we could find with ridiculous homemade ornaments and tchotchkes. That year, a cop showed up. Though we weren't technically doing anything illegal by cutting down the equivalent of a giant weed on the shoulder of the road, we panicked. Greer and Addy ran deeper into the field, trying to dodge the cop, and I hauled the entire scrappy tree back to the car myself.

Back then, I was almost a head shorter than both of them. The tree was as big as me. When we met up back at the car, I had already tossed it on the roof. We laughed until we cried. And from that day on, I was Pippy. Strong and stubborn, always hauling something heavier than I probably should.

"Don't be silly," I assured Greer. "This is temporary."

It was a lie. It wasn't my first lie to her. I'd been holding things back from her, and from Addy, for years. Not out of malice. Not because I wanted to deceive them. It was simply self-preservation.

I wasn't just shielding them. I was shielding myself. Because once I voiced the thoughts swirling in my head, they'd solidify. Keeping it unspoken made it feel manageable, containable.

We've been friends since we were 4 years old. No one knows me better than the Twins. They can read the shift in my voice before I even register it myself. They are my safe place.

This makes the withholding even harder to justify.

A hand brushes my shoulder. I turn back to Brett, a little startled by how natural his hand on my bare skin feels. He's waiting for me to say something. Normally, I'd feel guarded, walled up against the expectations of being exactly who a man wants me to be. But I don't feel the usual internal scramble, the quick mental scan for exits, the reflex to manage the moment. I just feel steady. Safe. Which is absurd because I don't know this man.

He appeared in front of me a mere 20 seconds ago. And yet, his presence settles something in me. Or maybe, it quiets something. The hum that's been running just beneath my skin all summer softens with him standing this close.

I shift on my barstool, perching upright, legs crossed neatly at the ankle like a good Southern girl, even though my fuchsia skirt has crept up a touch higher than intended. My sleeveless bubblegum-pink Isaac Mizrahi blouse is modest in cut but sheer enough to let the outline of my black bra quietly announce itself. It's a careful balance—sultry Barbie, executed with practiced precision, metallic silver stacked Chanel heels and all. He's still looking at me. Not hungrily. Not impatiently. Just open and waiting.

"Hi," I say, "I'm Morgan." I smile, surprised by my own calm.

"I'm married."

Chapter 2

THE CONVERSATION

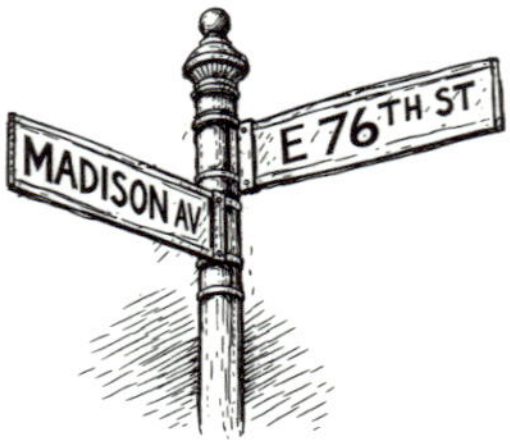

JUNE 18, 2009
10:32 p.m.—Bemelmans Bar at The Carlyle
Upper East Side, New York City

It feels easy to open up to Brett. It's been six years and 361 days since I was last single. Not that I'm counting. His eyes flick to my left hand in a quick, efficient glance to confirm that the platinum band holding a radiant, nearly perfect, one-carat diamond is in fact wrapped around the ring finger of my left hand. "Explain to me why you're here," Brett coyly asks with a smirk, "And he's not."

He shifts closer to me, not abruptly but slowly and deliberately—until the small space between us disappears. I can feel the warmth of him before he even touches me. The movement is subtle enough that anyone across the room might miss it, but to me, it feels enormous, like the air itself has changed. Then I catch it. His cologne.

It reaches me before he does. The scent is warm and clean at first, a flash of citrus and bergamot that feels almost bright, before settling in. Underneath it all is that unmistakable base of sandalwood, amber, and musk. It's the kind of scent that lingers in the air long after someone has left the room. Smell is my strongest sense. It bypasses logic and lands somewhere deeper. Scents transport me. For a split second, I can almost see the bottle in my mind, dark green glass, a red round top, but I can't place the brand. It smells like a grown-up. Not boyish.

Grounded.

I'd guess Brett is in his early 30s, not because of his face, which could pass for a younger Dennis Quaid, but because of his composure, the comfort in his posture, and the way he doesn't rush the silence after his question. He knows he doesn't need to.

"He's at home in Dallas," I reply in a voice steadier than I feel. "But I'm here for the summer. I can't seem to shake this city."

I realize I haven't stopped smiling. God, he's cute.

"So, what does your husband—spare me his name—think about you living alone for the summer?" Brett asks, still leaning toward me like he's afraid I might disappear if he looks away too long.

"I didn't exactly pitch it like that," I say, laughing gently and leaning into him. "He works on the East Coast quite a bit, and I'm in New York constantly for work, usually with my two business partners. We have a lingerie company." I pause, letting it hang for just a second. I watch as my last statement registers on his face. His eyebrows lift immediately, the reaction I was quietly hoping for.

"Of course you do," he says.

I laugh, shifting slightly on the barstool, crossing one leg over the other. The movement feels almost electric—my foot bouncing consistently against the brass rail, my fingers tracing the rim of my glass without realizing it. I can feel the energy in my body, the same restless current that makes me talk a little faster and smile a little wider.

Normally, this is the moment I excuse myself—politely, gracefully—before the conversation wanders anywhere near this level of familiarity. I would never let an interaction go this far, much less casually announce that I cofounded a lingerie company, a detail I knew would land like a lit match in a room full of gasoline. Yet, the girl inside me, the one running the show tonight, has other plans; plus, something about this particular man feels inexplicably safe.

I give Brett the condensed version of our company's story, how the idea for it was born in the corner booth by the piano, our booth, and explain how this place has long been a go-to for me and the Twins.

"I'm here so often that I practically have a punch card," I explain. "Aside from loving an old-school piano bar, I come here because I don't get hit on . . . well, usually." I give him a knowing smirk.

"And if a man does send over a drink," I continue, "it's mostly because I remind him of his granddaughter or because he assumes I can't afford to pay for it myself."

Brett studies me, amused, his head tipping back slightly in quiet laughter before he leans in again. Only now does it occur to me that I've never once brought my husband, Richard, here. As if some part of me knew to keep this corner of my life separate, I've quietly protected it as a small refuge where his expectations couldn't quite reach. A lucky instinct on my part.

"Do you believe in luck?" Brett asks, stopping me in my tracks.

"I certainly believe things that are meant to be will be," I answer.

"*Qué será, será*," he chimes back.

Our first jinx. Even if only in my mind.

"Luck got me here tonight," he continues. "I was finishing dinner at Nobu 57 when some friends called, telling me I must come uptown. I'm a downtown guy, but they insisted. It was pouring, so I hopped on the bus at Sixth Avenue and 57th, forgetting that it stops at 59th. I looked like a tourist, even though I've lived here since '96."

Brett laughs. It's contagious. And it makes me laugh, too, harder than usual. He's a little older than I first guessed. I do the math quickly in my head, trying not to look like I'm calculating. If I was a junior in high school in 1996 and he was already living here as a grown-up, then that makes him 37-ish. I've never given much thought to what a 37-year-old man should look like. But if this is the prototype, then I approve. There's something about him that isn't just handsome; it's settled. He's confident in a way that doesn't beg to be noticed.

"To be honest," he says, "I was about to call it a night, but a taxi pulled up as I stepped off the bus, so I jumped in. And now, here I am with you. Lucky."

The word lands purposefully, and it sparks.

How strange that we were on the same block earlier tonight before ending all the way up here. So many cross streets in this city. So many near misses. It makes me wonder if our paths have brushed before. I wonder if we've shared a sidewalk, a doorway, or a glance we didn't register. New York feels enormous until it doesn't. Sometimes, it feels impossibly small.

"I suppose that is lucky," I agree. It's forward and undeniably flirty, yet it comes easier than it normally would.

"Brett!" We turn as an excited feminine voice shouts his name. It's Shana—girlfriend of Suit Number One. "You made it!" she says. "And I see you've already met Morgan."

Earlier in the night, when I was chatting with Shana and the bankers, they mentioned they had a friend I had to meet. I caught snippets of them talking on the phone later, half-laughing, half-insistent, trying to lure someone out. I didn't give it much weight, especially since I had already told them I'm married. It's not like wedding rings are subtle.

How did Brett know I was the girl they'd called him about when he first walked in? By the time Brett arrived, the crowd had thickened, and a proper crush of blazers and silk dresses stood between me and his buddies, the self-appointed wine experts. I wasn't obviously "the girl" next to them anymore. Brett looks slightly confused, too.

"This is the girl you all called me about, begging me to come meet her?" he asks, gesturing vaguely toward the bankers. Then, he looks back at me. "She's married, you know," he comments. "That might have been useful intel, Shana."

He winks back at me. They laugh lightly, and something inside me recoils. Hearing him say it out loud feels different than when I said it myself. When he was speaking directly to me, my marriage felt distant, almost theoretical like a Yankees-in-Tara kind of thing, something to think about tomorrow.

But here, in the open, it changes shape. My marital status enters the room and settles—heavy. No longer mine to manage. Because the truth, suddenly visible from the outside, now seems unsavory. Icky.

I glance at my ring finger, thinking about the last time it was bare.

My "perfect" Father of the Bride moment, a sweeping white tent stood in my parents' backyard, strung with lights and heavy with summer heat. A killer band performed. All 11 bridesmaids lined up in timeless black column gowns with matching oversized pearl chokers. I wore a classic duchess satin, pintucked strapless gown with a full skirt. The veil so oversized it required its own handler.

All 300 guests were seated for dinner. Tables were drenched in pink peonies, Queen Anne's lace, and lily of the valley. Engraved linen invitations practically whispered forever.

My wedding was perfect in every visible way. But beneath all that perfection, there was a quieter truth, a secret hope I carried like a folded note in my bouquet. Deep down, I hoped my dad would pull me aside, before the double doors leading to the aisle opened, and ask, "Are you sure?"

I would have said, "No." I would have grabbed his hand, and we would have slipped out the back doors of our very "perfect" Bible Belt church and disappeared before the organ finished its prelude.

But he didn't ask, and I didn't offer. So, I stayed. I stayed for the packed sanctuary. I stayed for the 300 people who had dressed up and RSVP'd yes. I stayed because of the money my parents had already spent, because of how hard my mom had worked to make everything flawless for her only child, because I didn't know what else to do. Where would I go? What would I say? Who would I be? Standing at that altar felt less like a choice and more like the next expected step.

My entire senior year of college had centered around the wedding. I clung to it for all the wrong reasons. It was mostly a distraction for me, but maybe more so, it was a distraction *from* me. With all the planning, everyone closest to me was focused on guest lists for bridal showers, flower arrangements, and seating charts. There was little time to notice that I was at the lowest I had ever been—sleeping all day with zero energy or motivation to do anything, even the fun, senior year kinds of things. I hid out in my single room at the sorority house as much as I could without people noticing. I missed class after class. At a time when I felt so lost in myself, I welcomed Richard's attention, flawed as it was.

At 21 years old, practically a child bride, I walked down the aisle and said the traditional vows. And like a proper Christian girl, I lost my virginity that night. Not out of desire, but out of duty. For the nearly seven years that followed, I faked that part of my life—the enthusiasm, the fulfillment, the satisfaction. I learned the choreography of intimacy and a happy marriage and performed it well enough that no one questioned it. Faking became second nature.

I didn't even feel particularly guilty about it. In some ways, it felt encouraged. Southern women are trained to keep things tidy. Don't air your dirty laundry. Don't make others uncomfortable with your shortcomings. Don't disrupt the image. I'm quite sure that tending to one's own desires isn't exactly preached from the pulpit. But I took an independent study course years ago. Was I lying? Technically, yes. But I was also following the rules. A happy young lady has a full dance card, and she never lets anyone see her sit out. Or, God forbid, frown.

I suppose in his own way, Richard loved me, to the extent he was capable of loving anyone. Though if I'm honest, looking back, he fell in love with the idea of me, the polished outline I shared with the world. It was the version of me that fit neatly into photos for annual holiday cards and dinners with business associates. I checked the boxes. Pretty enough. Smart enough. Funny enough. Popular enough. But Richard didn't know all of me. Then again, I didn't know all of me either. Not when we met at 19 and not when we married at 21. I was still performing a version of myself I thought the world wanted.

But I'm beginning to like the girl sitting on this barstool at Bemelmans. I want to see where she might go, and what she might say and what she might do. Suspended in this amber-lit moment, shoulder to shoulder with Brett, a man who, by all logic, ought to feel dangerous, but instead, feels like someone who might actually see me.

Brett's gaze drops, unhurried, and glides from my metallic Chanel heels, up along the line of my calves, past my knees, to the hem of my skirt, which has conveniently migrated a few more inches north. When his eyes return to mine, there's no apology in them.

"Where were we?" he asks.

"Something about how lucky you are to be in my presence," I answer.

"Isn't that the truth," he says, with an amused smile. "Let me buy you another drink." He nods toward my nearly empty glass of Burgundy.

I give him a noncommittal hum, looking up at him thoughtfully. "I'm not sure you can afford it," I suggest. He tilts his head, confused.

"Your fancy friends picked it out," I continue sweetly, a playful smile tugging on my lips. "And you're unemployed, remember?"

Brett bursts into laughter, and it sends me into orbit. There's something intoxicating about being the reason for that sound. It makes me feel high.

"Maybe my unemployed comment was slightly exaggerated," he says. "The company I'd been with for a decade relocated to Atlanta. I chose to stay in New York, so I took a buyout." He pauses with a showman's grin. "A pretty good one."

I nod, pretending to evaluate him anew.

"Makes sense," I say. "Grown men don't usually volunteer unemployment without a footnote."

His eyes hold mine. "I'm feeling even better about the decision now," he says quietly. "If I were in Atlanta tonight, I wouldn't be talking to you."

He steps closer, more deliberate. His gabardine trousers tickle my leg as he leans slightly toward the bartender catching his eye with a small nod. Two more glasses appear without him saying a word. His knee still rests lightly against mine; I don't move away.

We chat back and forth for a while, comparing notes on our summers. He wakes early to run; I wake early to walk. He meets friends for happy hour; I attend fashion-house soirées and charity galas. He's exploring opportunities in Asia; I've just come back from visiting our factory in Thailand.

It's playful at first. Observational. Clever. Not exactly a conversation fit for a married woman in a bar, and somewhere around glass number three, it slips farther from appropriate banter. Brett asks why I got married at 21 and says he can't even picture it. He laughs, imagining who his 21-year-old self might have chosen. There's no judgment in his voice, just curiosity and a genuine attempt to understand the shape of me.

And I tell him. I don't hesitate. I don't edit. I don't protect. I tell him what it's like to grow up in a small town below the Mason-Dixon Line, where good girls finish first. Where you don't cause scenes. Where you don't test limits. Where you don't put yourself in the hot seat. Being "good" came naturally to me most of the time. I didn't like getting in trouble, so I simply avoided anything that might invite it. Short of sitting here, of course, flirting with this gorgeous man who just put his hand on top of my knee.

Brett's touch is warm. Casual enough to deny. Intentional enough to notice. The version of me I've always known would have gently moved his hand away, reclaiming the space and reinforcing the boundary. But I don't. It's been nearly 10 years since I've been touched by someone new and wanted it. Not accidentally. Not aggressively. Not by some entitled finance bro testing his luck.

This is different. The line—that invisible, sacred line I've held on to for almost seven years—has been crossed. And instead of panic, I feel heat. Instead of guilt, I feel want. I don't move his hand. Instead of leaning away, I lean in. His hand doesn't move.

"Now that you've grilled me about being a virgin child bride, it's your turn—20 questions," I suggest. My tone is teasing, but there's an edge to it now, curiosity laced with challenge. "You don't get to look at me like I'm some rare historical artifact and not expect a little excavation yourself. Let's start simple. Who were you at 21?"

I haven't checked the time or my phone in what feels like hours, but the room hasn't started to thin yet. Out of the corner of my eye, I see that Brett's group of friends is still here and a new blonde has joined them. He doesn't appear to notice or care.

Finally, the chair next to me opens. Taking the seat would mean putting space between us. Instead, he pulls it close to me, the legs of it touching my stool, before he sits down. Brett's body language is casual and comforting. His sleeves are now rolled up, and his poplin shirt is showing a few more wrinkles. The three glasses of red wine faintly tint his teeth and stain his lips, giving him an edge that feels just slightly undone. I suddenly wonder if mine look the same. Without breaking eye contact for too long, I reach into my clutch and pull out a tube of pink gloss. A small, practiced motion. Cap off. Swipe. Press lips together.

His eyes don't leave me. They track every movement, the slow glide across my bottom lip, the soft purse as I blend it in. It's a simple act. Ordinary. And yet, in front of him, it feels deliberate. Charged. I slide the gloss back into my bag and look up at him again, pretending I didn't just notice how carefully he was watching.

"So, new friend," I ask, "have you ever been engaged? Or close to finding the one?" Assuming the answer is yes but hoping he doesn't confirm.

"Nope, not once," he answers with a straight face.

"Bullshit!" I say, smacking his knee unapologetically. "Are you going to honestly tell me, that you, in your late 30s (yes, I did the math in my head), have never gotten down on one knee?"

Brett seems more shocked by me saying "bullshit" than by my question.

"Look at you, with the mouth of a sailor," he quips. "I'm serious though. Never close. Now, there might have been some that wanted me to marry them . . ."

He goes on to share a bit of his dodgy past. It seems his dating history leaves a lot to be desired, but none of it scares me. I might not voluntarily share it with my fair-haired grandmother, Bettie-Ann, but I can take it. He's not trying to impress me, and it's refreshing. Albeit slightly confusing, I'm not trying to impress him either.

"Well, aren't you full of yourself? Maybe they didn't want to marry you either!" I say, though somewhere in the back of my mind, a voice is saying that those girls must have been out of their minds if they didn't want to marry him.

"Who wouldn't want to marry Brett?" Shana chimes in, suddenly reappearing at my shoulder. I hadn't even realized she was back within earshot.

"Jaimie?" she adds, eyebrow raised. Brett gives her a look.

"Sounds like there's a story there," I say, turning back to him, interest piqued.

"There's always a story," Shana says, giving Brett's arm a squeeze. "Okay, you two, we're heading to our apartment across the street. Join us?"

The invitation hangs between us. It's tempting in theory, the continuation, the escalation. But something about shifting the setting feels like crossing into a different chapter. I hesitate. Before I can answer, Brett does.

"We'll keep you posted," he says easily, placing his hand on her shoulder, but his knee presses a little closer to mine as he says it. A small signal. We're not done here.

I've never loved the way "we" sounded more in my entire life.

"It was great meeting you, Morgan!" Shana says. "Let's stay in touch." She slips me her card. She mentioned earlier in the night that she was a lawyer at MTV, but the card makes it official.

Perhaps, it's just her champagne buzz making her extra friendly, but Shana comes in for the biggest hug, like we've known each other for ages. She's even tinier than I realized. I'm wearing pretty tall heels, but I feel like I'm towering over her. Sans the heels, I'm just barely 5'6". She must be 5'4" at the most.

After a few more hugs and goodbyes, Brett's friends head out the door toward The Gallery.

His friends are charming, energetic, and easy to like. But I don't want the group. I want him. And as if summoned by the thought alone, he turns back toward me, eyes finding mine again. His full attention is on me. It's almost midnight. Closing time looms.

Brett pats the seat of my barstool, motioning for me to sit back down. I hoist myself up the way you climb out of a swimming pool, hands pressing into the seat for leverage, trying to look graceful. My feet search for the brass footrest, so they don't dangle like a child's, as my skirt slides up a few more inches.

He notices. Now, we're back to just the two of us. The noise of the room fades again. The piano softens into background texture. We slip back into the good, the bad, and the complicated.

Up until tonight, our lives have existed on completely separate tracks. And though I've felt a bit of my darker side stretching its limbs all summer, the Puritan in me still has a surprisingly firm grip. After all, I announced I was married the moment we met. I'm not hiding anything. Not skipping the inconvenient pieces. Not pretending to be someone freer than I am.

"Just so you know," I say, lowering my voice, "since June of 2002, back when I became a child bride . . ." I attempt another wink. It feels awkward and terrible. "I haven't talked to another man for this length of time without my husband, Richard, somewhere nearby."

It feels both confessional and defiant. I've officially said my husband's name. Brett studies me for a moment, expression softening.

"We are just talking, friend," he says.

Friend. The word lands gently, but it doesn't cool anything down. If anything, it makes the air between us feel warmer. Now, I'm starting to think that I might just be a breath of fresh air to him, another night of killing time, with no strings attached. I've proclaimed that I'm taken. Perhaps this is heading (as it should) towards the friend zone.

"Seriously, what's it like to be a child bride?" he pokes.

"I guess I don't really know any other way," I admit. "And it's not all that unique when you're from my neck of the woods." Geez. Neck of the woods? Why did I have to make myself sound like backwoods Barbie?

It's not as if I grew up in the woods. Sure, Murray, Kentucky, is small, but it's a university town, which makes it more interesting and diverse than many small towns of its size. But it's the kind of small, Southern town with a church on every major corner, plus four off the downtown court square. It has local banks, not national ones. You can't go to the grocery store without running into people you know, so you never go without lipstick or with wet hair. I was raised to believe the Eleventh Commandment was "No wet hair in public." Only mildly more important was avoiding sexual scandals that might get the PTO moms talking. You can't recover from the reputation of small-town skank. "It will follow you forever," was what we were taught growing up.

I don't think for a second that my own mother, the PTO president a few years running, judged me for anything. That wasn't her style. But she knew others would, so she did her best to give me the knowledge and the tools for success, tools to get me out of there. And so far, they're working. Here I am with Murray far in my rearview mirror.

But then, Brett's hand slides from my knee to my thigh, and a rush of blood shoots through my body, making me aware that I'm starving. When did I last eat? Hors d'oeuvres at the party? I need a diner. I need matzo ball soup and string beans, and I need it now.

"I'm starving," I announce. "I've got to get food."

"OK, what sounds good?" Brett jumps on board immediately.

"No, go be with your friends!" I tell him. "I'm just going to hit a basic diner somewhere close by."

"You're not getting rid of me just yet," he says.

Brett subtly passes his platinum Amex card to the bartender, who's dressed in the signature red tuxedo jacket and black bow tie. With grey hair just starting to recede, I imagine this man has worked here since Reagan was in office. His actions are effortless and familiar. The man moves with complete ease, in what likely feels like his second home. He's been attentive, but never invasive. A true pro.

While Brett is looking down to sign the check, I study his hair. Fluffy waves that wing out above his ears are darker than chestnut brown, but not black. It's not as full or sculptured as JFK Jr's was, though, it's in the same lane.

He slides the signed check back towards the bartender, places the black enameled pen, stamped with The Carlyle in script, on top and smiles at the man, thanking him for a "top night."

Then, in one of the smoothest moves I've witnessed in years, Brett grips the base of my barstool, his hand grazing my leg in the process and gently pulls it back from the bar to let me out. It's understated and efficient. Chivalrous without being showy. I slide forward and step down with a slightly awkward hop, the heels higher than I remembered. I try to recover my composure as I head toward the door.

Halfway there, I realize I forgot my trench coat. I glance back, but of course, Brett already has it. It's draped over one arm, and the oversized umbrella from the Four Seasons is hooked casually in his hand.

He catches up to me in two strides and settles the coat over my shoulders. The satin lining slips against my skin, sliding off one side. Without hesitation, he adjusts it, slowly, deliberately, his fingers brushing my collarbone as he rights the fabric. His hand trails down my back, pausing just long enough in the curve of my waist to guide me forward. Not possessive. Not accidental. Intentional. He steers me toward the Gallery, with his palm warm against me, and I let him.

Down the stairs and around the corner, we pass the elevators and land in an empty lobby. It's a skeleton crew working the front desk; one solo attendant, suited in all black, gatekeeping the wall of key boxes, where the lucky guests store their golden keys when they're out.

I love how each specific role at the hotel is assigned a particular uniform, helping guests easily know who can help them with whatever service they might need. In a head-to-toe grey, double-breasted jacket and matching trousers, the bellman waves us towards the revolving door. He gives it a push, we accidentally stumble into the same tiny wedge of the door, and out we fall onto 76th Street. The rain has stopped for now.

"Shall we diner, my lady?" Brett sweeps a hand down the street.

"I suppose we shall, sir," I quip. We walk east.

Chapter 3

THE KISS

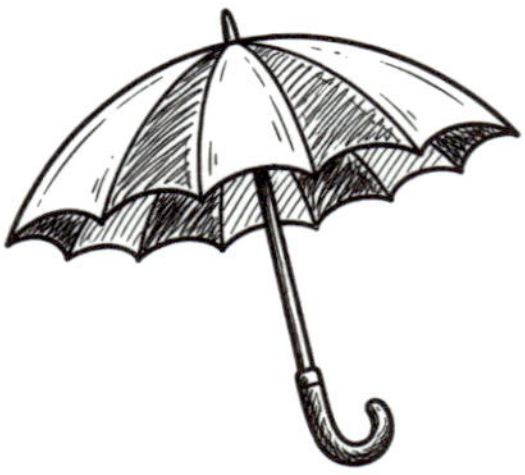

FEBRUARY 2009
Dallas, Texas

My mom is in town. She's not exactly a fan of Dallas either, though she does have a soft spot for The Women's Exchange, a glorious secondhand charity shop where we've unearthed everything from sterling Revere bowls to tortoiseshell keepsake boxes. Her visits usually revolve around treasure hunting: sifting through art, antique rugs, chinoiserie lamps, vintage jewelry, and mismatched Limoges plates that we insist we'll one day use properly. But today is less romantic.

Today, we're on a mission at TJ Maxx, with its fluorescent lights, red carts, and all. We're searching for a new toiletry bag and last-minute travel necessities. In two days, Greer, Addy, and I leave for a three-week work trip.

We'll start in New York for Fashion Week, marketing events, networking dinners, and any room that will have us. Then, we'll do the COTERIE trade show at Javits Center, one of our biggest wholesale moments of the year. It's a make-or-break few days where buyers decide whether we're expanding . . . or plateauing.

After that, we head east to Thailand for a factory visit, checking on production for our new shapewear line. Fit samples. Fabric tweaks. Factory floor walk-throughs.

Richard has been out of town all week, which makes it the perfect window for my mom to visit. He is due home today. She flies out tomorrow. Surely, we can all survive one night under the same roof, assuming I can deflect his comments, the digs, and the belittling tone he uses, not just on me and my mom, but also on his own parents. They're the kind of words that land lightly, but bruise deeply.

Like the time he nearly made my mother's head pop clean off, insisting, with unwavering confidence, that BMW stood for British Motor Works, not Bavarian. I had never once considered what the letters stood for, nor did I particularly care; but in that moment, caught in the crossfire of his condescending certainty and her rising frustration, I felt more divided than I had choosing where to spend Thanksgiving during my parents' divorce.

And the truth, the small, obvious truth, was that she was right. Not just factually, though she was, but in a deeper, quieter way. She had earned the right to be heard, to be trusted in her knowing. As his elder. As my mother. As someone who didn't need to raise her voice to deserve respect. But he didn't care. His intelligence reigned over all of us. He made sure of that.

It's ridiculous, but after years of incidents and having to choose a side, I now do everything I can to protect the perception of Richard in those moments. Perhaps it's emotional survival. Or maybe, I'm just trying to save face or to shield my mom from the embarrassment of the life I'm actually living.

Mom and I are wandering through TJ Maxx, half-heartedly scanning the lingerie section for no-show socks, when my phone lights up.

Richard.

It's 3 p.m. He should still be in transit. I answer. He's at our apartment. Apparently, he caught an earlier flight home. He's found the mess.

Before he even finishes his first sentence, panic floods my body. Flashes of our bedroom explode in my mind. Outfits meticulously styled and then abandoned. Shoes paired perfectly with tights and bangles. Bags draped over bedposts. Clothes hanging from bookshelves. Everything scattered like evidence.

I should have tidied up. I know better than to cut it this close. I need him off the phone before my mom can overhear his wrath.

"Of course, of course," I say quickly, overly agreeable. "We'll be right there. I'll get all that squared away." I'm vague. Neutral. Harmless. Anything to keep my mom from asking follow-up questions. I hang up and turn to her.

"You know what, Mom? I totally forgot I have a toiletry bag in our storage unit in the building," I lie smoothly. "I can make that work. Let's just head home."

She doesn't say anything. She doesn't have to. Her face says she knows, and somehow, that's worse than if she'd called me out.

"Can I at least check out?" she asks, attempting to hide her annoyance.

"Oh . . . sure," I say, not wanting to be rude, but, damn it, I know things are escalating by the minute. "I'll go get the car and pick you up right at the front to make it easy for you."

Knowing that shaving off any time at all might help my situation, I take my own cart to the front, putting away anything I can along the way to not leave a mess for one of the shop gals. Mom heads to the checkout with a frustrated look on her face.

On my solo walk to the car, my phone rings again. It's Richard. Ignoring him will only make it worse, so I answer. His tone is tight. Controlled. I can't quite tell if he's more irritated by the mess I left behind or by what it represents, the physical proof that I'm preparing to leave for a three-week work trip, that I might have a moment of joy without him, that I might taste success that doesn't include him.

By the time my mom slides into the passenger seat, I can feel her watching me. The air in the car is thick. She's irritated, and I'm already calculating how to soften it. I default to the oldest script in the book.

"He's just tired," I say lightly. "He works so hard." Even as the words leave my mouth, I know how hollow they sound.

I apologize and make an excuse to go home and clean. I'm always apologizing, even when no one has asked me to. Mom doesn't respond right away. But I can see it in her jaw, the way she stares straight ahead, chewing on the inside of her bottom lip with her hand resting on her chin. Long orange-red nails on her tan hands. She's angry. Just not at me.

June 19, 2009, After Midnight, 76th Street, NYC

Outside, after a long rain, the city smells different. Still gritty but rinsed, refreshed, it's like the sharp edges have been polished just enough to feel invigorating instead of exhausting.

The streets are wider up here, calmer than where my summer apartment sits in Midtown. They're free of the usual parade of glossy black garbage bags sagging at the seams and stacks of waterlogged cardboard boxes collapsing into themselves. Instead, there are tidy patches of manicured greenery tucked carefully at the base of each tree surrounded by small iron fences with polite little signs reminding residents to "curb your dog," as if manners extend even to the sidewalks.

Brett shifts positions without announcing it. He's no longer trailing slightly behind me; he's moved to my right, taking the street side. The polite position. It's the one any gentleman is supposed to know. Brett seems like a gentleman, but I find myself wondering if he actually knows the etiquette, or if it just comes naturally to him. Brett's home state of Ohio borders Kentucky, after all, but that invisible line, when the North becomes the South, comes with a rule book Southern girls and boys are handed at birth. Walk on the street side. Walk her to the door. Open it for her. Don't swear in front of her mother.

I'm trying to keep a careful, intentional distance between us, but I secretly love that Brett keeps closing it. When we approach the first crosswalk, I brace for him to reach for my hand. He doesn't. Instead, he pauses and gestures toward a puddle spreading across the curb.

"I'll stay on the outside," he says casually, "so you don't get any rain spray on that head-turning skirt."

He steps closer to the street, positioning himself as a shield from passing cars. He knows the rules, or maybe, he just knows me.

It's been a while since I've been with a boy, well . . . a man, who knows the rules but isn't also wearing the full good ole boy "starter kit"—pressed khakis that have seen more SEC tailgates than board meetings, a brown leather belt purchased in 1998 and still going strong, driving loafers without socks, a pastel button-down shirt in something aggressively named "Seafoam" or "Regatta Blue," and, optional but preferred, a monogram.

For the first time, I glance down at Brett's feet: Ferragamo loafers. Sleek. Intentional. City. Not New Balance. Not something that has ever stepped foot on a bass fishing boat.

A small, private footwear victory—stamped with my approval. Not that he needs it. We get stranded in the middle of Park Avenue, misjudging the timing of the traffic lights. The begonias are blooming all along the median, perfectly planted, unapologetically manicured. I don't think I'll ever outgrow the quiet sense of wonder that comes with crossing this boulevard. Park Avenue feels less like a street and more like a statement.

Most of the windows above us are dark, likely owned by a far more settled crowd than the one inhabiting my current Midtown building and its revolving door of college students and temporary tenants, all living loosely defined timelines.

Yet, a few apartments still glow. Through the lit windows, I imagine custom lampshades pleated in Schumacher or Brunschwig & Fils textiles, casting that perfect, honeyed diffusion light that designers chase but rarely achieve. Symmetrical curtains trimmed with silk tassels frame each pane like a stage set. I can practically see the floors, intricate mosaic inlays or, at the very least, a timeless herringbone. Nothing basic for a Park Avenue apartment.

For a second, standing in the middle of this iconic street with Brett beside me and traffic waiting on all sides, I feel suspended between worlds, the temporary and the permanent. The curated and the chaotic. The girl who sublets. And the woman who owns.

I grew up in a beautiful home. My mother knew all the right colors to paint the rooms, all the right prints to pair together, and to only splurge on good Oriental or kilim rugs, but the paints were Behr, dupes of Farrow & Ball, and the fabrics were Waverly, the more accessible arm of Schumacher, created for families just like mine. Champagne tastes with a middle-shelf bourbon budget.

For a Thursday night, even at this hour, the city is exceptionally quiet, and I'm oddly aware of how loud my shoes sound when they hit the pavement. Does Brett hear it, too? I fear I sound like an elephant barreling my way toward Lexington Avenue.

I'm trying to follow his amusing story, something about his dad, a commercial airline pilot, flying one of the first planes to take off after 9/11 because he had a penguin on board, but all I can hear is the sharp, unforgiving clack of my sample sale Chanels striking the pavement. Each step ricochets off the buildings. The sound feels indecent on a street this dignified. I'm half-expecting lights to flick on in the lower floors of these immaculate Park Avenue apartments, older women in quilted, powder-blue robes appearing at the windows peering down with narrowed eyes. Judging. Sensing. Surely, they'd know, with their cultivated intuition and decades of cocktail-party observation, that the man beside me is not my husband. They'd sense something slightly improper is unfolding below their tasseled curtains. My heels crack against the crosswalk again. Confession by footwear.

Rather than wait for another red light, we turn down Lexington Avenue and walk south a few blocks, still in search of an open diner and still deep in conversation about everything and nothing at all. Brett watches my every move. Even in the moments when I look away, I can feel his eyes on me. He's sometimes focused on my lips as I talk, sometimes at my waist as I move, sometimes at my hands as I wave them around feverishly, like every other woman in my family, all in the name of better storytelling.

As we approach 74th Street, he lengthens his stride, stepping just ahead of me. Then, he turns quickly. I'm suddenly inches from him, no scaffolding overhead, no metal bars separating the sky from the street, just open night above us, wide and unprotected.

Brett steps into my space, and I feel it everywhere. His chest nearly brushes mine, the fold of his shirt, damp from the humidity. The warmth radiates off him. The faint trace of his cologne cuts through the air. My pulse moves to my throat. His hand slides firmly against my lower back, drawing me forward as if gravity has shifted. For a split second, I think he's going to kiss me. And I don't move, not at first.

Then, conditioning kicks in, and I dip backward, just enough for his lips to miss mine by inches. My smile is uncontrollable, breath shallow, body still angled toward him.

He exhales, mocking his agony but lacing it with truth. "Denied," his voice low now. Closer to a murmur than a joke.

"Friend," I say, though it comes out softer than intended. "I'm married. You remember, right?"

"I was trying to forget," he answers, and that smile—devastating and boyish—spreads slowly across his face. His hand hasn't left my back. In fact, it presses me slightly closer, his thumb grazing the curve of my waist. He doesn't pull me in. He doesn't step back. He just holds me there, suspended. What frightens me most is not that he almost kissed me but how badly I wanted him to. Clearly, the friend zone isn't a concern. What might happen next is. But I don't feel worried at all. I feel safe. Maybe delusional. Which is almost more alarming.

I've been faithfully married to Richard for almost seven years, but I was with him for nearly three years before that. I've given him nearly a decade of loyalty, of showing up, of doing the right thing. And yet, I don't feel safe with him anymore.

With Richard, everything is conditional. Fragile. At any moment, his contempt can surface, over something silly. Things that feel microscopic to me are monumental to him: crunching loudly while eating, wearing a dress he doesn't approve of, leaving a cereal bowl out, staying on the phone too long with my mother, or dancing on stage at my best friend's wedding.

With Richard, the temperature shifts without warning. The last time it did, it shook something loose in me. It shook me enough to leave, at least physically. I still haven't had the courage to officially say the words out loud. Not to my family. Not to the world. Not even fully to Brett.

I'm a coward. I know it, and, yet, here I am, standing inches from a man I barely know, feeling steadier than I have in years. This should terrify me. It doesn't.

"Morgan," Brett says, "I think we might be striking out, but I have a spot in mind on the West Side that I think you might like. There's no matzo ball soup and string beans, but it will have fried chicken which feels right for a Kentucky girl."

I'm short of breath but not for any physical reason. Trying for casual, I respond, "I'll do a lot of things for fried chicken. Even ride across town with a stranger . . . "

We've made it all the way to Third Avenue in search of the perfect diner, but somehow, in the wee hours of the morning, we find ourselves hailing a cab instead.

Brett opens the cab door for me, one hand holding my trench coat, the other resting on the top of the door, ensuring that he's coming with me. The streetlight catches the faint five-o'clock shadow along his jaw. I'm not sure how I'm only noticing it now.

He slides in after me. And suddenly, we're in a tiny, dim cocoon. Just the two of us. The city is muffled outside. Even through the satin of my skirt, the seat is tacky against my legs. Sliding over is awkward. I make it three-quarters of the way across before physics intervenes. Every bump in the road brings our bodies back together.

Through the park, under the bridge, everything goes pitch black. The kind of black that feels intimate. I know Brett wants to kiss me. I can feel it in the way his voice lowers, in the pause between sentences. I try not to make too much eye contact.

Meanwhile, he's telling me about college, Case Western Reserve University. I've heard of it, vaguely. In my mind, it exists somewhere between "prestigious" and "nerd school." Certainly not a label ever applied to the University of Alabama, my alma mater.

The fact that he graduated from a relatively unknown, smarty-pants school does something unexpected to me. It makes my insides warm. He's hot and . . . decent. That's the word. There's something deeply attractive about intelligence without theatrics. No airs. No chest-thumping boasts about an Ivy League pedigree. He's just sharing stories about cross-country meets in freezing Ohio wind, late nights in the library, and calculating how high he had to keep his GPA so he wouldn't lose his academic scholarship.

He drops in a few details about his parents. Says he'd actually been set to attend the University of Michigan but pulled out at the last minute when he realized it would cost them significantly less if he chose Case instead. He says it without self-congratulation. Just fact. Responsibility at 18 years old.

I try to picture myself at 18, making a financial decision for the greater good of my family. I can't. I was a mess from the divorce. It was so fresh then. I knew my first choice of Wake Forest was out of reach, too far, and too expensive. I understood that much. Kentucky would have been free. But staying close, somewhere that still felt like home? That was not the plan. I wanted distance. I wanted anonymity. I wanted a place where no one knew me or my parents.

So, Roll Tide it was.

Not to mention the fun of it all, waiting for me, tucked inside a large, beautiful campus. SEC football. Cocktail dresses to games. Mixers. Sorority houses the size of the White House.

The cab lurches to a stop at Amsterdam and 77th. Brett pays in cash. Actual folded bills, tucked perfectly into a sterling silver Tiffany's money clip. It screams gift from an ex-girlfriend.

Cash is a currency I rarely carry, and I'm perpetually punished for not having. All summer long, taxi drivers have been playing the "my credit card machine is broken" game, dodging merchant fees like it's a competitive sport. Most of my life is funded by credit these days. Floating. Swiping. Not looking too closely at bank statements, assuming I look at all. But tonight isn't about balances.

I step onto the sidewalk. The sky has shifted, heavier now, dark and moody, but I feel light. Giddy. But not just because of him.

"Here she is," Brett announces dramatically, gesturing toward the glowing sign. "The iconic Chirping Chicken."

We fold in half laughing. After all that Park Avenue grandeur, after nearly kissing under the bridge, we've landed at a fluorescent chicken joint.

"A cab ride for this?" I ask, the corner of my mouth curling. "It better be finger-licking good."

He promises it won't disappoint with far too much confidence.

Resting my hand on his shoulder, looking up at him, I say, "This chicken could be as dry as the turkey in *Christmas Vacation* . . . and this night still wouldn't disappoint."

There it is. My biggest flirt of the evening. He catches it without hesitation. No deflection. No nervous laugh. He just smiles, slow, satisfied, like he knew I'd get here eventually.

My cheeks flush hot. It would be wrong to blame it on the wine.

Usually, fluorescent lights at this hour make me self-conscious. It's far harsher than the glow of Bemelmans, but I give it one fleeting thought and move on. Brett's too much fun to consider vanity.

This place is cute in its own way. Less classic diner with chrome and vinyl booths, more neighborhood joint built for speed and grease. Counter service. Trays. The red plastic kind that feel straight out of a middle-school cafeteria, or, if we're being honest, a low-security mental institution.

Apparently, the Upper West Side requires access to fried chicken at all hours, because this place stays open well into the night. That might be its most attractive feature so far. More time. With him.

I order the special platter and a drink.

"Make that two," Brett says, without even glancing at the menu.

The man behind the counter, apron slightly dusted in flour, hands us two thick, clear plastic cups stacked upside down, the wavy, opaque kind that survives being dropped by generations of children. Growing up, the cups were always red, stamped with the Dr. Pepper logo. This always puzzled me. In the South, we only drink Coke products. Everything is Coke. Sometimes, it is actually Coke or Diet Coke, preferably, but "Coke" really just means soda in the South. The one thing it never means is Pepsi.

I smile at the memory, turning the cup upright. Brett watches me.

"What?" he asks.

"Nothing," I say. "Just thinking about how complicated Southern beverage terminology can be."

He laughs.

And just like that, we're standing in line for fried chicken, holding cafeteria cups, talking about soda semantics. Park Avenue feels a world away. But somehow, this feels more intimate.

The cashier hands me a silver stand stamped with the number 11 and tells me to pick a seat. There are exactly five tables in the entire place. All two-tops. Light brown faux wood laminate with basic black pedestal bases, identical to those in the first restaurant I ever waited tables in, complete with the same plastic cups.

Honestly, it was the only restaurant I ever waited tables in. I love to work. Maybe too much. But waitressing, while lucrative for a 16-year-old, was not my calling. I dropped trays. Forgot sides. Smiled too hard when I messed up.

I scan the room for a place to sit. Brett is gone. Bathroom? Or did he bolt? A flicker of panic rises. Why would he bail now? Yes, I denied him one kiss, but he's the one who suggested fried chicken as a consolation. And he doesn't strike me as the "quit after one try" type.

I claim a table anyway. The metal chair is cold and unwelcoming. The surface is crowded—napkin holder, saltshaker, vinegar bottle, crushed red pepper flakes. It's busy. Like my dad's grandmother's countertops. Jars and condiments permanently stationed as decor. Always a little sticky.

For a split second, I imagine myself sitting here alone with two massive plates of fried chicken. And then Brett walks back in.

"Sorry to disappear on you," he says, sliding into the chair across from me. "I saw they were cash only and needed to hit an ATM."

Of course, he didn't abandon me.

The simple fact that he thought ahead and went to the ATM, without fanfare, doesn't go unnoticed. Richard used to excuse himself to the bathroom right as the check arrived when we'd have dinner with my parents. I always offered to pay, anyways, of course. But that wasn't the point.

Brett adjusts awkwardly on the hard seat, long legs negotiating limited space.

"Number Eleven!" the counter boy shouts. Brett stands and retrieves our trays, returning with two heaping plates.

"You know," he says, as he sets one tray down in front of me, "I usually order grilled and just hope they accidentally bring me fried. Occasionally," he continues, lowering his voice just enough, "the world works in mysterious ways, and fried chicken appears." He looks at me. "Like it was meant to be . . . "

The line is absurd. And yet. Here we are.

I am hungry in a way that surprises me. Food actually sounds good. My eating has been . . . unpredictable lately. Sporadic enough that my mom has noticed.

The chicken smells divine. Steaming, crispy skin crackling, heat rising into the fluorescent air.

As I go to take my first bite, my lip catches on my tooth, dry, uncooperative, like it's forgotten how this works. Oh shoot.

"I never got us drinks," I say quickly. "I'm so sorry. I got distracted when you disappeared on me. What would you like?"

"Please don't apologize," he says easily. "I've got it. Tea? Water? Soda?"

Oh Lord. If he doesn't like a woman who apologizes for things that don't warrant apologies, then we're already headed for couples counseling. Apologizing is practically a core competency for Southern women. We say "I'm sorry" almost as much as we say "y'all."

On any given day, I probably tell friends, family, and total strangers "I'm sorry" at least five times every waking hour. And lately, with my nonexistent sleep schedule, I have a lot of waking hours. A hundred apologies a day doesn't feel like an exaggeration.

Short of telling Richard I'm sorry for being out with a man who is not him, and feeling more alive than I ever do with him, I'm not sure most of the other apologies are necessary.

I'm sorry you're standing in front of the soap dispenser, and I need it. I'm sorry it rained today, though, I am not God. I'm sorry the line is long. I'm sorry your coffee is too hot. I'm sorry I exist in a way that mildly inconveniences you.

"I'm sorry," I say again.

Oh, my God. I just apologized for apologizing. It hits me in real time how reflexive it's become. The tally has been climbing for years now. Far beyond what's socially expected of a "nice young lady." With Richard, apologizing for simply being myself has become muscle memory. For my tone. For my laugh. For my timing. For my ambition. For my moods. For taking up space.

And here I am, sitting in a fried chicken joint well after midnight, apologizing to a man who just told me not to apologize. He smiles at me, soft but direct.

"You don't have to do that," Brett says.

And something inside me tightens, not in fear but in recognition. It's exhausting trying to live up to a version of myself that Richard constructed in his head. More exhausting to admit that I helped build her. When Richard and I met, I was desperate for something solid to stand on so I wouldn't fully disappear. So, I handed him a curated girl—agreeable, light, uncomplicated.

Richard fell in love with the façade, and now, I resent him for believing it. Every crack in that façade feels like a letdown to him, like a reminder that I'm not quite what he signed up for. Not shiny enough. Not steady enough. Not enough.

It might be the very thing that has me here tonight, with my elbows on a laminate table, actively gnawing on a fried chicken leg across from the most engaging man I've ever met. A man who, despite the fact that I am tearing into poultry with alarming enthusiasm, seems to find me fascinating. Both of us have too much fine red wine in our systems. Burgundy bravado replaced by grease-stained fingers and paper napkins. Grease to the rescue.

Brett and I lean back in, picking up the thread of conversation from our barstools at Bemelmans like no time has passed. Only now, there's hot sauce on our knuckles and no pretense left to maintain.

He asks follow-up questions. Real ones. About my business. About Thailand. About why I chose college at Alabama over Kentucky. He listens in a way that makes me feel expansive instead of scrutinized. There's no evaluation in his eyes. Just curiosity. I catch myself mid-laugh and realize something almost dangerous: I'm not performing. I'm just . . . here.

Messy. Greasy. Honest. And somehow, it's enough.

"So, you were seriously a virgin on your wedding night?" Brett asks, revisiting my earlier confession, still trying to compute it.

Somehow, the topic felt far less exposed in the velvet darkness of Bemelmans. Under unforgiving lighting, with my mascara pushing hour 10, it feels harsher. If I resemble Uncle Fester at this point, Brett's kind enough not to let on. Because in his gaze, I've never felt prettier.

"That didn't come out right," he adds quickly, setting his hand on the table, not quite reaching for mine, but close. Searching, maybe.

My hands are in my lap, mid-bite, puny paper napkin draped perfectly across my skirt. When I glance down, I notice a grease spot blooming across the satin. Unavoidable. Worth it. For the first time in my life, I wish my table manners were worse so my hand would already be there for him to find.

"I'm not saying it's a bad thing," he says, genuinely. "I just don't think I've ever met anyone your age who 'saved herself for marriage,' as you put it."

"I thought you said you grew up Catholic," I respond. "Isn't that, like . . . the whole thing? Virgin Mary and all?"

His head tips back, laughing.

The truth is, I don't actually know that much about Catholicism. The Bible Belt of my youth was a sampler platter of denominations: Southern Baptist, regular Baptist, Presbyterian, Church of Christ, nondenominational mega churches with fog machines and rock bands, and, of course, Methodist. Like me.

There was one Catholic church in my hometown, but I'd never stepped inside. Odd, considering I'd been to most of the other churches at one point or another for youth group swaps, Wednesday night revivals, or friends' Confirmation ceremonies.

Growing up, church was a one-to-three-times-a-week affair for me. And like most things in my life, it came with high highs and low lows. Youth group at First Methodist and First Baptist was half God, half hormones. Super Bowl Sunday parties with the cutest boys in school. Ski trips to the questionable slopes of Gatlinburg, Tennessee. We worshiped Jesus while side-hugging our crushes. Innocent, mostly. The occasional make-out session, sure, but better in the back of a church van than in the back of a boy's Pathfinder, right?

For me, church was a happy place. Loving. Judgmental, at times, but manageable. First Methodist drew the lawyers, the doctors, and the bankers. Faith for golfers. Not like the Church of Christ where my grandmother attended. No instruments. No alcohol. No women leading prayer. The only woman I ever saw at the front of that church, aside from baptisms, was a sweet girl who got pregnant on prom night and was made to confess before the entire congregation. The boy wasn't beside her. He didn't have to stand there. That image never left me.

I always told myself I was "saving myself" out of obedience. For God. For faith. For virtue. But if I'm honest, and apparently tonight I am, it was probably less theology and more fear. Fear of small-town shame. Fear of being that girl. Fear of derailing the bigger life I swore I'd have. One beyond Murray, Kentucky. One beyond expectation. One not possible for most teen moms. So, I abstained.

OK . . . abstained-ish. I glance back up at Brett, heat rising in my cheeks again.

"Let me clear this up for you," I say, ready to lay it all out for him, right here at the Chirping Chicken. "Yes, I was technically a virgin on my wedding night, but . . . "

I pause. "I wouldn't label myself a saint. Other bases had a go from time to time."

"Got it," he says. "A bit of a technicality then. Are you sure you are not Catholic?" He laughs.

"Yes, a technicality," I confirm, looking directly into his eyes. "But for the record, it does matter to me. My faith, that is. I'm kind of a mess at the moment, but my faith doesn't waver."

"I get it; faith is critical," he says unfeignedly. "But also, you don't seem like a mess to me. For the record."

I wasn't expecting this. Flirtatious quips? Sure. Somewhat braggy comments about his success? Of course. That's what all NYC dudes say. But faith is critical? Shocking.

"This isn't a mess?" I tease. "A married woman, covered in fried chicken grease, out with a stranger at almost three in the morning?"

"Believe me," he says, "I know a hot mess when I see one. You're far from it. You're basically perfect, short of being married. Plus, I'm not a stranger anymore. We've covered too much ground."

"OK, friend," I say in a slightly facetious tone, "this night has been unexpected and, honestly, pretty wonderful." My head tilts down, but my eyes flash up to him. "Because of you."

Brett blushes. For the first time all night.

"But I think it's time for me to go back to my real life," I tell him. The chicken has sobered me, though not completely, and I'm aware that tomorrow brings responsibilities and visitors to town. Visitors who will ask me what I did last night.

I want Brett to fight me on it. For a moment, it seems like he might. But then, he looks at me in a way that I've never been looked at before. Like he sees me as no one ever has. He looks at me with the kind of genuine care that takes decades to build. But here we are. Only hours in, and he appears to want nothing but to help me get wherever I need to go, to do whatever I need to do.

"Let's get you a cab then," he says softly, standing as he gathers both trays without asking.

He stacks them neatly, deposits the trash, slides them into the rack above where they'll be wiped down with an old white rag stitched in odd red thread, sprayed with a mystery cleaner of mostly water and vinegar in an unlabeled bottle, spreading germs in the name of sanitation.

I head toward the door. Full of fried chicken. Full of disappointment. I don't want the night to end, but I know where it could go from here. And I know I cannot follow.

Brett pushes the door open and holds it for me. The space is small. I feel his breath warm against my neck as I pass. My shoulder brushes his chest.

Outside, the city is silent. No taxis cruising. No post-party girls laughing too loudly as they stumble home. No sirens. It feels staged. Like someone forgot to cue the extras.

Brett raises his arm, and a cab appears out of nowhere.

Unfortunately. It's downtown bound.

Time slows.

I walk toward him, toward the taxi, studying him like I might not see him again. His shirt is even more rumpled now. His five-o'clock shadow darker. His eyes glossier. His hair slightly wild from running his hands through it all night. I feel suddenly painfully aware of myself, smudged mascara, rain-flattened hair, lips dry from forgetting gloss. He holds open the taxi door.

Every word between us has been effortless. But now? What do you say to cap off something like this? I turn toward him, waiting. Wanting something cinematic. A line ripped from a rom-com. Something about fate. About souls stirring. About how meeting me has changed everything.

Cold raindrops begin to fall. And his arm wraps around my waist. Fast. Feverish. He pulls me in with a decisiveness that steals my breath. My feet tangle. I steady myself by grabbing his shoulders, then his neck. His hair is thick beneath my fingers. His shirt soft, unstarched. Warm.

Strong hands press firmly at the small of my back as he looks at me, really looks. His eyes close first. Then, he leans down. His lips hover over mine for the briefest second, close enough that I can feel the heat of them. And then, they're there. Soft. Deliberate. Testing.

I don't flinch. I don't retreat.

I deepen the kiss. Not frantic. Not sloppy. Intentional.

His weight shifts into me, and instinctively I dip backward, surrendering to the pull. My hands slide through his hair. Down his back. We stumble, twisted, breathless, and, together, we tumble into the open taxi door.

Chapter 4
THE GREAT TAXI ESCAPE

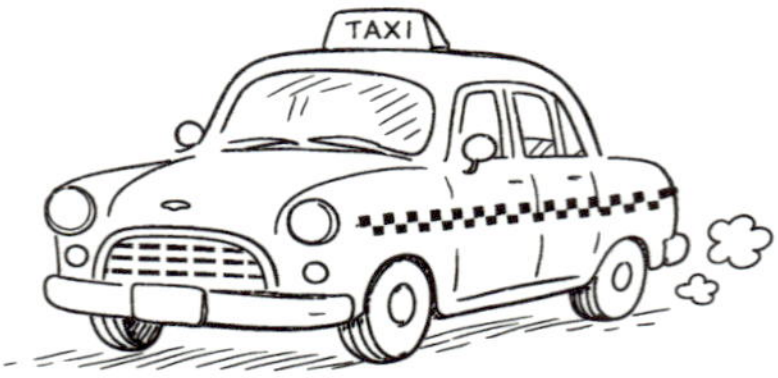

JUNE 19, 2009
Sometime between 3 a.m. and 4 a.m.
Upper West Side, New York City

I trust fall into the back seat of the taxi, certain Brett will catch me. His hand slides firmly down my lower back, steadying my descent as the black vinyl gives beneath me. The seat is slick with rainwater; the air inside is thick and humid. My skirt inches modestly across, but I need help getting over the middle-seat hump. The backs of my heels knock awkwardly against the metal door frame before my body fully lands inside, rain tickling my ankles. Brett's right knee slides inside the space between mine, nudging my skirt up higher, not aggressively just inevitably. His arm, braced under both of us, tightens around me and guides me deeper into the seat. For a second, he hovers above me. One arm planted. The other reaching back to pull the door shut.

The taxi seals around us with a dull thud.

Everything feels damp. Charged. The windows fog instantly, beads of rain racing one another down the glass in distorted streaks. The city lights outside blur into watercolors.

Brett leans forward and gives the driver an address. I barely register it. The sound of it is distant, like adults speaking in the background of a Charlie Brown cartoon.

I'm far more focused on Brett. On the way his chest rises and falls. On the way his hair curls slightly at the temples from the rain. On the weight of his body still angled toward mine.

What will he do next? And how many times has he done this before? This certainly is a first for me.

Not the kissing. Not even the back seat. But the surrender. The feeling of choosing something without calculating the fallout first. He looks down at me, rain-damp, breath slightly uneven, eyes darker now. Of all my NYC taxi-cab adventures, this is the best yet.

The sound of the windshield wipers gets louder and faster at the same rate of my breath. Brett's body on mine, bracing himself so his weight doesn't crush me beneath him. His left hand, wet from the rain-soaked door handle, feels cold against my right cheek as he strokes my face and slides his hand to the back of my neck, pulling me up, towards him, higher until our lips brush. He falls deeper into me. Every kiss in rhythm. He tastes faintly like fried chicken and red wine—a strangely intoxicating combination. My leftover perfume masks the musty smell of the cab. His five-o'clock shadow tickles my skin and sends a shiver down my spine to my toes.

When his mouth leaves mine, it doesn't go far. He trails slow kisses along my cheek, soft at first, then with growing hunger, as if memorizing the shape of me. He brushes my ear, a gentle graze that makes my body freeze, then continues down the curve of my neck.

His hand follows, exploratory. It glides down from my collarbone, lingering at my rib cage as though he's tracing something delicate, something worth studying. I arch instinctively toward him, closing whatever space remains between us. And I feel the evidence of his excitement against me.

His hand tightens at my waist, firm but careful, pulling me closer. His thumb presses lightly at my hip bone while his fingers anchor at my back, steadying both of us in the shifting cab. There's confidence in the way he touches me, like I've never felt before.

I'm trying to keep up. To match him. To make my touch feel just as certain, just as knowing. Following his lead feels instinctive, like my body understands something my mind is still scrambling to process. My right hand slides around his neck, fingers threading into his hair. It's softer than I expected. Longer, too. I hold him there, anchoring myself as much as him.

The small buttons of his shirt press through my sheer blouse, firm against my skin. My outfit is twisted beyond recognition now, satin bunched, blouse pulled, everything slightly off-kilter. My left hand is trapped awkwardly between our bodies. I wriggle it free, clumsy and eager, wanting to touch his face, his jaw, his chest—anything I can claim as mine in this moment.

Brett's touch is intoxicating. His every movement feels amplified, deliberate, electric, like he's tuning my nerves to a higher frequency. And yet there's a strange duality. I've almost become familiar with the feeling as if I'm both inside the moment and hovering above it. Watching myself.

From this imaginary bird's-eye view, it's obvious: I'm inexperienced. Hesitant in places Brett is not. Reacting where he initiates. Learning as I go. The fact that Richard and I were both virgins when we married once felt like a virtue badge. A box checked. A comfort. Right now, it feels like seven years of untouched potential.

It's startling to realize how little I've actually learned about myself. How much has been routine. Obligation. Performance. This feels different. Not just because of Brett. But because of me. Because, for the first time, I'm not trying to be good. I'm trying to be honest. And honesty, it turns out, is far more freeing.

Earlier when Brett jokingly peppered me about being such an "old" virgin, I didn't think about it in the context of rookie foreplay skills. It didn't occur to me that I would need to.

When I shared my lack of experience with him, he certainly didn't shy away from sharing his own plethora. Not in a braggy, big man on campus way. He was vulnerable. He spoke honestly about what it was like to be a single, 30-something man in Manhattan, with a good job and good hair. Turns out, it doesn't take that much to be a panty-dropper here. I was fascinated by it.

Maybe, in retrospect, Brett was a little braggy. But he camouflaged it with his wit and charm. Confident, but not cocky. Such a difference. He did tell me about his two serious-ish relationships, lasting a total of three years collectively. But his life in the Big Apple has been primarily centered around being a singleton, racking up quite the "number." It's not hard to do a little first-grade math: X number of weekend nights times X number of years in the city unattached = holy man-whore.

Man-whore. That's the kind of name-calling my 21-year-old self would have used. I've lived a little since then. All journeys are different. Mine seems to be taking quite the detour at the moment. It's "Captain Obviously" clear that, just because you save yourself for marriage and do all the things you're supposed to do, doesn't mean you won't end up in the back seat of a Manhattan taxi with a hot, strange man on top of you, kissing your neck with his hand between your thighs, traveling slowly up your skirt.

My previous tendency to judge didn't come from my parents. It's more so from organized religion, not to be confused with faith. My parents were not the shame-wielding, rule-thumping type. Quite the opposite. They were level. Kind. Reasonable. If anything, they worried I judged myself more harshly than they ever would.

Certainly, some of the judgment and the constant reminders to remain pure and chaste came from church, specifically from the youth group. But the message didn't stop there. It followed us to school as well. During our senior year of high school, the Twins and I were approached to lead a new club called PSI—an acronym for Postponing Sexual Involvement. Our task was to speak to middle school students, encouraging them to save themselves for marriage.

Officially, the program claimed no religious affiliation. The stated goal was simply to curb Kentucky's overwhelmingly high rate of teen pregnancy. But growing up deep in the Bible Belt, it was impossible not to recognize the unmistakable undertone shaping the whole effort.

Both girls and boys attended the meetings, but the PSI videos we showed on VHS were crystal clear—the message was intended for girls. As if the shame of gaining regular weight wasn't bad enough. Heaven forbid the weight gain was caused by an out-of-wedlock pregnancy.

My parents didn't sit me down with a purity contract and ring ceremony. They didn't tape Bible verses to my mirror. The "virgin thing" wasn't pushed on me by them. In reality, I sometimes think they were quietly puzzled by my abstinence. Especially when I was dating Richard. I imagine my dad, in his understated way, thinking, "Are we sure this is healthy?" And my mom, scanning the situation with her mother radar, wondering if it shouldn't be harder to wait.

In retrospect, resisting temptation with Richard should have been more difficult. But the "good girl" identity fit me like a pressed Easter dress—structured, flattering, and slightly restrictive.

The inconvenient truth? It wasn't heroic restraint. I didn't want to sleep with Richard, which, when you think about it, makes the whole thing far less saintly and far more telling. In 2001, the cultural messaging around me was crystal clear: Be pure at heart. Guard your body. Save it. Protect it. But then . . . ding, ding, ding! Once the wedding ring slides on and the vows are exchanged, you're expected to flip a switch. Overnight, you're meant to transform into this enthusiastic, sexually available wife, who somehow knows exactly what she's doing and is delighted to do it. Years of careful instruction about purity and restraint vanish the moment the bouquet is tossed. It's a rather abrupt transition for a girl who spent most of her life being told not to give it up.

There's shame in wanting sex before you're "supposed to." And then, there's shame in not wanting it constantly once you're married. It's really a no-win system. Shame before. Shame after. Gold star if you manage to feel nothing confusing in between. I internalized this script so thoroughly that I didn't stop to ask whether it made sense for me. Not until much later. Not until the back seat of this taxi, apparently.

Regardless of how many women Brett has known biblically, there is nothing remotely seedy about him. Earlier at Bemelmans, while I was talking about my marriage, carefully airbrushing it into something far less cracked than it actually is, mostly to avoid embarrassment or admit failure, Brett told me, without any bravado, that he isn't married because he hasn't found "the one."

He didn't say it in a cliché way but in a measured, almost reverent way. His parents have been married nearly 40 years, and in his mind, their relationship sits on a mighty tall pedestal. A gold-standard, framed-and-lit, museum-level pedestal. It's a tough comp. And one he feels he can't match . . . yet.

I, on the other hand, have become quite adept at editing the truth about my marriage, depending on the audience. Close friends. Family. Casual acquaintances. I can spin a tidy narrative in seconds. It's second nature after so many years of practice. The thought of truly opening up now feels exhausting. Where would I even begin? And with whom? Greer? Addy? My mom? My best friend from college, Brandace? How would I explain it after all these years?

Greer would be the trickiest, but not because she'd judge me. She absolutely wouldn't. She'd understand immediately. The issue is that she would go straight into solution mode. Type A meets Type A. Flow charts would appear. Strategic plans would be drafted. And there's the tiny complication that her husband is technically Richard's boss now.

We moved to Dallas because Richard decided being an attorney in New York was "too stressful" and "too cutthroat." Apparently, I was the only one "getting to enjoy the city." Not entirely untrue. Third-year associates work inhumane hours. I'm not saying his complaints were invalid. I just never had a flicker of desire to leave New York.

But after connecting Richard to Greer's very successful father-in-law, the founder of a large Dallas-based company with national reach, the move felt inevitable. I still kick myself for making that introduction. Richard is crazy smart, and he interviews exceptionally well. He's possibly the best first-impression man I've ever met. Unfortunately, the longer you know him, the less sparkle remains. Longer when you have a wife who protects your image.

I tend to love people more over time; I appreciate their quirks, their layers, and the oddities that make them human. Maybe, I just bring out the worst in Richard. Regardless, Greer is off the table. I'm not ready to open Pandora's box with her, yet.

Addy is out for a different reason. She's too good. Genuinely good. I've known her since we were toddlers, and I've watched people mistake her kindness for something performative more times than I can count. It used to infuriate me. Now, I realize people are simply missing out on something rare. If I told Addy, her heart would crack first. And then mine would. She would worry about my future, about my happiness, about my soul. I don't think I could survive the look on Addy's face, our resident sweetheart, sticky with kindness and optimism.

My mom? That's loaded. I've suspected for years that she doesn't love Richard, or even like him for that matter. She's far too guarded to say it outright, but in the last year, it's become obvious. She's seen the missteps. The tone shifts. The way I over-explain things. But still . . . I don't know what Mom's reaction would actually be.

First question? Money. "Do you have cash stashed?" she'd ask. "Ratholing," she calls it. And I would have to admit that I don't.

There was a time when I did have a secret stash. Mom would send cash and tell me to tuck it away. "Just in case," she'd say, as if hurricanes and husbands required the same emergency planning. For a while, I listened. But lately? My spending has not been . . . prudent.

If I like a shoe, I buy it in every color. If I wander into a vintage store, I come out with armfuls of '80s party dresses I absolutely do not need. The stash, and then some, is long gone.

Honestly, confessing my lack of a "rathole" to my mom might be harder than admitting I need out of my marriage to survive. That said, I'm her only child. And she is a worrier. I'm not sure she could carry the weight of knowing about my darker thoughts. The ones that creep in when the lights are off and the house is quiet. That information would live in her chest forever. No. I can't tell my mom.

Which leaves Brandace. A.k.a. "Bran." She's a safe space. Always has been. We met the first day of sorority rush, sitting on the steps of the Chi Omega house, both pretending we weren't terrified. She's always been the kind of friend who can sit in silence without trying to fix you. I almost told her. Just last month.

We were in New Orleans for a college friend's bachelorette party. After one final round of hurricanes at Pat O'Brien's, the rest of the group called it a night. But I needed more time with her. We only see each other once a year, twice if we are super lucky. I would've stayed up until sunrise just to catch up with her.

We were starving, but our options were limited, so we landed at a 24-hour all-you-can-eat buffet at Harrah's Casino. Nothing says emotional breakthrough like a heat-lamp-warmed meal. The casino had tipped into gross territory. It hadn't started out great—hideous carpet, aggressively colorful furniture—but now, it felt sticky in spirit.

Bran and I sat with basic white plates piled high with cheesy hash browns, chicken fingers, mashed potatoes, overcooked green beans, and fries that had clearly lost the will to live. We didn't dive in right away. There was a warm-up lap, recapping the night, dissecting everyone's questionable dance moves, updating each other on jobs and trips, and the usual adult-life bullet points. And then, I felt it. The moment.

I was just about to say it: "Bran, I'm going to leave Richard."

Then, Bran said, "I have to tell you something." Her news was big. Life-altering big.

It was clearly not the moment to "Carrie Bradshaw" her. (I always hated how Carrie would hijack everyone's vulnerability with her own.

Samantha's cancer announcement might've been the only time she didn't.) So, I swallowed it. Pinned my confession to the corkboard of "later." That night had one storyline. And it wasn't mine.

With no one to tell, I pushed it down again. Like I've done so many times before. But Brett made it easy to open up. I found myself saying things to him I hadn't said out loud to anyone. The cracks in my marriage slipped out between sips of wine and bites of chicken. I told Brett about renting my own apartment in the city for the summer, husband excluded, and he instantly knew that was off. It struck me again how odd it was that the people closest to me didn't question the move, the apartment. They didn't press, didn't probe.

Maybe, I missed my calling as an actor. It's probably more lucrative than the panty business during the biggest financial crisis of my lifetime. Apparently, jet-setting lingerie is one of the first casualties of a recession.

All I know is this: my "faking it," emotionally, domestically, sexually has landed me here. Back in my favorite city.

With very few questions asked.

I'm not faking anything right now. And I have the unsettling suspicion I'd never need to with Brett. His attention is singular. Focused. Devoted to the moment. To me. His hand moves gently, gliding under my satin skirt, slow and exploratory. I shift on impulse, lifting slightly from the seat to give him room. His fingers curl, testing. Each small movement pulls the fabric higher.

My breath shortens. The world narrows. When my skirt lifts too high, and his fingers cross the line where lace meets skin, charged tension snaps through me. More than desire. Suddenly, it's gone too far. His touch deepens, and in one dizzying second, my body reacts before my brain can catch up. I jolt upright as if struck. My feet slam against the taxi's rubber floor mats. Both hands fly to my forehead in panic.

What the hell am I doing? This isn't you, Morgan. You are a good girl. You do the right thing. You don't torch your life in the back seat of a taxi. I look up. Traffic light ahead.

"Stop!" I shout. "Right here is fine."

I tug my skirt down, adjust myself, and grab my clutch from the damp floor. The cab screeches to a halt somewhere on the East Side. I have no idea where we are. My sense of direction is tragically unreliable.

It takes Brett a beat to understand what's happening. He's not angry. He's concerned. I hadn't given him a clear boundary. I hadn't signaled retreat. And yet, something deep inside me knows this is the line.

Honestly, the line blurred the second Brett and I locked eyes at Bemelmans. But this? This is irreversible territory.

There's no elegant exit from the back seat. Only to go over him. So, I do the least elegant thing possible. I swing my leg over his.

For three seconds, I'm straddling him, close enough to feel his heart beat and the undeniable proof of where we are headed. I sink into him just long enough to memorize it.

And then, I kiss him. One last kiss. Not frantic. Not sloppy. Just perfect.

When I pull back and reach for the door, Brett's arm tightens around my waist. His silent protest. He doesn't want me to go. But he knows I have to. He squeezes my hand as I pull away.

I tumble out onto the street and shut the taxi door quickly, before my resolve cracks. The light turns green. Through the rain-streaked window, Brett's hand presses flat against the glass. A quiet goodbye. The taxi pulls away. I don't know his last name. He doesn't know mine. Somehow, this makes it hurt more.

Chapter 5

THE MORNING AFTER

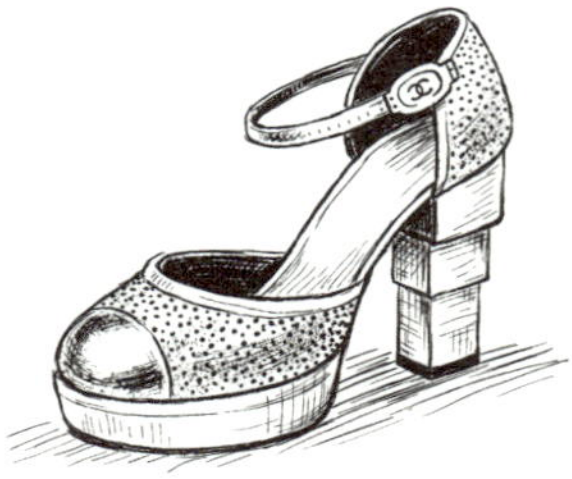

JUNE 19, 2009
9 a.m.—My Temporary Apartment
Midtown, New York City

I wake to tingling feet, like I stepped into a bucket of Pop Rocks. They're fully asleep, draped uncomfortably over the arm of an unfortunate brown microfiber sofa with a thick-ribbed texture, tufted with fabric-covered buttons. It's the kind designed to trap crumbs in its dimples forever, no matter how aggressively you vacuum.

My head feels heavy. Not sharp pain. More like a slow internal drumbeat, thumping from the inside out. Something tugs at my right hand, and my fingers feel cinched tight, as if they're wrapped in an invisible rubber band. I blink awake to a white popcorn ceiling.

Normally, I find popcorn ceilings offensive, the lazy contractor's solution to covering flaws in commercial-grade buildings. But here, in this apartment, sprinkled generously with design crimes from what appears to have been a 1980s renovation spree, I can't bring myself to judge.

Vertical blinds that never fully align. Closet rods hung so close to the shelf above that I skin my knuckles every time I change outfits. Faded cookie cutter parquet floors. And yes, that aggressively textured ceiling.

But this place? She's mine. All 654 square feet of her. A place carved out just for me. Temporary, perhaps, but earned. I would never criticize her. Not her blinds. Not her popcorn ceiling. Not her cramped closets. Not when she represents something far bigger than aesthetics.

Freedom.

And I don't intend to take a single square inch of her for granted.

August 2001, Dallas, Texas

In a crowded Italian restaurant, which he absolutely cannot afford, on a small dance floor, flanked by intimate booths and a piano player tucked in the far corner, Richard gets down on one knee.

White tablecloths and waiters in pressed shirts surround us. One other couple drifts nearby, lost in their own orbit. Their closeness with one another makes me feel the sting of envy. Though I'm not exactly sure why.

Richard is looking up at me. Words are falling from his mouth. All kind. All wonderful. But they swirl around me, never landing fully. The whole thing seems rushed and oddly timed. This place is beautiful, but it's random. We have no sentimental connection to it.

He stops talking and opens a small black velvet box. Inside is a one-carat radiant diamond set in platinum and flanked by round sapphires, my birthstone. It's exactly what I had described once to him in passing. He's a thoughtful gift-giver. He has been since we started dating a little over 18 months ago.

I'm meant to leave tomorrow, headed back to Tuscaloosa for my senior year at the University of Alabama. Sorority rush starts in three days. I'm the president. I have to be there early. No exceptions. I came to Dallas to help him move in, to get him settled before his first day of law school. His parents are here, too. They never miss an opportunity to offer a hand. They're generous and kind in a way that makes his life smoother. Endlessly supportive. The kind of parents who show up with extra towels, a toolkit, and snacks you didn't ask for.

I look down at the ring, sparkling in the candlelit room. My eyes shift to Richard's face. I smile to calm his nerves. He's off-kilter. Uncalculated. I can feel it. Why is he doing this now? Sure, I've had an inkling a proposal might be coming, but it's unlike him to do anything on the fly, without total control. Typically, everything is planned to a T. By him. With his comfort in mind.

I might have pictured it a little differently, something more open, maybe including more of the people who matter, but that would have introduced variables. More moving parts. More unpredictability. This way is cleaner.

Just the two of us. His parents waiting neatly at a hotel, folded into the evening at the appropriate moment and distance. My parents not told at all, their presence always a bit too complicated, a bit too real for Richard to comfortably manage.

And the timing, too, just before I return for my final year of undergrad feels intentional. As if asking now keeps everything tidy and in place before anything has the chance to change.

My heart beats faster. I have 30 seconds or less to make the most finite decision of my life. Saying yes means a whole string of things. I'll be a lawyer's wife. Just like my mom. I'll design other people's homes while fussing endlessly over ours. I'll belong to a man who has no idea about the darker thoughts that plague me, thoughts now infiltrating daily.

Is saying no even an option? What's the alternative life if I refuse? I think he loves me. A part of me genuinely loves him, too. I don't know if I'm in love with him. I'm not even sure I fully understand the distinction. I just know that, in the beginning, he felt interesting. Different from the endless loop of the fraternity scene. A GDI (God Damn Independent) as they say at Alabama. It was a breath of fresh air to be taken on proper dates, outside of football stadiums and basement band parties. I got swept up in it. And then, suddenly, a year had passed.

I had only just wrapped my head around the idea of having a long-distance relationship. Him in law school, me finishing my senior year. That felt like a stretch already. And now, he wants me to commit to so much more?

A deep breath.

"Yes," I say. I'm 20 years old. What else should I say?

He stands up to hug me. I hold onto him. He feels shaky. The whole thing feels surreal. My outfit is all wrong. The room is clapping. Cheering us on. Clinking their glasses and requesting us to kiss. We do. Quick. Dry. Routine. We walk back to the table. Waiting for us is a delicate dessert with an intricate chocolate garnish that reads "Best Wishes & Congratulations!" in fine script.

One thought is running through my head: What dessert would they have placed on the table if I had said no?

I thank the server more than once. His eyes are kind. You can tell he's a lifer. And he can tell that I'm not 21, but he serves me champagne anyway. Trying to calm my inevitable cold feet, I think.

That night, we stay at a Super 8 hotel just off the highway. His mom booked it. She always does her best, but aesthetics simply aren't her strong suit. Brutal fluorescent lighting. Carpet that knows things. The smell of cleaning solution and old smoke. A quilted floral coverlet in a shade of mauve that was likely discontinued a decade ago. An old television with maybe 10 channels. And, of course, a popcorn ceiling. I stare at that popcorn ceiling longer than I stare at the ring.

Something about that feels like an omen.

June 19, 2009, 9 a.m.—My Temporary Apartment, NYC

My current home is far from charming prewar vibes, but I couldn't care less. It actually reminds me of the slew of apartments I toured before finding the gem on 61st. I didn't know what prewar meant back then. Of course I'd heard it mentioned in movies over the years, and I knew it implied something important. Now I get it. Prewar signals plaster walls, gorgeous moldings, heavy French doors with layers of lacquered paint, transoms, and window seat nooks designed for reading *Vogue* cover to cover, warm on the radiator that lies beneath.

But that little "gem" came with a roommate. This one doesn't.

Perhaps her location isn't particularly charming, sandwiched between corporate glass and generic storefronts, but she offers easy access to Bryant Park and the New York Public Library, two of my favorites. Not to mention, the 42nd Street subway hub is dangerously convenient. I can be almost anywhere in the city in minutes.

Though, truthfully, I prefer to walk. It feels so good to be in motion. To move with intention. To let the city carry me block by block. Assuming, of course, that I choose my footwear wisely.

Greer and Addy are convinced I don't have nerve endings in my feet, based on the length of time I can survive in absurdly tall heels. They're not entirely wrong. Pain tolerance has never been my issue. But even I have limits.

Speaking of shoes . . . mine are still on. From last night. Or this morning. Time feels irrelevant.

I force my stomach muscles to cooperate and push myself up onto my elbows. Red rings circle my ankles with tiny interlocking Cs pressed into my skin like a luxury brand's version of a cattle mark. Proof of commitment. Or poor planning.

I close my eyes, and it all flashes back in fragments.

My heels stepping in rhythm down the avenues of the Upper East Side. Ferragamo loafers beside them. The way Brett's hand felt firm at my waist. The way he pulled me in like he wasn't entirely sure I was real. The weight of him, the certainty in his touch. The way his lips lingered on mine. The way I wanted him more than anything.

I sit all the way up.

The room tilts.

My fingertips are ridged and pruned, deep lines pressed into them from gripping a thin white plastic Farmers Deli bag for far too long. I must have fallen asleep or passed out while clutching it like a security blanket.

The sun is unapologetic. It floods through the plate glass sliding door that leads to my precarious balcony, the kind that looks glued on as an afterthought, like a small architectural shrug jutting into the sky with no visible support.

The vertical blinds hang stiff and beige beside it. I never close them. I don't care to look at that much beige.

When you're an impressionable 18-year-old interior design major and your favorite professor announces, with theatrical disgust, that vertical blinds are reserved for trailer parks, you remember. My mother, gentler but equally firm, relegated the blinds to dental offices and roadside motels, two places best avoided.

So, I keep them pulled back as tightly as they'll go, trying to will them out of existence.

I peer into the deli bag: a half-finished zero-calorie orange Vitaminwater, a six-pack of Light & Fit vanilla yogurt, and saltines. None of which I remember buying. Though I rarely leave a market without saltines. The problem is that I didn't need any of these items. This exact assortment sums up the summertime contents of my little galley kitchen.

I have only the faintest memory of stepping into a poorly lit bodega somewhere between the taxi and here. The details are smudged, like my make-up.

I swing my feet off the arm of the sofa. They hit the floor hard, still slightly asleep. The stacked heels, stunning with their uniquely mirrored details are architectural masterpieces and absolute torture devices. My ankles are over carrying their load. My body is jittery from exhaustion, from adrenaline, from something unnamed.

For a moment, I don't move. Last night feels both wildly reckless and impossibly tender. And now, in this bright, unforgiving morning light, I have to decide what to do with it. I set the thin white plastic bag down and unbuckle each shoe. It feels glorious. I pick the bag back up to take my purchases to the fridge.

When I jumped out of the cab last night, I had no plan. None. Other than stopping things before I crossed a line I wouldn't be able to uncross. Though, if I'm honest, that ship had already sailed.

I didn't want to leave Brett. I didn't want to stop kissing him. I didn't want to step back into the version of myself that plays by all the rules. But I could see the ending in my mind, the inevitable next step, the full unraveling. And it terrified me. Not because I didn't want Brett. But because I didn't want to become someone I swore I would never be: an adulterer.

I've never cracked open *Merriam-Webster* to read the technical definition, but I feel certain what happened in that cab qualifies. Maybe not legally. But spiritually? Emotionally? In the eyes of the Lord?

Absolutely.

In Richard's eyes, I'd already be condemned. Wrath. Cold, cutting wrath. Deserved wrath, a voice inside me whispers.

Shame enters, but then, Brett's laugh cuts through it. The warmth in his eyes. The way he looked at me like I wasn't fractured or fragile or failing at life. The way he held me like he didn't want to let go.

Watching the cab drive away made my chest ache in a way that felt unfamiliar and ancient all at once. Did Brett feel it, too? That sharp pull when the light changed? Is he waking up wishing I hadn't jumped out? Or was I just another almost? Another story for him to tuck away and laugh about later?

I'll never know. And that not knowing makes my stomach twist.

After the taxi disappeared around the corner, I stood still for a moment, the city suddenly too quiet. I had no idea what street I was on. Typical.

I squinted at the street signs, trying to piece together my route like a scavenger hunt. I walked a few blocks, replaying every second in my head, before ducking into a bodega for guidance.

Maybe, I needed water. Maybe, I needed food. Maybe, I just

needed to pause long enough to remember which way Bryant Park was. Left or right? Back toward safety, toward the version of me that still gets to say she stopped in time.

At the Farmers Deli, a young man with gorgeous skin and bizarrely blue eyes, pointed me in the right direction after I made my purchase.

It's not the first time I've shopped in that bodega. It has one of the best fresh flower selections out front, overflowing with peonies, ranunculus, and English roses in unexpected color assortments, never boring, and wrapped in pretty paper. Classic, not cheesy. I hadn't bought flowers often this summer, but I did get a few bundles to make an arrangement for the apartment when my mom visited last week.

About 48 hours earlier . . .

It doesn't matter what city I'm living in, New York, Dallas, or London, when my mom comes to visit, her trip is always a careful blend of sightseeing and survival management. We'll stroll charming streets, pop into museums, and comment on window displays.

We'll hit up our usual spots, like Daffy's to dig for designer European treasures. Mom is always tickled by their tagline: "Bargains for Millionaires." The brands are often obscure, but it doesn't matter because the quality is the point—cashmere, silk, and French seams.

I'll make sure to get us to her favorite spots too: street corn from Café Habana, chocolate sandwiches from City Bakery, and cheesecake from Carnegie Deli.

And then, without fail, she'll quietly assess the state of my pantry like an undercover nutritional detective.

On this particular visit, her attention zeroes in on my yellowed oak kitchen cabinets and the echo inside them. She opens one cabinet. Closes it. Opens the fridge. Pauses. "Morgan . . ." she says lightly, which is how Southern mothers begin interventions, "You have no food."

I'm leaning against the counter, barefoot, one heel hooked against the cabinet, absently peeling the label off a water bottle in slow, thin strips. The kitchen still smells faintly like my shampoo, steam lingering from the shower, mixing with the cold, clean air spilling out of the fridge.

"I've been eating out," I say, reaching for the bottle, taking a sip like evidence. "I've been meeting friends. Trying new places all over town." Technically true.

She doesn't argue. Just gives me a slow once-over. Not dramatic. Not even disapproving. Just . . . taking stock. Collarbone. Wrists. The way my skirt hangs.

Mom came prepared. She always does. Out of her carry-on comes a box of Kraft spaghetti mix and a tiny can of tomato paste, both wrapped in a plastic grocery bag like contraband. She sets them on the counter with quiet authority.

"They don't have the right one here," she says, already moving. "Only Kroger in Murray carries it."

I smile, watching her, knowing better than to challenge the geography. Next—a fresh bag of Mint Milano cookies. She taps the bag once, like punctuation. "You can't trust small city markets."

Manhattan, apparently, still unproven, like a frontier town.

At some point earlier, while I was in the shower, she must have slipped out. Now, she's unpacking more: Fiber One cereal "for your yogurt," cans of tuna that seem to multiply as she pulls them from the bag, berries in their clear plastic cartons. Raspberries. Blueberries. Blackberries. She lines them up on the counter, like edible jewels.

I find myself drifting closer, picking up a blackberry, rolling it between my fingers before eating it. It's cold, slightly tart. Real.

She moves through my kitchen like she's done it a hundred times before, opening drawers, shifting things just slightly, making space where there wasn't any. Deli meat. Mayo. Cheese. Ground beef for the spaghetti.

She doesn't ask where things go. She decides.

I watch her from the edge of the room, arms folded now, the water bottle forgotten on the counter. There's a rhythm to it. Efficient, but gentle. Nothing wasted. Nothing rushed. She's not saying much. She doesn't need to. This is how she loves. Acts of service.

She organizes everything inside my refrigerator. The same white, textured model every upper-middle-class kid had in their garage growing up. The "overflow fridge." The "drink fridge." The one that hummed louder than necessary. Now, it's mine. My only one.

She closes the door, then opens it again, adjusting something I can't see. Steps back. Considers. Satisfied. "You need to eat," she says, finally, the afternoon before she leaves. "That Laughing Cow cheese is really good on a saltine. Or a celery stalk."

Not accusatory. Not dramatic. Just practical. Loving. Direct.

On the morning she left, she kissed my cheek at the curb outside my building, overtly hesitant to leave. It's only now, staring at the deli bag on the floor and the uneaten berries in the fridge, that I realize she wasn't just stocking my cabinets. She was desperately trying to balance me. And I'm not sure I let her.

I really thought I nailed it for her this trip. I slept at the right hours, kept my stories measured, even let silence hang in the conversation instead of filling every inch of air the way I sometimes do when my mind is racing. I ordered sensibly at lunch, walked instead of darting ahead, and resisted the urge to narrate every idea that popped into my head. From the outside, it must have looked calm, balanced, even.

But a mother's intuition doesn't get distracted by the sights of the city or a well-priced *prix fixe* lunch. She scans deeper.

With her suitcase zipped and lipstick freshly applied, she paused in the doorway and softly asked, "Do you want me to stay?"

Not do you want more time together? Or, do you need me? The exact unspoken question hung there between us. It wasn't that I wanted her to leave. I never want her to leave. But I didn't feel fragile. I didn't feel like I was unraveling. Quite the opposite.

"I'm good, Mom," I said, maybe a little too brightly. "Really."

I had a touch of a summer cold. A scratchy throat, slightly swollen glands, but otherwise, I felt electric. Alive. The city felt wide open. My apartment, however imperfect, felt like a cocoon. My days stretched long with endless possibilities. I wasn't sinking. I was soaring.

She studied me for a second longer than usual, like she was deciding whether to trust the performance. Then, she nodded. "Okay," she said. "Call me if you need anything." As if I ever wouldn't.

I watched her cab pull away, feeling light. Independent. Entirely capable. Excited for 48 hours of alone time before Richard arrives for his weekend cameo.

My calendar is conveniently, beautifully full. The Young Patrons Party at the Whitney Museum tonight. Bvlgari on 57th and Fifth tomorrow. Diamonds and philanthropy, a pairing that feels very on brand for this city. I will wear something fabulous. I will smile. I will do my best to sparkle appropriately.

Richard has been in Philadelphia all week. The plan is simple: he'll take a train up for our anniversary dinner and fly back to Dallas at an ungodly hour on Monday so he can be at his desk on time.

We have reservations Saturday night. Seven courses to celebrate seven years. If that isn't poetic, I don't know what is.

A tasting menu that will likely stretch three hours, maybe four, if there's a wine pairing. Tiny, precious plates arriving at polite intervals. Waiters describing foam and reduction and heritage grains. Us nodding. It sounds, at this exact moment, about as appealing as being clipped by a delivery truck on Madison Avenue.

Not entirely because of Richard. Lately, long, drawn-out dinners make my chest tighten. Too much sitting. Too much expectation. Too much nowhere to go. I don't manage feeling trapped well.

When I feel cornered, something feral kicks in. I get restless first. Leg bouncing. Fingernails tracing patterns on my skin. It starts small, a repetitive scratch along my forearm or thigh. Absentmindedly.

Until it's not. Until the scratching turns deliberate. Harder. Deeper. A sharp line of sting that cuts through the fog in my head. When skin finally breaks, when there's the faintest bloom of red, something in me exhales. Releases. Like letting steam out of a pressure cooker. I've never let Richard see that part.

It would become evidence. Exhibit A in the case against me. More proof of instability. Hiding it felt less like deceit and more like protection of my independence. Afraid I would never be left alone again if anyone knew.

Truly, what's one more secret? Add it to my pile . . .

The scratching. The suffocation I feel in Dallas. The fact that my illness isn't exactly "managed" at the moment. The growing, undeniable truth that I don't want to be married to him anymore.

But I can do this: Seven courses. Seven years.

Thankfully, I still have 48 hours until the performance resumes.

As I add last night's yogurt and saltines to the supplies left by my mother, I spot my YSL clutch. Thank God.

Up until this second, it wasn't outside the realm of possibility that I'd left it in the cab. Or at the Chirping Chicken. Or on the sidewalk. Although, in hindsight, the groceries I bought are a promising sign I'd managed basic object maintenance.

My lips feel like sandpaper. I press them together and wince. I hope that's not how they felt to Brett last night. Shit, Morgan. Why does that even matter? You'll never see him again. Getting into that taxi was mistake enough. What a ridiculous thing to even entertain.

I flip open the dark green pebbled patent leather clutch and dig around for my lip routine of choice: Softlips for moisture and Lip Venom for plump, a combination I've treated like a science experiment all summer.

Before my fingers find the tiny white tube, they brush against something heavier. Stiff. Textured. I pull it out. A thick piece of linen paper. A business card. My eyes adjust.

Shana. Of course. I had completely forgotten. At some point during her enthusiastic attempt to lure Brett and me across 76th Street to her apartment, Shana had pressed the card into my palm.

"I just got them today!" she'd said, beaming. "I got a promotion. I'm dying to give them out. Take one!"

"She's been working so hard for years," Josh had added, the proud boyfriend chorus. "Youngest legal associate at a major media player!"

I remember feeling genuinely happy for her. Proud, even, in that girl-code way you are for women you've just met but instantly respect.

And now, here it is. Her name. Her number. Her email. Crisp. Clean. Innocent. But somehow, this simple square piece of paper feels heavier than it should. Like it carries voltage. Because it isn't just Shana's card. It's a thread. A thread that, if tugged, leads directly back to Brett.

I stare at it longer than necessary, my thumb tracing the raised embossing of her name. Sure, I could throw it away. That would be the responsible thing. The Christian thing. The married thing.

Instead, I stand there in the middle of my little box in the sky, barefoot and hungover and still faintly smelling like rain and wine, holding in my hand the key to a door I thought would stay locked. And for the first time since I jumped out of that cab, I realize this story might not be over.

Chapter 6

THE SEVEN-YEAR ITCH

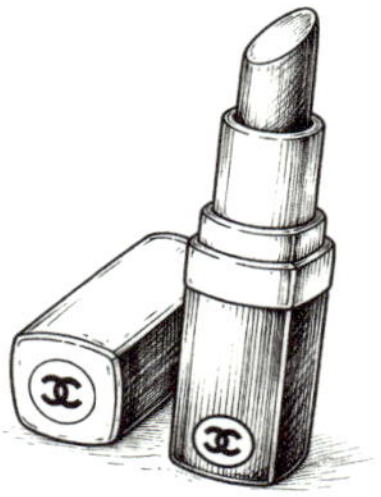

JUNE 22, 2009
7:30 a.m.—My Temporary Apartment
Midtown, New York City

I shut the door behind Richard as he leaves and lean against it for a second, listening to his echo settle. My little haven is mine again. He'll be on a plane back to Dallas in a couple hours. Weekend complete. Wedding anniversary celebration successfully performed. Lines delivered. Smiles exchanged. Photos probably passable, if anyone had taken them. Seven years, toasted.

Oddly enough, Richard and I had a genuinely nice time together. Dinner at Daniel on Saturday night, upscale and immaculate. Three Michelin stars and not a crumb out of place. The kind of dining experience where every fork has a purpose and the cheese cart is as large as a studio apartment.

I excused myself more than once to the ladies' room to answer a handful of light, flirty text messages from Brett. Harmless on the surface. Charged with risk underneath. Back at the table, I nodded thoughtfully over amuse-bouches and a variety of tiny protein courses. Tiny portions are my ally. You can rearrange, sample, sip water, and no one questions anything. Not that Richard would have noticed.

He doesn't track my bites. He doesn't clock what disappears, or doesn't, from my plate. His attention operates in larger themes—optics, timing, presentation.

We walked miles that weekend. Uptown, downtown, through neighborhoods we used to call ours, like happy tourists in a city we already knew by heart. Per my request, of course. Movement helps. Motion disguises an abundance of symptoms.

And underneath it all, bouncing inside me, is anticipation. The possibility of seeing Brett again. I can't help but think that's what allowed me to not only endure the last 48 hours but to actually enjoy them. The hope around the corner.

I glance down at my wrist. My silver Cartier Tank catches the morning light. A gift from Richard for our first Christmas as a married couple. Classic. Timeless. Engraved on the back: "I Can't Wait . . ."

He was so pleased when he gave it to me. I remember pretending I understood the deeper meaning of the engraving. I never asked what, exactly, he couldn't wait for. Maybe, it was a lifetime. Maybe, it was success. Maybe, it was children. And maybe, if today goes sideways, it will become: "I can't wait . . . to divorce you."

The thought should terrify me. Yet, it doesn't. Apparently, I'm comfortable with risk now. I glance at the watch again. I have exactly two and a half hours to get ready for my first date with another man on my seventh wedding anniversary. The apartment is quiet. My pulse is not. I turn on some MGMT.

June 19, 2009, 10 a.m.—My Temporary Apartment, NYC

I look at the business card in my hand. To text or to email? Email feels formal. Measured. Like I'm submitting a résumé. Texting is easier. Casual. Breezy. As if I'm not detonating my entire life before lunch. I pick up my BlackBerry and type in the number on the card.

Hi, Shana! It's Morgan from Bemelmans last night. So great meeting you! Like an idiot, I left something behind in the cab riding back downtown with Brett. Any chance you could connect me with him?

It's shameless and transparent. I left nothing of value in that taxi, except maybe my dignity. I hit send anyway. I'm sure she'll see straight through it. A woman like that doesn't miss subtext. But she's the only card I have to play, figuratively and literally.

Then, I wait. And wait. An hour passes. I imagine scenarios. Did she message him first? Did she ask if it was okay to give me his number? Did he hesitate? Did he laugh? Would he actually say no? Is there a world where I felt everything and he felt . . . what? Curiosity? Entertainment? A pleasant Thursday night?

This whole summer has felt like Technicolor, oversaturated and sped up. Every color brighter. Sunsets on rooftop bars: flaming orange. Taxi cabs: electric yellow. Fruit stands: reflective rainbows. Last night, Brett was a glowing neon sign. But now, I'm worried that my condition romanticized the six hours we spent together into a life-altering event? Was it even real? Finally, my phone dings. The sound is sharp. Buzzy. Shana's name flashes across the tiny screen and my stomach flips.

So great to meet you, too! Blah blah blah. *We love The Carlyle.* Blah blah blah. *I drank too much.* Blah blah blah. *Brett would love to hear from you!*

My breath falters. Not he said you can text him. Not here's his number if you want it. He said, "Would love." Present/future tense. Eager. Open. Shana included his number.

Just like that, the door I've been pretending not to stare at swings wide open. I spent six short hours with a stranger, and my entire internal compass feels recalibrated. Like someone adjusted the dials on my life, and suddenly, there's another frequency available, one where I don't shrink. One where I don't apologize. One where I don't have to edit myself into something smaller. It feels like the stuff of Kermit the Frog dreams. Rainbow arcs and reckless optimism.

My thumbs hover over the keypad. This is the moment. If I text Brett, I step forward. If I don't, I step back into the script already written for me. My heart pounds loud enough to rival the tiny buzz of the BlackBerry in my hand. And for the first time in a long time, I realize I want to choose. But what do you say to a man who unraveled you in mere moments without sounding unhinged? Or worse, too eager? That I forgot my umbrella?

Technically it's true. I left the stolen Four Seasons umbrella in the taxi. A truly elite umbrella, I might add. Sturdy. Windproof. A champion of precipitation. And given the way this summer in New York has leaned biblical with the amount of rain, I should probably mourn it more. But Brett and I both know I don't care about the umbrella. He'll see right through it.

I can't say umbrella. Credit card? Sure. I'm going with that. In this situation, a tiny white lie feels like a socially acceptable bridge. Something to reconnect us without screaming, "I cannot stop thinking about you!" Just type already. My thumbs move before my courage can catch up.

Hey there, taxi cab companion! It's Morgan from last night. Sorry about making a break for it. Yikes! I think I dropped a credit card behind in the chaos. Any chance you found it?

Message sent. I stare at it, waiting.

"Taxi cab companion? Yikes?" I physically wince. I have never been the cool girl. Cute girl? Yes. Nice girl? Absolutely. Student council. Dean's list. Organized. Polite. Quadruple check. But mysterious, hot, and aloof girl, who says three words and leaves men spiraling? Hard no. Capital N. Squared.

I toss my BlackBerry onto the sofa beside me and pace the length of my apartment, the hardwood cool under my bare feet, like I'm awaiting jury deliberation. My heart is beating faster than the situation deserves. I can practically hear my own pulse in my ears.

Brett is probably laughing. Reading my message aloud. Filing me away as "sweet Southern girl who briefly lost her mind in a taxi."

Maybe someday, he'll tell the story to his beautiful, sophisticated wife. "One summer night at Bemelmans, I met this adorable, married librarian type, who almost had a one-night stand with me but didn't quite have the nerve . . ."

My BlackBerry buzzes. The sound slices through the room like a fire alarm. I freeze. Then, I grab it. A new message. It's from Brett.

Hey! I was hoping I would hear from you. I don't have your credit card, but I wish I did so I had a reason to see you again. ;)

A small wave of warmth rolls through my chest. My shoulders drop. I hadn't realized how tightly I'd been holding them. He wrote back without hesitation. No overthinking. No "per my last email" energy. Just smooth. Direct. That wink. Intentional, made of a semicolon and parenthesis. I type back before I second-guess myself.

You don't seem like the type to let a girl without her credit card starve. Sounds like a proper reason to see me.

I pause. Okay, Morgan. Not terrible. Flirty. A touch self-aware. Not entirely unhinged. Brett's reply comes quickly.

Obviously not. Remember the chicken?

I smile at my phone like an idiot, heat creeping up my cheeks. Hearing the tone of his text in my head. I send a simple colon parenthesis smile. Then . . . nothing. Three minutes. Five. Seven. My confidence wobbles.

The ball is officially in his court now. He has to ask. I already broke at least 12 Southern girl commandments by initiating contact with him. Girls do not call boys. Girls wait. Girls are pursued. But I can't just sit here staring at my BlackBerry like it's going to hatch.

I walk to the fridge and grab a Diet Coke, selecting the one shoved farthest to the back. The coldest. The chosen one. I crack it open, carbonation spraying, the can already sweating in my stuffy kitchen where the air vents don't reach, and I take that first aggressive sip. The sharp, carbonated burn hits the back of my throat and fizzles down my chest like tiny fireworks.

Mid-bubble bliss, my BlackBerry buzzes again.

How does breakfast 10am Monday sound? Gemma inside The Bowery?

I like it. Assertive. Specific. Time and place with no ambiguity. The Virgo in me practically purrs. What I don't love is that it's only

Friday. Not even midafternoon. Monday feels like a decade away. I was selfishly hoping for something sooner—before Richard, my "roomie," arrives tonight.

Another BlackBerry buzz. My body follows suit. I'm sweaty. The caffeine of the Diet Coke starting to stir inside me.

I wish we could do dinner tonight, but I'm in Atlanta. I probably would have missed my flight if you hadn't jumped out . . .

I vaguely remember Brett talking about this—something about a last-hurrah visit with the team that moved South—the ones who didn't take or receive the same fancy buyout plan.

A soft laugh escapes me before I can stop it, echoing off the empty apartment. I'm relieved. I didn't hallucinate the chemistry. He felt it, too. I type back carefully, the phone warm in my hand now.

Sounds perfect. I'll be the blonde, dripping in bangles.

Monday morning at The Bowery Hotel . . . on my seventh wedding anniversary. Why not? I take another sip of Diet Coke and feel the fizz travel all the way down my body—detached from reality. The fun girl from the bar is making a big play to stick around.

June 22, 2009, 8 a.m.—My Temporary Apartment, NYC

I should have booked a salon blowout. I love that New Yorkers just go and get their hair washed and dried. No cut or color. I hate washing and drying my hair. Mostly the drying part. Plus, I never learned how to correctly use a curling iron without crimping the ends of my hair. I imagine I'm the only person under 65 years old who still uses hot rollers and a teasing comb in Manhattan.

I can't see Brett without clean hair though. I want it to be bouncy and smell fantastic. Oh, how I wish they still made Salon Selectives, specifically the one in the coral bottle. It's my favorite shampoo smell of all time. Tan lines, youth, summertime fun, and innocence in a bottle.

Unilever really screwed the pooch by discontinuing it a few years ago. Bumble and bumble will have to do.

The shower in this apartment is a black hole. The only lamp hovers uselessly over the potty, frosted and dim, like it's embarrassed to be there. The thick, commercial-grade shower curtain seals off what little light exists. Far too dark for precision grooming on a morning that feels . . . pivotal.

The 1980s ceiling vent roars overhead, like a jet engine attempting and failing to clear the steam from the mirror. With rollers perched strategically in my hair like a suburban crown, I balance on the bath mat and reach for Richard's shaving gel. I quickly clear the vanity mirror with a hand towel.

I haven't used shaving cream since I was 12. It was the first time I shaved my legs, off the back of a boat on Kentucky Lake, balancing one foot on hot fiberglass, razor in hand, pretending I knew what I was doing. There was definitely blood. Band-Aids, too.

I can't have bandage-clad legs today. So, I lather slowly, deliberately. No rushing. No shortcuts. There will be no nicks. No forgotten strips. No rogue shin patches catching the light at an unfortunate angle.

I bend and inspect the front of my knees. Then the backs. Ankles get extra attention, those sneaky long hairs that hide in the little dip between bone and calf muscle like they've signed a lease there. I drag the razor carefully along my shin bones, studying the curve. Meticulous. Focused.

It's ridiculous, really, this level of care going into something Brett may never consciously notice. But I'll know. And that matters.

Steam curls around me. The vent groans. My reflection in the mirror is blurry and flushed. I rinse the razor and set it down like a surgeon finishing a procedure. No cuts. No blood. So far, so good.

All morning, I've been telling myself that it's only breakfast between two new friends, but the precision with which I just shaved my legs suggests otherwise.

I keep my makeup simple. Mostly because that's all I know how to do and also because it's early morning on a Monday. No eyeshadow, just rosy blushed cheeks. Pink, plump lips. Volumizing mascara. And bronzer, with a touch of shimmer.

With "New York Groove" blasting from my laptop speakers, I dance across the parquet floors toward the bedroom. The sight of the solid oak double bunk beds makes me laugh. Every single day. It's impossible not to giggle. I'm 28 years old, allegedly a grown-up, living in what is essentially summer camp housing for overachieving undergrads.

This apartment only fell into my lap thanks to a sweet college friend Evie. Her husband, James, the vice president of fundraising at a local college, knows how to monetize every square inch of Manhattan real estate. During the academic year, these apartments are student dorms. In the summer, they become "charming furnished sublets." Charming is generous.

The irony is not lost on me: Evie is the reason that Richard and I met in the first place. We had no natural overlap. No fraternity connection. No shared classes. No accidental run-ins. Without Evie's introduction, our paths would never have crossed.

And now, Evie's husband is the reason I have an escape. She is the alpha and the omega of our love story.

Ace Frehley's voice pours through the room as I swing open the closet in the bunk room, the sacred space where I keep my favorite pieces, separate from the rest of my life. I start assembling today's ensemble. The goal: elegance with a little edge . . . and cute. I'm not trying to be someone I'm not.

I step into a Jet Set Lingerie black lace thong, with our logo, a cheeky pair of pilot "wings," stamped front and center. The logo is our nod to vintage flight attendants and jet-set dreams.

At Bemelmans, when Brett asked me what I did for work, he didn't just nod politely at my reply. He leaned in. He asked real questions. About Greer and Addy. About how we started our lingerie company.

About the initial napkin sketch we made in the corner booth of the bar. About trade shows and margins and manufacturing in Thailand. He listened like it mattered. Like he wanted to be a part of it, an entrepreneur, to start something himself or, at the very least, to be released from the hamster wheel of private equity and corporate finance.

When I told him how we dress as vintage flight attendants for trade shows and selling events, complete with pillbox hats and red lipstick, his face lit up. When I took a package from my clutch to show him the brand's panty-with-wings logo, conceived on a red cocktail napkin in that very room, he laughed and told me his father had just retired after 40-plus years as a commercial airline pilot.

"Wore his own set of wings," he grinned, "just not on his man parts."

I nearly aspirated Burgundy. I had to swallow hard to keep red wine from shooting out of my nose. Maintaining cool was already a stretch.

The first time Brett saw the official logo, it was printed neatly on the Jet Set Lingerie case. Now, as I smooth the lace against my hips and glance at my reflection in the mirror, I wonder, am I prepared to show it to him again? This time, on me.

It's my 30-minute warning. Game-time decisions must be made.

I put on an ivory silk blouse with at least a dozen pintuck pleats at the jewel neckline. Its bold puffy sleeves fall above my elbow and add a lady-like touch. My black bra underneath peekaboos perfectly through the sheer silk.

For the skirt, only the GOAT of my wardrobe will do. A black mini, fitted at the waist with tailored box pleats, creating a full silhouette and a short hemline. Made of rich black faille taffeta with a French grosgrain waistband, hand-embellished with tonal beads and stones.

If I recall correctly, Brett is tall. Definitely taller than Richard. Which means I need height. Sultry, not circus act. I don't want to feel clumsy. I reach for my black patent leather and metallic gold spectator wedges. Four inches of stability. Goldilocks perfection. I can walk Manhattan end to end in these without a wobble.

Next stop: the bangle bar. It sounds glamorous. It's not. Five abnormally tall stainless-steel IKEA toilet paper holders standing upright like minimalist sculptures, stacked high with color-coded bracelets. Golds. Pinks. Lucite. Enamel. Resin. Some designer. Some flea market. Some unidentifiable but essential.

It's wildly inconvenient when I want one from the bottom of the stack. I've nearly dislocated a wrist more than once. But after years of failed jewelry boxes and tangled travel disasters, this setup is the most efficient chaos I've managed.

My bracelet game cannot miss today. At Bemelmans, Brett was fascinated by my stack. Not politely intrigued, genuinely curious. He asked about the origin of specific pieces. He noticed the way they chimed when I moved. I don't think he's ever encountered someone with such a committed relationship to arm candy. Certainly not someone who engineered a "bar" to house them.

I love bangles. Always have. Three per wrist is baseline. Perhaps today requires more.

I start with Chanel, courtesy of Addy's first PR job and the holy grail of sample sales. Without her access, I'd maybe own two secondhand tops from INA, where half the Upper East Side's PR girls offload their hauls to cover rent. No one enters fashion for financial security. That's clear.

I build each wrist carefully. Weight. Texture. Sound. A full stack on both sides, balanced but intentional. I grab my quilted black clutch and pack it strategically: ID, one credit card, $40 cash, Lip Venom, oversized vintage black sunglasses with fluted gold trim, keys, Altoids, concealer, and a Jet Set Lingerie case for good measure.

I head to the bathroom for a final check. Teeth. Lipstick. Hair. I brush my teeth one more time, maybe too aggressively, and when I look up, my lipstick is smeared just slightly beyond the line. The gloss has migrated. My mouth looks . . . uncertain.

I stare at myself in the mirror. The rollers are out now. Hair soft and full. Eyes bright. Bangles gleaming. I blot carefully. Reapply. Press my lips together. Better.

9:42 a.m. Not great. I'll be late. But okay. Let's do this.

The humidity smacks me in the face as soon as I step outside. Even my freeze-hold Spray & Play can't keep a curl in place with this sticky heat. Messy hair and dewy skin is a look I've struggled to master over the years. Perhaps a little help from Mother Nature is all I needed.

I hail a cab easily and hop in. Luckily, traffic seems to be moving, but inside the taxi, it's *en fuego*. I crack the window to circulate the air and slide over to let the air vent blow up my skirt. My thighs are already sweating. Is it the heat? Or the thought of Brett?

The taxi breezes through green light after green light. I'm making great time.

"This is it, sir," I tell the driver. "Just pull to the right after the crosswalk." I pay in cash, a rare act for me. My bare legs stick to the cab's vinyl seats as I lean toward the door to open it.

After the fifth thank-you to the man who drove me just over 30 blocks (I tend to over-thank as much as I over-apologize), I shut the door and head to the crosswalk. I anxiously wait for the crossing signal's big red hand to change. In those remaining 17 seconds, counting down, I examine myself from shoe to blouse. The off-white pintucks mirror my virginal white wedding dress. Was it subconscious?

The little white figure appears on the signal. I stroll towards Gemma. Standing in front of The Bowery Hotel's double doors, on my seventh wedding anniversary, I imagine the tall, dark, devastatingly handsome man, who is not my husband, waiting somewhere on the other side.

And suddenly, in my mind, I'm somewhere else. Seven years ago. In front of two very different double doors. Heavy. Ornate. Framed in lush pink and white florals and glossy greenery. The entrance to our very traditional church. A string quartet warming up inside. The 300 guests fanning themselves in cherry-stained wooden pews, trimmed in lacquered white.

It was one of those Kentucky summer days that feels like you're walking through a rainforest. Ninety degrees. Ninety-five percent humidity. The kind of heat that makes silk cling and mascara slide.

At the last minute, I abandoned the soft, romantic curls we had practiced for months and opted for a tight, slick chignon. In theory, it was timeless. Elegant. Audrey Hepburn-approved. In reality, it made my round, baby face look even rounder.

But on that suffocating evening, I couldn't imagine adding big, fluffy curls beneath an even bigger, fluffier cathedral veil. I was already drowning in satin and expectation. I remember standing there, in front of those double doors, with a bouquet of lily of the valley in hand and a veil pinned so tightly that my scalp ached. The image rushes in so vividly it nearly steals the air from my lungs.

She was me. Of course she was. But I barely recognize her now. She was lost. Hollowed out. Retreating quietly from friendships, one by one. Skipping college parties in the name of her "future." Depressed in ways she couldn't articulate. Channeling all her energy into peony counts and calligraphy fonts so she wouldn't have to examine the more pressing questions. Am I okay? Am I happy? Is getting married to Richard the right thing to do?

She buried herself in napkin samples and seating charts because those were solvable problems. Mental health was not.

A sharply dressed woman brushes past me, snapping me out of my tragic trance. She exits through Gemma's leaded-glass doors, intentionally antiqued but undeniably new. The whole building is like that. Designed to look storied. Seasoned. As if it has witnessed decades of romance and scandal, when, in fact, it only opened a couple of summers ago. Manufactured nostalgia.

I've been here before. Once with Greer and Addy. Once with a law school friend of Richard's. The place is charming in that carefully curated downtown way. Dark. Just enough mystery. Smart choice on Brett's part.

I catch my reflection in the glass as the door closes behind the woman. No veil. No bouquet. No 300 guests waiting for me to perform permanence. Just me. Bangles stacked. Lips freshly painted. Heart racing for entirely different reasons.

Seven years ago, I walked through double doors because I didn't know how to say no. Today, I'm about to walk through another set because I finally know how to say yes. Because the spark inside me has officially grown too big to control.

Sitting at the first seat of the bar, more like a counter for the breakfast crowd, Brett has the New York Post in his hands, flipped open to the sports section. His face is familiar, which surprises me seeing as our first meeting, just a few days before, is hazy in my mind, undoubtedly caused by a mix of nerves, wine, and lack of sleep.

Just as I begin to panic that he might not recognize me. That, in the daylight, I might look less sparkly, he spots me. Our eyes lock. And then, I see it. His mouth forms a silent, unmistakable "wow." The knot in my chest dissolves. He stands, no hesitation, and walks toward me.

"Good morning!" he says, genuinely bright.

Brett looks exactly right. Classic jeans. Casual white button-down, sleeves rolled just enough. Loosely tucked in that perfectly imperfect way that suggests he didn't try, even though he absolutely did.

"How are you?" he asks, smiling like he's been waiting for this all weekend.

"Good morning to you," I reply. "I'm great. How was Atlanta?"

I say it as if I routinely keep tabs on his travel schedule. As if we've been doing this forever.

"Hot," he answers. "My back is completely sunburned and . . . "

And then he's off to the races. A rapid-fire account of rooftop drinks, a last-minute golf outing, a friend who forgot sunscreen, a cab that got lost, a shirt sacrificed to aloe vera. He talks quickly, animated, slightly breathless. I find myself leaning in, physically and mentally, trying to keep pace. Although he's not talking any faster than I've been talking all summer.

Did he talk this fast the night we met? Or is he just nervous? There's something endearing about the possibility that I'm not the only one vibrating slightly out of rhythm.

Mid-sunburn saga, he gestures toward the dining room and asks, "Should we grab a table? Get you some coffee?"

The hostess leads us across terra-cotta tiles that echo faintly beneath my wedges. Brett's hand rests lightly at my lower back, just enough pressure to guide, not enough to claim. My entire body registers it anyway. Ten seconds. 17 steps. I count. That's all it takes to cross the room. But it feels like something ceremonial.

Gemma is exactly what it wants to be: curated old-world romance. Candles stacked and melted into thick, waxy monuments. Brown leather banquettes softened by time. Rustic chairs that look rescued from a Tuscan farmhouse. Wrought-iron chandeliers casting a golden wash over everything.

It's a bustling Monday morning. Suits and sunglasses. Laptops open. Espresso cups clinking. Conversations pitched just low enough to feel important. These are technically "meetings," I'm sure. Though most of them are likely recaps of weekend escapes to the Hamptons.

We slide into a corner booth. We are not here for business. And suddenly, I realize I'm not entirely sure what we are here for. Is it closure? Or temptation? Does Brett want to give me a test run? Or are we trying to uncross a line we already crossed?

He's still smiling, that same open, curious expression from last week. Whatever this is, it's not accidental. And it isn't casual. The waitress appears like a small mercy, cutting through the tornado in my head.

"Anything special to drink this morning?" she asks, tone lifting just enough to suggest that "special" does not mean chamomile.

"Ladies first," Brett says.

Damn. Why is basic chivalry so disarming? Now, I have to set the tone. With a beverage. Is this a date? Is it a meeting? Is it a moral crisis disguised as brunch? What is happening?

Focus, Morgan. It's just a drink.

"I'd love a breakfast tea, with a side of whatever non-dairy milk you have, please," I request.

The lie floats out smoothly. Polished. Proper. What I would actually love is a Bloody Mary with an aggressive floater on top, three olives, and a salty rim. Something to quiet the buzz in my chest. Something to blur the edges. But instead: tea.

"Hmmm . . ." Brett pauses, just slightly. "I guess I'll just continue with black coffee then."

There's a flicker there. A recalibration. Did he clock my restraint? Did I just shift us into weekday-conference-call territory?

I ordered poorly. Note to self: listen to the new girl inside you. The one who kissed a stranger in a taxi and lived to tell about it. The one who texted first. The one who is sitting here on her seventh wedding anniversary wearing naughty lace beneath silk.

The uptight, gold-star, goody-two-shoes version of me needs a brief sabbatical. Look where she's landed us in comparison. Seven years of hiding. Seven years of agreeable. Seven years of shrinking into the appropriate shape. Seven years of "staying in her box."

The phrase "stay in your box" isn't metaphorical for me. I've seen the box. Richard has drawn it more than once. The most recent time was at a Thievery Corporation concert. It was downtown Dallas, standing room only, concrete floors slightly vibrating beneath our feet. I had actually been excited for it. I love live music.

About three songs in, I started to feel it, the rhythm sliding under my skin, the lights bouncing off the walls. I closed my eyes and let myself sway. Nothing wild. Nothing scandalous. Just hips shifting, shoulders loosening, hands lifting slightly above my head. I think I teased our friend Beau about wanting to get on stage.

Richard leaned in close, his mouth brushing my ear. "No stage," he said, half-laughing when Beau was in earshot. Richard followed with a strong, "I mean it!" when Beau wasn't.

I smiled, trying to soften it all. Then, Richard stepped back, looked down at the floor between us, and with the toe of his leather driving shoe, traced a slow, deliberate square on the concrete.

"There," he said, tapping the imaginary boundary. "Stay in your box." He grinned like it was a joke, like we were sharing a private, clever moment. "So, you don't embarrass yourself." But that wasn't what he meant. He meant: so you don't embarrass or outshine me.

The bass pulsed. The crowd surged. Colored lights flashed across Richard's face, turning him blue, then red, then green. I remember looking down at the invisible outline and feeling something small inside me comply. I tightened my elbows. Brought my hands down. Contained my hips. I swayed in place, two inches of movement in any direction. A well-behaved concertgoer.

I told myself Richard was protective. Loving, even. That he didn't want people looking at me. That he just preferred subtlety. But that square on the floor followed me. Invisible lines marking the perimeter of acceptable Morgan.

"I'm really glad you texted me, even if it was against your better judgment," Brett says, chin tipped down, eyes lifting up at me with that slow, devastating wink.

"Everything about this breakfast is pretty PG," I toss back, light and playful. "I don't think I need to be so worried now."

"I assure you," he says, leaning in just slightly, "no one has ever rated me PG."

But the conversation stays easy. Safe, even. The kind that doesn't need to reach for anything deeper to feel full.

He tells me about his mom—how hard she worked to keep everything moving. Two boys, endless practices, a full-time job, meals somehow appearing in the middle of it all while his dad was off flying routes as a pilot. There's a warmth in the way he talks about her, a quiet admiration that doesn't need to be dressed up.

And then his dad—how present he was when he was home. Family dinners that actually happened. Pancake breakfasts that felt like an event. Showing up to every baseball practice when he wasn't in the air, as if he could make up for the time away by being fully there when it counted.

I can see it as he's telling it. The rhythm of it. The kind of childhood that feels anchored. I meet him there and share the lighter parts of mine, the easier stories. Summers on my grandparents' house boats, the lake stretching out around us, cousins everywhere, sunburned shoulders and long afternoons that didn't need structure. Twilight golf, chasing the last bit of daylight. The frosting of it all. I leave the rest for another time. And he doesn't push.

We stay there, in the easy back-and-forth, the kind that feels like a first crush and like something more grounded, warm, familiar, just enough to feel like we're beginning to understand each other without having to say everything all at once. His dark hair falls into his eyes, hazel, not just brown. There's warmth in his skin, olive and sun-kissed, not burned. He looks leaner than I remembered. Athletic. No puffed chest, no performance. Just . . . contained strength.

Heat blooms low in my stomach. My thighs press into the leather banquette, and I'm suddenly hyperaware of my body again. The space between us feels charged, like the air right before a summer storm.

"Well," I say, pushing back from the table before I do something reckless like drag him across it, "on that note, Mr. Big City, I'm going to excuse myself to the ladies' room." I need oxygen.

As I weave through the restaurant toward the back hallway, my mind betrays me. I imagine Brett following. Pushing open the restroom's door just as it swings shut. Locking it. Pressing me against cool tile. His mouth at my neck, deliberate. Then finding mine. Not subtle. Not careful. Not boxed in. I want him here. In public. In daylight. Consequences be damned. I catch my reflection, cheeks flushed.

We drift through the rest of breakfast in rhythm. Oatmeal for me. A safe, predictable, and beige choice to calm my tummy. A gorgeous omelet for him, folded and golden and unapologetic. I eat half. He cleans his plate. Teas and coffees multiply. There's laughter. There's silence that feels loaded instead of empty. There's flirting that borders on something else entirely.

By noon, Brett and I stand outside Gemma, our eyes still adjusting to the sun. It's awkward in the way only real chemistry can be. Magnetic. Unsure.

Based on our breakfast conversation, I know he lives two blocks away. Two short east-to-west blocks. The knowledge hangs between us like a neon sign. This is not my average Monday. But is it his?

"Want to take a walk?" he asks.

I nod, because speaking feels dangerous.

Three blocks in and the city conspires against us with jackhammers pulverizing Bowery, dust in the air, men in neon vests shouting over machinery. Not exactly an aphrodisiac. We veer west onto Fourth Street to escape the noise and stop dead in front of Astor Wines & Spirits. The windows are a shrine to bourbon. Bottles stacked floor to ceiling, amber and gold catching the sunlight like stained glass in a Kentucky cathedral.

Something in me loosens.

"Based on the other night, you might think I'm a champagne or red wine girl," I say, stepping closer to the glass. "Not true. Bourbon's my drink. Pappy Van Winkle if I'm feeling spendy. Woodford Reserve if I'm feeling elegant. But middle of the day on a Monday, in this heat?" I turn to him. "Maker's Mark with a splash of ice-cold Diet Coke. Don't you think?" His smile widens.

"Know of any place around here we might find that?" I add, letting the challenge hang.

"I certainly do," he says, already pushing open the door.

Inside, the store is cool and bright. Labels glow in rows of color: ruby, emerald, gold. Sunlight filters through the windows and turns the bourbon bottles into a sea of caramel. We move easily now, shoulder brushing shoulder, fingers grazing as we walk the aisles. We've crossed an invisible threshold. He grabs a fifth of Maker's Mark without hesitation.

Half a block later, we're in Gristedes for limes and Diet Coke. When we step back onto the sidewalk, supplies in hand, Brett turns to me and extends his free hand.

"I've got the perfect bar in mind," he says.

His palm is open. All I have to do is take it.

Chapter 7

THE BOY & HIS BAR

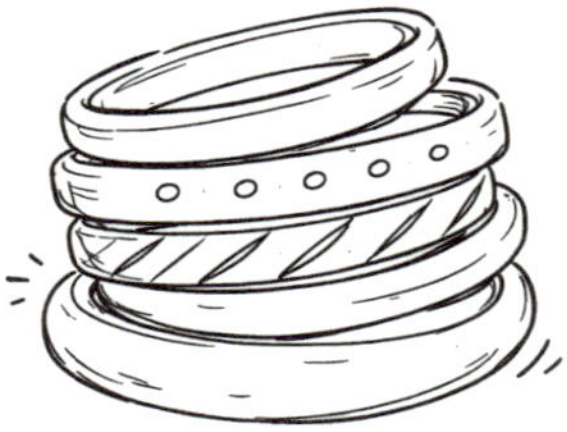

JUNE 22, 2009
Midday—West Fourth Street
Greenwich Village, New York City

One block later, we're standing on the corner of Mercer and West Fourth in front of a building, not a bar. It's 10 floors or so, stacked in old apricot brick and wrapped in soft sage trim. It's Brett's apartment building, I presume.

"Is this spot okay with you?" Brett asks, gesturing towards the sliding doors. There's something disarming about the way he says it. Not cocky. Not assuming. Genuinely checking.

I tilt my head, surveying the façade like a real estate agent. "Well, I haven't seen the inside yet, but it's a lovely prewar property," I tease.

He laughs, that easy, boyish laugh that undoes me. "I'll take that as a yes," he says.

He greets the doorman by name. It's familiar and relaxed. He motions toward the elevator.

"I could have sworn you mentioned living on the second floor," I say, arching an eyebrow. "Or was that part of the wine haze?"

"Good memory. Second floor," he confirms.

My brain is bizarre these days. It forgets to eat lunch but remembers the exact floor a man lives on. What it absorbs and what it skims over make no sense. The elevator dings.

"Do you always take the elevator for one flight of stairs, Mister

I-Run-Ten-Miles-a-Day?" I ask, poking at him.

"I was trying to be polite," he shoots back, eyes dipping briefly to my shoes. "Don't think I haven't noticed your footwear. And the sticks balancing on them."

"These sticks," I say, lifting my chin, "can absolutely handle one singular flight of stairs. Show me the way."

He pivots smoothly, pushing open a heavy gray stairwell door with his shoulder, bourbon and Diet Coke tucked securely under one arm. I start up the stairs first. And, of course, I steal a glance back. He doesn't try to be subtle. He stays five steps below me. Not two. Not three. Five. A respectful distance that is absolutely not accidental.

His eyes are locked on my "sticks." So I climb a little bit slower than necessary.

The stairwell is stark and echoey; our footsteps bounce off concrete. My bangles chime softly with every movement. The air smells faintly of dust and old paint. At the top landing, I pause and let him catch up, because there's something about him opening doors for me that feels . . . like an old habit now.

He pushes through into a hallway with soaring ceilings and strange, misplaced columns. It's industrial, structural, unapologetic. We curve around one of them and stop in front of a door that is wide and tall and unmistakably loft-like. He reaches into his pocket for his keys. And I think, fleetingly: Well, here's hoping he's not a serial killer.

He swings the door open and steps aside, one hand extended in a half-bow that is equal parts gentleman and showman. At first glance, the apartment screams one thing, and it's not "unemployed." There is absolutely more to his story. The three words that do flash through my mind? Metrosexual bachelor pad.

Southern men love to weaponize the term metrosexual, usually while wearing pleated khakis and socks with sandals. It's always said with a smirk, like caring about how you present yourself is somehow suspicious. But let's review the evidence: a single man in a chic loft, who trims his nails, owns tweezers, irons his shirts, and shines his shoes. In what Emily Post universe is that a flaw?

The ceilings soar, 20 feet at least with white-on-white exposed beams that make everything feel even taller. The space is mostly open. From the foyer, I spot a legitimate bar straight ahead, stocked better than half the gin joints on the Lower East Side. To the right is a glossy, recently renovated kitchen. To the left are tall double doors leading to rooms I cannot see.

It's not my aesthetic—the dark marble counters and deep Shaker cabinets with very masculine lines—but it's undeniably handsome. Intentional. There is zero trace of a woman's touch, and I find an odd thrill in that. No decorative hand towels. No scented candles. No "Live, Laugh, Love" casualties.

I peek inside a cabinet and nearly laugh out loud. An entire shelf is devoted to takeout menus, rubber-banded soy sauce packets, and plastic cutlery. The man has curated a museum of singlehood. This guy is aggressively unattached.

"Would you care for a quick tour?" Brett asks.

"Of course." My interior design brain shifts into high gear. I trail him like a highly curious HGTV host, asking about materials, layout changes, and contractor disasters. He lights up explaining the renovation. He shares about the walls he knocked down, the beams he exposed, and the bar he insisted on building himself. There's something deeply attractive about a man who cares about where he lives. I save my sharpest commentary for the bathroom.

"Is that a television embedded in your vanity mirror?" I ask, leaning closer. "I guess the 60-inch flat screen in your bedroom, a mere 10 feet away, isn't convenient enough?"

He answers earnestly, "I hated watching the Yankees' highlights backwards in the reflection while I was shaving." I blink at him.

"Well, obviously, I hate that, too," I say, making a face that's equal parts adorable and skeptical.

He pauses and then finally catches it. A slow grin spreads across his face. "Got it," he says. "You're teasing me. But as a season ticket holder, I take my Yankees very seriously." There it is again, that quick wit meeting mine in the middle.

The apartment is impressive. The renovation is thoughtful. And the bar is dangerously well stocked. But what feels most interesting isn't the square footage or the soaring ceilings; it's the way Brett keeps watching me watch his space. Like I'm the real tour.

Like the kitchen, the bathroom isn't exactly my vibe, a little stark, but I can appreciate the intention behind it. Tankless toilet. Seven-head shower system. Clear vessel sink perched atop the vanity.

"Did you use a designer?" I ask, running my fingers lightly along the marble edge.

"Yeah," he admits. "Mostly for paint colors and to help execute." At some point, he casually references Farrow & Ball, and I nearly smile to myself. Most men have no clue about paint brands. Brett says it like he's ordering coffee.

Floor-to-ceiling windows stretch along the entire north wall of the living room, overlooking Fourth Street, currently wrapped in the city's favorite accessory: scaffolding. I swear there are more buildings in New York draped in green metal than not.

The sectional sofa is enormous. Neutral and soft. Six people could nap comfortably on it. The whole room feels like an upscale boutique hotel collided with Tom Hanks' loft in the movie *Big*. Elevated furniture is layered over serious rugs, and then . . . full-sized arcade games are tucked playfully in the corner. No trampoline, unfortunately.

The living room flows seamlessly into the main bedroom through a massive, cased opening framed with double French doors. The opaque glass softens the transition, privacy without heaviness. The floors—pickled hardwood laid in a herringbone pattern—steal the show for me. Thoughtful. Unexpected. Understated. Second highlight, of course, being Brett.

His California King bed, absurdly large by Manhattan standards, is dressed entirely in white. The bedding is crisp yet fluffy, with the kind of duvet that has clearly been pressed by someone who is paid to care. There are signs of a professional housekeeper everywhere.

But signs of a woman? Nada. Zero throw pillows. That, to me, is the loudest tell of all.

The headboard is low and modern, upholstered, flanked by two sleek bedside tables. On each sits a mounted dark horn on a heavy brass base.

A kudu? Maybe. I'm not entirely sure. But the symbolism is . . . unmistakable. He catches me looking.

"They're meant to be funny," he says, smirking. "The finishing touches to my cliché bachelor pad."

I scrunch my nose at him, with my little bunny wrinkles I've had since childhood. They crease on both sides of my nose. I know, one day, some glossy med-spa doctor will suggest freezing them into submission. I'll say no. I love my bunny wrinkles. Brett wrinkles his nose back at me. I have a feeling he might love them, too.

The end of the tour lands us at his bar, the crown jewel wedged between the foyer and the sweeping living space. The ceiling dips here, making the spot more intimate, because above it floats a sleeping loft accessible by a narrow spiral staircase. It adds several hundred square feet of intrigue to the already generous main floor, though technically it can't be called a bedroom. No doors. No walls. If someone added a few glass block tiles, red suspenders-and-power-ties vibe, this place could pass for a renovated *Wall Street* movie set.

Brett pats the top of one of the barstools. "Will this do?" he asks.

His mood is light. Easy. No undertone of control. No subtle correction of my posture or tone or volume. He isn't trying to contain me. He isn't measuring me against some invisible standard. Blissfully unaware of the decades I've spent trying to be perfect, he somehow makes me feel perfect without trying. Either he's wildly in denial about the fact that I'm a nearly adulterous disaster . . . or he likes me exactly as I am.

"It sure does," I reply, sliding onto the stool. "Also, a friendly reminder for the bartender, just a splash of Diet Coke with the Maker's. No need to overdo it."

He laughs, slicing limes with practiced ease. While he builds our drinks, I wander again, scanning for clues. No framed ex-girlfriends. No gallery wall of "the guys." Just one photo of him with a taller version of himself, a man with long hair and the same jawline. Brett's brother, I assume. And another photo of Brett with two people who must be his parents—the resemblance immediate, unmistakable.

The absence of clutter is almost louder than clutter would be. He's not lonely. But he hasn't let someone in.

"Should I put on some tunes?" he calls from the bar area. "Any requests?"

"I'm a little old-school. Michael Jackson maybe? Otis Redding? Or Dolly Parton is always a winner in my book. Or Phoenix, if you want something fresh," I suggest.

At breakfast, Brett told me how music is one of his muses. Not in a pretentious way. Not boastful. It was jolly. Almost simple except for his library of knowledge. I felt an immediate urge to show him I wasn't just politely nodding along—that music has always been a quiet thread running through my life, too—everything from the classic hymns of my childhood to records my mom played to whatever spins in smoky New York bars late at night. I want him to know that I can meet him there, that I'm a girl who understands how a song shapes a mood, a memory, even a moment between two people. It matters to me that he sees my range, that I can keep up with whatever soundtrack he carries around in his head.

Michael's "Human Nature" filters through the speakers a moment later, smooth and atmospheric. It's a solid choice. Plus, choosing it over Dolly rules out one very specific theory: a gay man would never miss an opportunity to listen to Dolly. Greer, Addy, and I confirmed this theory years ago at her concert at Radio City, where we were three straight girls swallowed by a sea of impeccably dressed men screaming every lyric.

I circle back toward the bar to evaluate ice cube size and Coke ratio like a bourbon sommelier in wedges. On my way, I pass through the bathroom again. And that's when I see it. Two robes. Hung neatly on hooks behind the door. One large. Plush. Masculine. One smaller. Cinched at the waist. I stop.

The music pulses from hidden speakers peppered about. Ice clinks in glasses.

Two robes. With monograms. My stomach tightens, not with heat this time, but with awareness.

"These drinks aren't going to drink themselves, ya know," Brett says, laughing at his own cleverness.

"True, sir. Very true," I giggle back. "Plus, bourbon melts ice faster than a hair dryer," I shout from the bathroom. "I'm on my way!" Trying to shake the sight of two robes off my Etch A Sketch of a brain.

Bellied up to the bar, we toast ourselves and the fabulous Monday we have created. The first bourbon goes down fast. Too fast. But, damn, it's good. He quickly prepares a second one, returning to me in under a minute.

"You're a quick study I see," I say, placing my hand on his, as he sits the lowball on the bar.

"Didn't want to waste any of my time with you," he says.

Halfway through our second bourbon, something shifts. The conversation deepens, not heavy, not confessional in a therapy-session way, but personal. Thoughtful. Still playful. Still quick. It's everything I want conversation to be—soft, curious, layered, tempting.

We trade stories about where we came from, the shape of our childhoods, the quiet way family leaves its mark on you. He brings up his dad again and the travel. He shares how they always found fun ways to see each other, using standby passes to meet him in whatever city he landed, sometimes for a baseball game or sometimes just for dinner. Not just when he was a kid, but well into adulthood. There is something steady and intentional in the way he says it, like showing up is never a question. I decide to go deeper than I did over breakfast, sharing my version more carefully, the edges a little less clean—how my relationship with my dad is complicated, messy in the wake of divorce, something I am still learning how to understand. It isn't dark, but it is honest. And in that space, sitting next to each other, knees touching, with drinks in hand, it feels like we are letting each other in, for real.

The bold girl who's been simmering under my skin all summer officially takes the mic. She doesn't ask permission. She doesn't overthink. Before I can censor her, she leans forward and asks, "So what's the deal with the his-and-her robes in there? Because I see zero signs of female life in this entire apartment . . . but where I come from, Down South, monogrammed robes mean something. Something big."

Brett bursts out laughing. Not defensive. Not irritated. The kind of laugh you give when someone catches you off guard in a way that feels endearing. Because asking the question, bold as it is, reveals something softer. It shows I care.

"Yes," he admits, grinning, "it did belong to a woman. An ex-girlfriend, to be specific. We broke up seven or eight months ago. Back in the fall." He shrugs lightly and continues, "She wasn't the one. Never was. I've been meaning to box up the stuff she left, robe included, but I've had more fun things to do with my time."

And with that, and a look that is dangerously close to an invitation, he hooks his foot around the leg of my barstool and pulls me closer. My legs are still crossed toward the bar, but he turns fully toward me. Then, without breaking eye contact, he places both hands on the seat of my stool and swivels me so I'm facing him. I uncross my legs to fit into the narrowing space. There is almost no air between us now. I realize I've stopped breathing.

For the last hour, I've been waiting for him to close the distance the way he did in the taxi, decisive and sure. But here in his apartment, he's been almost restrained. Respectful. Letting me set the rhythm. Now, our noses are inches apart. Instead of grabbing my waist or pulling me in, his eyes drift to my wrist, the soft clink of my bangles catching his attention. He studies them for a moment, then looks back at me with that same curiosity, like the jewelry is just an entry point. It's the kind of look that says he wants to know everything and plans to take his time getting there.

"I need to understand this bracelet situation," he says, affectionately taking my right hand.

Not what I expected. But somehow even more intimate. He lifts my wrist between us, studying it like it's rare artwork. His thumb grazes the inside of my arm as he rolls the first bangle between his fingers.

"This one?" he asks, sliding the black resin cuff with gold metal embellishments off my arm.

"Vintage Chanel," I answer. "It's a heavy one, right?"

He nods, slowly. Interested. He sets it on the bar and removes the next bangle, his fingers traveling deliberately along my forearm.

"And this?" he wonders, as the baby pink pearlized Lucite band tickles down my arm.

"Night market in Bangkok," I whisper. "Picked it up earlier this spring."

Another one slides free. His knuckles brush my skin.

"That one?" he asks.

"Garment District," I quietly tell him. "Right here in New York."

The white enamel, lined with gold, is warm from my body heat.

He takes his time. Each bracelet removed with intention, stacking them neatly beside our bourbons. "This is a favorite," I confide, tapping the last one remaining, my voice lowering without my permission. "Found it in the Marais. Paris. Last year. The most perfect shade of chartreuse. I love its asymmetry—like it's not trying to be perfect."

With every answer, my voice grows breathier. He's not just undressing my wrists. He's unraveling me. By the time the last bangle slips free, my arms feel strangely bare. Exposed. His fingers linger at my wrist a moment longer than necessary.

After he slides the last bangle from my wrist, his hands don't leave me. They settle on my knees instead. Gently. Deliberately. He nudges them apart just enough to fold in closer, and suddenly, the little space between us disappears. His palms glide up my thighs, slow and certain, pushing up my skirt, until they reach my waist. With a subtle pull, he draws me forward. I don't resist.

In one fluid motion, I'm perched against him, my body aligning with his like it was always meant to fit there. His hands anchor at my waist, firm but not possessive.

Our lips meet. Not tentative. Not rushed. Deep. The kind of kiss that feels both urgent and inevitable. Soft and hungry at the same time. His mouth moves with confidence, but there's playfulness in it, too, like he's still discovering me even as he claims the moment.

After 30 seconds in, my body is molten. The room fades. The music dulls. The bourbon disappears from my bloodstream, replaced by something far more intoxicating.

Brett's mouth trails along my jaw, down the curve of my neck, and my breath betrays me. My hands grip his shoulders, fingers tangling in his hair as if I might float away without the anchor.

He lifts me effortlessly, and I wrap my legs around him without thinking. He carries me through the French doors into his bedroom, kissing me as he goes, my mouth, my cheek, the hollow beneath my ear, like he can't decide where he wants to land and so he chooses everywhere.

We barely make it across the threshold before he lowers me onto the bed. Not carelessly. Not rough. Just decisive. My skirt slides higher as I fall back against the crisp white duvet, and for a moment, he simply stands there, looking at me.

He unbuttons his shirt first, slow enough that I feel every second of it. Then his jeans. Then the rest. No bravado. No theatrics. Just comfortable in his own skin. Lean and defined in that effortless runner's way, all long lines and smooth strength.

When he leans over me again, the energy shifts from spectacle to closeness. His hands return to me, guiding, not grabbing, adjusting me higher against the pillows with an ease that suggests he knows exactly what he's doing, but isn't in a rush to prove it.

His lips continue down my neck, and his hands trace up my torso, lifting my arms over my head to pull off all my pintucks. There's nothing abrupt about it.

The air conditioner blows behind us, cool against my overheated skin. I shiver. Not from the temperature, but from the contrast of it. He leaves my bra in place, fingers brushing the scalloped lace as though it's something delicate, something to be respected. He eases the fabric down just slightly, enough to press a soft kiss first to one side and then the other, slow and lingering.

He reaches toward the nightstand without breaking the rhythm of the moment. There's something almost endearing about the practicality of it, a small interruption in the poetry. The motion is efficient, familiar, clearly not his first time navigating this choreography of protection.

For a fleeting second, that realization pricks at me. He carries the ease of experience, while I carry the wonder of newness, and yet, there is something beautiful in the contrast. He handles it smoothly, practiced, and the tiny detail of it, the normalcy, grounds the moment.

When he comes back to me, fully present again, the earlier wave of insecurity dissolves beneath the warmth of his attention. Whatever routine he may have learned before this moment, what happens next doesn't feel recycled. It feels immediate. And entirely ours.

We cross into something deeper, and my body responds before my mind can interfere. Something inside me unlocks, something startling and new. It isn't just physical. It's seismic, as if I've been hit with a tidal wave of satisfaction. And I realize, I do like sex.

Before I can spiral into shame, Brett takes me again. And then again. Time blurs in the kind of way it only does when you aren't checking clocks or weighing consequences. One moment folds into the next. We lose track of where we begin and end, far more than once. A few hours pass like minutes.

Eventually, breathless and undone, I slip off the bed in search of something to wrap around myself. His white button-down hangs over a chair, no longer crisp. I button only a few buttons and head toward the kitchen for water, still floating somewhere between here and elsewhere.

That's when I glance at my BlackBerry.

Missed calls. Texts. The time. 5 p.m. Shit! It's Greer. She's at my apartment, waiting downstairs with her massive suitcase. Undoubtedly annoyed and pretending not to be. Addy will be there any minute.

"Oh, my goodness!" I gasp. "I have to go. I'm so late. How is it 5 o'clock already?" I'm scanning the room for my things. "Greer is downstairs at my building. I'm at least 30 minutes away at this hour."

"Okay," Brett says calmly, already moving, gathering my blouse and handing it to me. "We've got this. Can you call your doorman and let her up? He might not give her a key, but he'll at least let her drop her bag."

He thinks in solutions. I love that about him.

I text Greer something about being stuck at the dentist. Vague. Plausible. She responds immediately. She appears to buy it. A few minutes later, she's upstairs. Crisis postponed.

I'm not ready to leave.

"I don't want you to go," he says softly. "Are you sure you have to?"

"Pretty sure you'd be hard to explain," I answer, attempting lightness. "I'm married. Remember?"

His smile fades into something almost boyish. "I kind of forgot," he admits. "I was willing it not to be true."

I meet his smile, feeling the pull of it, and in his gaze, I wish he were right. I wish I was free to be who I am with him, no strings, no past, no illness, just this. I step into the bathroom to wash my face, reapply lipstick, and finger-comb my hair. I study myself in the mirror. There is no version of me that looks like I just came from the dentist. As I slide my bracelets back on, he watches from the doorway.

"It was more fun taking them off," he teases. He dresses, lacing his shoes.

"Do you have somewhere to be, too?" I ask.

"Did you think I wasn't walking you out?" he asks, smiling.

We head down the stairs together, side by side this time. Silent. The kind of silence that isn't empty, it's heavy with the understanding that whatever just happened cannot be neatly folded away.

This was our moment. Now, I must go back to my life. I don't have a plan for how to survive that life, but I have Greer and Addy. They are my people. I will tell them . . . eventually.

As we head outside, the door automatically opens, and Brett steps aside, letting me go first. The city acts as if nothing just occurred behind the apartment's walls. I know he wants to kiss me goodbye. I want that, too.

But New York, for all its size, can surprise you with coincidence.

So instead, he takes both of my hands in his and squeezes, once, twice, three times. A code. I walk toward the corner. I can feel he's watching. I turn back fully, memorizing him.

"This isn't really goodbye, right, Kentucky?" he calls out.

"We'll have to see, Ohio," I answer.

I turn right. Wrong direction. Of course. I wait half a beat before pivoting, hoping he's already gone inside. Then, I hustle toward the subway, wedges clacking, heart racing.

I don't think I can shrink back into the girl I'm supposed to be. I don't think I want to. As I swipe my MetroCard, hoping the train will be faster at this hour, my BlackBerry buzzes.

It's Brett.

Best. Monday. Ever.

Chapter 8

THE WEEK OF SNEAK, PART I

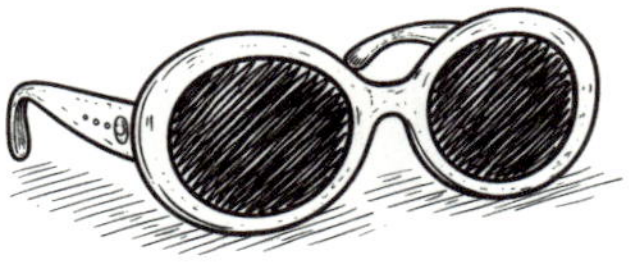

JUNE 22, 2009
6 p.m.—My Temporary Apartment
Midtown, New York City

When I get back to 41st Street to meet Greer and Addy, I brace myself for their annoyance or, at the very least, confusion. Silly me, I should know better by now. Whether it's been two days or two months, which, let's be honest, it never is, our reunions are always the same: hugs that lift you off the floor, high-pitched squeals, and ridiculous accents deployed as affection.

We've been calling ourselves blood sisters since we pricked our fingers at The Ritz in Paris like dramatic little lunatics. Being genuinely mad at one another is almost unfathomable. And if irritation ever does creep in, we can usually trace it back to one of four culprits: low blood sugar, sleep deprivation, excessive alcohol, or too much time apart.

They're already inside my apartment when I arrive, exactly as Brett predicted and helped orchestrate. Suitcases exploded open. Shoes kicked off. Making themselves completely at home, just as I'd hoped. Limes sliced. Diet Cokes cracked. Dolly Parton playing.

"Pippy!" they sing in unison the second I walk in. "You're here! How are your teeth?"

Oh no. My teeth. I hadn't thought about my fictional dental emergency since I sent them the text. I give them the breeziest summary imaginable, something about a bad filling, a quick fix, nothing major. Keep it moving. Keep it light.

"Pip," Greer begins, squinting at me, on the verge of a laugh. "Do they serve bourbon at your dentist's office now? You smell like it."

My stomach bounces. "That's hilarious! Must be the fluoride," I say, laughing a little too quickly, too loudly. Face reddening. I'm still a little tipsy. Before either of them can dig deeper, I pivot.

"So!" I announce, bright and animated, clapping once. "What are the plans for tonight? And more importantly, what are we wearing?" Distraction by fashion. Works every time. Their eyes light up instantly. My favorite risk-taking style-makers are ready to turn any random Monday into a runway. For a moment, just a moment, it feels simple again. Three girls. Music on. Closet doors flung open. No husbands in sight. And no one asking the questions I'm not ready to answer.

"I booked us a table at Bagatelle for 9 p.m.!" Addy cheered. "So put on your dancing shoes!" For a pregnant gal, she's still a ball of fun.

I don't even pause. I just slide on my comfiest pair of metallic platforms, and shout over the music, "Done and done!"

The kind of energy buzzing through me isn't meant for sitting still. And it's not like my day could get any more ridiculous: Sex with a stranger, drinking bourbon before noon, and openly lying to my oldest friends in the world about the state of my pearly whites.

The next few days move at hyper-speed. Mornings are all business: Jet Set Lingerie spreadsheets, acquisition conversations with "big players," production calls to Bangkok about shapewear quantities and fabric weights, and mapping out fall trade shows while factoring in Addy's impending maternity leave. We speak in margins, markups, and MOQs before noon. Afternoons mean power lunches at Jean-Georges or the Four Seasons, where we pick at delicate plates, share a side of fries, and pretend we won't miss a beat once Addy's baby arrives. We speak bravely about balance and support systems and Skype-in factory visits. We are naive enough to believe very little will change.

By 5 p.m., we are freshly glossed and re-dressed, slipping into charity events inside designer boutiques and art galleries with champagne flutes in hand (for me and Greer) and air kisses at the ready. And by midnight, we are somewhere darker and louder. Bungalow 8 feels different with a baby bump in tow, but comfort keeps us returning. The music still hits. And if our outfits feel tamer or our hair isn't quite as coiffed as it once was, we make a pit stop at Beatrice Inn.

Somewhere in the margins of all that, between limes and lip gloss and line sheets, I send dozens of texts to Brett. Flirty. Honest. Curious. Some long, some saucy one-liners. With the Twins in town, seeing him is impossible. The anticipation stirs me even more, as if I wasn't stirred enough. The logistics of how we'll carve out time feels like a secret puzzle only the two of us can assemble. The Twins head back to Dallas and Knoxville early Friday morning. Brett and I plan a late-morning coffee date for then. I feel like I might combust if I don't see him soon.

Greer and Addy keep me from igniting. There is a sweetness to our last few days in the city together like we are unknowingly savoring something that's already beginning to slip through our fingers. Everything feels just a little more meaningful, the laughter lingering longer, the stories deeper, the small rituals suddenly worth remembering.

On our final night together, as we primp for the last NYC supper of the summer as a trio, I almost tell them everything. There is no chance they haven't noticed the uptick in my texting. I keep confirming it's Richard, which is laughable. Richard and I rarely have that much to say unless it involves a misplaced document or an electric bill. Last year, in a new apartment, I forgot to set up autopay with Reliant Energy. A few months lapsed, and the power cut off on him while I was in Paris with the girls. It was an honest mistake but a terrible look as I frolicked up the Champs-Élysées, while Richard sat in darkness. I deserved his frustration, but I'm not sure I deserved his condemnation of my character. In seven years of paying every bill, this happened only once with our utilities.

While applying my eye makeup, staring at my reflection in the mirror, I test the waters with Greer and Addy. I confess, "I met someone at Bemelmans . . ."

Their heads snap up in unison. I describe him first. A young Dennis Quaid. That earns immediate attention. I tell them I crossed a line. One I had never even tiptoed toward before. I pause for their reaction. Their faces mirror each other instantly, eyes widening in perfect sync, mouths parting just slightly, already invested in my story.

I feel safe to share the bar conversation I had with Brett and the way he rested his hand on my leg and how I didn't move it. Didn't flinch. They don't gasp. Don't scold. So, I continue.

I tell them about me leaving the bar to get food. About Brett following. About him trying to kiss me in the street. Another pause. They glance at each other for a split second and then back at me, their faces softening, like I'm okay in their hands.

"I let him!" I blurt, covering my face dramatically. A rainbow of bangles dig into my cheeks. I freeze, but just for a moment. And then, I give them the cinematic version: the rain beginning just as our lips touched and the way it felt like a movie.

"Morgan!" they shout together in twin harmony. Their lipstick application halts. Their voices equal parts shock and intrigue.

I take a breath, place my eyeshadow palette back in my makeup bag, and give them the version I know they can hold. I tell them a more constrained story that won't keep them up at night. I conveniently edit out the scene in the taxi, replacing it with the earlier moment when I did push him away. Technically true. Just . . . reordered.

But what I don't say lingers louder. I don't tell them about the electricity of that taxi ride, how the whole world seemed to narrow down to the space between us. I don't tell them how his hands on me felt unfamiliar in a way that made me feel more like myself, not less. I don't tell them how, for a few suspended minutes, I felt awake. And I definitely don't tell them the lack of remorse that I feel. They won't hear the aliveness. They will only hear the risk.

Greer and Addy's reaction to my curated confession is even kinder than I expect. Curious. Concerned. Protective. Fearful. The undertone, however, is clear: I cannot see him again. Under no circumstances. And I am to tell no one. That part will be easy.

"We didn't exchange numbers or last names," I assure them, as I slip on a pair of yellow, crocodile-embossed secondhand Manolos. "Nothing to worry about."

In the moment I'm referring to, that was also true. But all these half-truths add up to full lies. Strangely, I don't feel worried. I feel hopeful. Finishing touches of lipstick applied and handbags carefully paired with our outfits, we leave for dinner, slipping back into normalcy like nothing major has shifted. A little drama shared between sisters. A kiss in the rain. Life moves forward. At least, that's what I tell myself.

June 26, 2009, 8 a.m.—My Temporary Apartment, NYC

While I'm genuinely sad to see Greer and Addy leave, because New York is at its best when we are together, I am restless. Electric. I hardly know Brett, yet four days without him feels like a month.

He and I attempted a secret visit late last night when the girls unexpectedly met up with friends from college for a post-dinner drink. It was a risky idea. I didn't care. I parted ways with Greer and Addy, taking a taxi in the opposite direction. Traffic was insane. At dinner, we learned that Michael Jackson was found dead in his home. You could feel the loss permeating the entire city. Droves of people came out to honor the King of Pop. Every cab window was rolled down, and the sounds of "P.Y.T.," "Thriller," "Rock with You," and "Man in the

Mirror" meshed in the air to create the perfect, chaotic harmony. The traffic. The timeline. It just didn't work. Brett and I would have to wait.

By the time Greer and Addy leave for the airport, I am racing the clock. There isn't time for my usual meticulous primping. I slip into a sunshine-hued racerback tank, finished with delicate bias trim and elegant darts. After the monochrome restraint of the last outfit Brett saw me in, I am craving color. God forbid he thinks I'm one note.

I choose a vintage royal blue silk mini skirt with edgy pockets. It's easy, slightly relaxed. Platform gladiator sandals in brushed silver add just enough edge. I stack a rainbow of bangles, slide on orange sunglasses I'd picked up on St. Mark's Place, and fasten a small white Chanel crossbody over me, just big enough for the essentials. The silver hardware echoes my shoes.

We are meeting at Think Coffee on Mercer Street. This time, I'm acutely aware of how close we'll be to his apartment.

I take a cab instead of the subway. No arriving overheated and flustered. I get there a few minutes early and open the door to peek inside. Brett isn't there. There isn't a single seat available anyway, so I step back outside, heat pressing down on me, my curls already surrendering. Panic rising inside. What if he isn't coming? Five seconds into that spiral, I hear a whistle. I hesitate before turning, just in case it isn't meant for me . . . that would be embarrassing, but then, I hear Brett's laugh. I look. He is wearing yellow, too, a fitted pique polo and tailored blue pants. Likely Paul Smith. We're "twinning!" I throw my head back laughing.

"I recognized those sticks from a block away," he teases.

Something about how casual he looks, softens my nerves. There is no playing hard to get. Not for me. I reach out without thinking, resting my hand on his chest. He covers it with his for a beat too long. Married or not, neither of us is pretending this is neutral.

Since the café is packed, we start walking, deeper into Greenwich Village, drifting through quiet streets lined with townhouses that once held poets and now belong to hedge fund managers. An hour disappears.

When we loop back toward West Third, Brett gives me a look and opens a heavy gray pub door. I enter without hesitation. The place is dim and tucked away, sticky floors and tufted booths. It smells like decades of spilled whisky. Brett chooses the most secluded corner.

"Our usual?" he asks.

I love the sound of that. "Obviously."

Two bourbons and a round of our "this or that game" we'd been playing via text all week. His hand finds mine beneath the table like it has a mind of its own. It doesn't take long to admit, without saying it, that we want more time, but not here.

We backtrack to Mercer, walking faster this time.

The second time through Brett's apartment building feels different. Familiar. There is no lingering. No small talk. In the stairwell, before we even reach his front door, Brett turns me toward him with the ease of someone who knows exactly what he is doing. My back meets the wall; his hand squeezing the side of my waist. The kiss is urgent but sure, like it has been waiting all day.

Inside, the pace accelerates. Clothes fall somewhere behind us, forgotten. The world narrows to breath and touch and the sound of air conditioners running overtime in the background. Later, under cool bed linens drenched in the scent of dryer sheets, we talk. Laugh. Hide from the chill of the blasting air-conditioning units. The intensity softens into something sweeter. And then, suddenly, it is 5 p.m. Borrowed time. Richard's train will arrive in just over an hour.

I bolt for the bathroom to shower and collect myself. Brett follows quickly and steps in behind me. Steam rising, fogging the glass. He pulls me back into him, and for a moment, I forget entirely about schedules and trains and consequences. It feels like an '80s Cinemax moment, the kind they only showed after midnight. Hot. Impulsive in a way that makes me laugh at myself.

I don't mean to get my hair wet, but with that much motion and that many shower heads, there is no avoiding it. Now, I'm scrambling. Thankfully, a hair dryer remains, a ghost of someone before me and a reminder of Brett's colorful dating history. We rush to get out the door.

"I'll ride with you," Brett says. "More time."

I don't argue. We kiss through 30 blocks of traffic, the late afternoon light catching the shimmer on his skin from my bronzer.

"I'm leaving you with fairy dust," I laugh, climbing out at the corner near my apartment building.

He grins, glittered and glowing. "When do I see you again?" he calls.

I have no idea. My calendar is a war zone. "Tuesday?" I suggest.

"Consider it yours."

The cab pulls away, as Brett's hand waves from the window.

I rush upstairs to my apartment. Re-entry mode. Wiping saltine crumbs off the counters. Placing scattered bangles back on their bars. Hiding piles of handbags in drawers. Making space in the closet for Richard's things. Straightening towels. Pulling sheets tight. Lighting a candle to camouflage the dorm room odors. Erasing evidence, not just of Brett, but of joy. Of Greer and Addy. Of Mom. Of any version of me that isn't controlled and contained.

Ten minutes to spare. My phone lights up. Three missed calls from Mom. I'll call her back. But not now. God forbid Richard walks in while I'm talking to her. I'd have to invent something. Like always.

Another weekend with Richard under my belt. But this one came with an unexpected buffer. Greer's husband, Rhett, decided to meet her in the city instead of flying back to Dallas, so she changed her flight and stayed. In my rush to meet Brett on Friday morning right after the girls left my apartment for the airport, I missed the flurry of texts from Greer about the switch, which, in hindsight, was probably suspicious. Thankfully Rhett arrived early enough in the day that she didn't press me too hard about my whereabouts. The two of them were off having a grand time, staying Uptown at a gorgeous five-star hotel.

There was a time when that would've stung. When I would've compared, calculated, and felt left out. But I was floating too high. Nothing could touch me. For good measure, and to survive with my composure intact, I added an extra Zoloft or two to the mix. Chemistry as a coping mechanism. A little pharmaceutical insurance policy.

My texting with Brett, on the other hand, had moved well beyond careful. I stopped slipping into bathrooms. Stopped angling my phone away. I responded wherever and whenever, whether I was at dinner, on the couch, or in Richard's direct line of sight. My boldness surprised even me. Or maybe it didn't.

The Atlanta Braves were on a hot streak, and Richard was consumed with watching the games. I've never been grateful for baseball in my life, but that weekend, I could've sent the entire roster a thank-you card. Every inning bought me more freedom. Every pitching change, another text message sent.

On Saturday night, my crazy leveled up. Richard and I were at a Korean BBQ spot on 32nd Street, just the two of us, the air thick with smoke and sesame oil, the sharp bite of kimchi clinging to everything. Outside, bad karaoke spilled into the streets, neon signs blinking over hostess bars and private singing rooms. The whole block pulsed off-key. My phone buzzed. Brett. He was at a karaoke bar one block away.

Without hesitation, I texted him that Richard and I could head over and book the private room next door to his. We could "accidentally" cross paths. Slip out. Meet for a minute. I didn't exactly text "make out," but it was implied. It felt brilliant in the moment. Efficient. Chaotic in a delicious way. Brett's response came fast.

Morgan, no. I love the idea of seeing you, kissing you, but that is insane.

I stared at the word "insane" longer than necessary. I didn't like hearing no from him. Was it really that wild? It felt . . . manageable. Bold, yes. But impossible? I wasn't convinced. Or maybe, I just didn't want to be.

Your loss ;) I shot back, forcing breezy where there was none.

The truth, I was disappointed. Not just because I wanted to see Brett. I did, but because part of me wanted him to be just as carefree. And he wasn't. For someone whose stories made him appear to be footloose and fancy free, with a significant focus on the "loose" part, for his entire 30s, this was a surprising response. Why hold back now? To protect me? Or because he's having too much fun with someone else? Or maybe, I've exaggerated what is happening between us. Or maybe, it's nothing. Or maybe, I'm just too much. Yet again.

June 30, 2009, 8 a.m —My Temporary Apartment, NYC

When Monday comes and Richard doesn't leave, my happy little "dorm" apartment starts to feel like a prison cell. What once felt scrappy and charming now feels neglected and dim. The popcorn ceiling presses down. The vertical blinds look institutional instead of ironic. The absence of a garbage disposal suddenly feels like a personal attack. Before Richard's arrival, there was ample hot water. Now, it gives up halfway through my shower, leaving me shivering and annoyed. Dishes stack faster than I can tolerate without a dishwasher to hide them in. I had avoided using dishes all summer to eliminate this problem, and now, with Richard in my space, everything is a nuisance. He has invaded my retreat with stress, expectations, and rules. His complaints seep into every corner of the room, leaving the air thick and impossible to escape: There is not enough space for his toiletries in the tiny vanity. The iron is cheap and gets brown water stains on his chinos. My clothes take up too much of the rack in the closet.

The apartment's lighting, though always bad, now casts a permanent gray wash over everything, like the space itself is disappointed in me for letting Richard inside, for not having the courage to just leave—for real.

With Richard working from my summer home, tapping away on his laptop at the tiny table, the air feels thinner. I have to get out. Not to mention, I can't do any real work around him. Jet Set Lingerie is a full blown trigger now. The mere mention of the brand that he once championed, mostly because it connected him to Rhett, became "off-limits" before I even left for New York. Too much time. Too much risk. Too much me.

Richard is sick of it. Sick of hearing about production delays in Bangkok or wholesale margins or logo placement. Sick of the way my eyes light up when I talk about it. So, I obey . . . no more mentions.

I don't dare tell the girls this part. It's too embarrassing. Like the fact that, when we needed a contract reviewed, I asked my dad to look at it instead of my own husband. Because Richard refused. Flat out. Said he didn't want to "get involved." Said it was my responsibility. As if I were asking him to cosign a massive loan instead of glancing at legal language that he reads for a living.

So, I sent it to my father. I told Greer and Addy that Richard had "given some feedback." I said it casually. Like, it was obvious. Of course, my lawyer husband would help. The lie slid out easily. I keep thinking my affair is the biggest betrayal here. But it started long before. Not to mention the financial betrayals I've been hiding for years.

With Richard here, I invent reasons to leave. Errands. Meetings. Fabric sourcing. Coffee catchups that don't exist. I dress like I'm headed somewhere important, bangles stacked, sunglasses on, and then I just walk. For hours. Midtown to SoHo. SoHo to the Village. Ducking into coffee shops to answer emails, text Brett, take "work calls" with Greer and Addy, trying to avoid the allure of retail, of spending. Failing most of the time. Movement feels like oxygen. My phone vibrating, blood in my veins.

My mom is texting more than usual, too. Little check-ins: *How's your week? You sound off. Call me when you can.* Like she knows. The way mothers always do. I keep our conversations short. Surface level. I'm afraid, if she hears my voice for too long, she'll detect the cracks.

My first Monday with Richard stretches endlessly. Every hour feels like three. By dinner, I'm certain this is the longest day of my life. When Tuesday finally arrives, I'm surprised by how sleep matters less and less.

Time with Richard is usually draining for me, the kind of emotional exhaustion that seeps into my bones, but I'm still in motion. Still operating at a frequency slightly too fast. Tonight, there is a big charity event at The Gramercy Park Hotel. Richard isn't invited. Not technically, and not incidentally either. It's one of the few perks of this New York summer, rooms and rooftops that belong to me alone.

Since Richard can't attend, he's made plans with a few college friends who happen to be in the city. We've already seen them once this summer at the "Welcome to New York" party I threw for myself back in May. I framed it like it was for both of us, of course. A joint celebration. A fresh start. What a façade. But then Richard left the morning after that rooftop soirée, the best party I've thrown in years, and didn't return for weeks. Anyone paying attention could have spotted the truth. If they'd looked. But no one did.

I leave the apartment before Richard does. Summer events start early, positioned on Tuesdays and Wednesdays only, strategically avoiding competition with Hamptons' shares and Montauk sunsets. The city empties out on weekends, so influence stays midweek.

The plan is simple. I'll arrive right when the party begins. Make a lap. Track down Patrick McMullan for a photo op, proof of attendance for the girls. Smile wide. Chin up. Shoulders back.

Thirty minutes in, Brett will be outside. We'll slip away. And then, we'll have the whole night. A proper date. Our first real dinner date.

Chapter 9

THE WEEK OF SNEAK, PART II

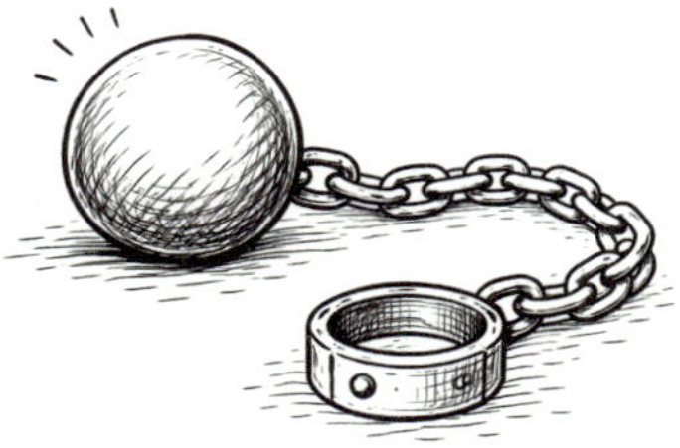

JUNE 30, 2009
6 p.m.—The Gramercy Park Hotel
New York City

Exactly 30 minutes after arriving at the event, I glide back through the Gramercy's outdoor space, the pergola wrapped in ivy, black-and-white curtains pulled back like stage drapes. Early evening light filters through in amber streaks. In my nude patent Louboutins, a sample sale purchase with one heel slightly higher than the other, I descend the handful of stairs into my favorite room on the roof—the one crowned with hundreds of Edison bulbs suspended from the ceiling, glowing low and golden. It's tucked among a maze of spaces that unfold one into the next, some open to the night with garden string lights draped overhead, others more enclosed and moody. French doors cracked just enough to let the air slip in. Cabana-style curtains frame each turn giving the whole place a sense of quiet intrigue, as if every corner holds a slightly different version of the evening.

The room looks like an art installation. And given Ian Schrager's penchant for filling the hotel with pieces by Warhol and Damien Hirst, you'd assume it was. It's not. Just design. Fabulous, nonetheless.

The elevator ride down feels endless. Butterflies riot in my stomach as the vintage dial ticks floor by floor. I smooth my lavender satin D&G pencil skirt, an INA treasure, definitely paid for on credit, and slit scandalously high in the back. A taupe faux-silk tank from H&M tones down the look. A dark burgundy belt from an old Betsey Johnson dress (purchased solely for the belt) cinches my waist. Clear Lucite bangles. Vintage metallic brushed-gold Chanel clutch. Thoughtful, but not overworked.

The revolving doors spin. And he's there. Like Jake in the final scene of *Sixteen Candles*. No Porsche. Though, Brett once owned one.

Lavender was the right choice. If only I'd thought to add a flower crown for the full Molly Ringwald effect, I could reenact the '80s film. I wish, absurdly so, that someone was nearby so I could subtly point and whisper, "It's him," the way Molly's character does to her dad. For obvious reasons, I can't. But it feels like a movie anyway: The sounds of the city. The faint trace of santal exiting the hotel lobby. The warmth of Brett as he leans in to kiss my cheek. Suddenly, I'm nervous.

The last time felt illicit. Dive bar. Urgency. Heat. Cliché in the most dangerous way. This feels different. Brett's holding flowers of all shades of pink. He's in a blazer and a white shirt, unstarched but fresh. Ferragamo loafers, no socks. Effortless summer polish.

"Peonies are apparently out of season," he says, smiling, "so I went all pink." He learns fast.

"They're stunning. Thank you," I say, feeling my own pink rise to my cheeks. My brain empties. Nothing clever surfaces. I tilt my head slightly, attempting coy, likely landing somewhere closer to facial twitch.

"Shall we?" He extends his hand. "I picked somewhere we can walk, not far. I knew you'd be wearing shoes like that." His eyes drop to my mismatched heels. "After dinner, I thought we'd stop at POP."

"Stop rhyming, I mean it," I blurt, quoting the movie *Princess Bride* before I can stop myself.

"Anybody want a peanut?" he sings back instantly.

We collapse into laughter. And then, just as quickly, the laughter softens—not because the joy fades, it doesn't, but because something lands between us. Something feels real, which makes this infinitely more complicated. How could it possibly work? My life is a maze with no visible exit. There is no clean path from here to there. And yet. Brett and I were meant to meet. I just know it.

He takes my hand, and we head south toward Union Square. He chose Olives, a Todd English restaurant, classic, clean lines, and tucked inside the W Hotel. The space glows in that warm, flattering way restaurants in hotels always do, like everyone inside is just a little more important than they are outside.

Brett's hand rests low on my back as he guides me to the table. The hostess is stunning, the kind of pretty that makes you assume she's auditioning for something bigger than seating diners. An actress. A Rockette. Something luminous. I assume Brett notices, too. But when I glance back, his eyes are on me.

At the table, I study the menu carefully, though nothing on it makes me hungry. Everything reads delicious; nothing sparks my actual appetite. I decide I'll match whatever Brett orders. Meanwhile, he is laser-focused on the wine list. The intensity is almost comical. Either he's a connoisseur or completely bluffing. After a long pause, he selects a 2001 Sangiovese. Confident. No hesitation. Then, he orders for us but pauses midway. "Would you be okay if I order a mix of things for us to share?" he asks me.

"Sounds delightful," I reply, secretly relieved not to have to pretend to choose.

He leans closer, hand warm on my knee, and asks, "Nervous?"

"Very," I admit.

"Me, too," he says. "Something about it being a real date, I think." He smiles. "And now, I know what I have to lose. When you were just the 'married chick' . . ."

"What?" I gasp, my voice jumping an octave. "The married chick? That's what you've been calling me?"

Brett laughs. "Not me," he says. "My friends, including Josh. I talk about you too much. Everyone's invested."

I laugh at the absurdity of it all, at the speed of this, and the version of myself sitting here. The nerves dissolve. Over rare filet with creamed spinach, roasted Brussels sprouts, and wood-fired fish, Brett and I tell each other everything. The biggest revelation: China.

His recent job opportunity is moving quickly, faster than either of us expected. A due-diligence trip is scheduled in two weeks. 6,000 miles are suddenly realized. We'd been dreading my lease ending before my trip to Miami for Greer and Addy's 30th, a weekend already shaping itself into something celebratory and slightly unhinged, but now, it looks like he might leave first. I catch myself calculating time zones and flights like a woman with no sense of reality.

"I'm sure we can handle distance and time change," Brett says lightly. "Then, we just have to figure out the marriage thing." He laughs.

"Oh right," I say. "That minor detail." What is happening?

As the check comes, his phone rings. He apologizes and steps away, mouthing that it's the friends staying in his loft tonight. I watch him while finishing my wine, his back turned, shoulders tense. When he returns, something's off.

"They're arriving four hours earlier than planned," he says carefully. "Any chance you'd turn this into a double date?"

He wants me to say yes. I don't want to share him. Our time already feels borrowed. But I look at his face and cave.

"Well," I say lightly, "let's go meet these lifelong friends then."

Like I'm not married. Like this is normal.

As we stand, he hesitates.

"One little thing," he says sheepishly. His eyes make their way to my wedding rings. "Any chance you could take those off?"

The words land harder than they should. Not because he's wrong. But because, for the first time tonight, something real and irreversible edges into the fantasy.

July 1, 2009, Morning—My Temporary Apartment, NYC

I wake up without shame. Richard is asleep in the bottom bunk across the room, mouth open, head tilted back, wearing a gray striped pajama top wrinkled from days spent crumpled inside his suitcase. The air feels stale. Used. It was after 4 a.m. when I got home.

Brett rode in the taxi with me. Walked me right to the door. Kissed me goodnight, technically good morning. Part of me wished Richard had been standing behind the revolving door, watching.

I want to get caught. I need to get caught. I'm a boiling pot with water about to spill over the sides. The only shame I feel is that I'm too much of a coward to detonate my own life.

In 13 short days, Brett has become the catalyst. The spark. He has ignited the thing that was already smoldering inside me long before he crossed the room at Bemelmans, and it's the push I needed to acknowledge it. Whether I ever see Brett again or not, something has to change.

Richard stirs. I consider pretending to be asleep, but it's too late. He sees my eyes are open.

"When did you get in?" he asks.

"Late," I say lightly. "I didn't want to wake you. I ran into Amy Sacco at the event, and we ended up at Bungalow talking business." I leave it there. I already know he doesn't want to hear about it.

Our conversation topics have narrowed significantly in the last few years. What remains is: sports (which I barely understand), politics (which I barely care about), and food (which lately I barely eat).

"But what time exactly?" he presses.

"I don't know," I reply. "I texted you. When you didn't respond, I figured you were out or already asleep. I came home not long after."

Lie. I was out for hours after I texted Richard. But I knew he was asleep, and there was no barrage of "Where are you?" messages to indicate otherwise. Thankfully, he lets the matter go.

He makes coffee. I crack open a Diet Coke and break off three little Toblerone pyramids for breakfast. He showers with the bathroom door closed, likely scratching the itch that I won't. I steam the outfit I plan to wear later and hang it back up before he emerges.

He dresses quickly: light blue button-down; flat-front khakis; and brown suede Tod's driving loafers, a Christmas gift from his parents.

We barely speak. To fill the silence, I play MGMT on my laptop. We have tickets to see the band in Brooklyn tomorrow. I'm excited about the music, less excited about trekking all the way out there with Richard, farther away from Brett, as if geography could solve our problems.

Richard places his scratched white coffee mug, part of the sad mismatched set that came with my digs, in the sink, grabs his briefcase and extra keys, and gives me a limp kiss before heading out for the day. Our bodies don't touch. No smiles exchanged. The version of me who would smile through anything is starting to slip.

"See you tonight. Don't forget, we're grabbing a drink with Charles from the firm," he calls over his shoulder, walking out the door, as it starts to slowly close. Like a repelling magnet, I'm halfway to the bedroom when I shout back, "Oh, right. Just text me the place we're meeting." The malaise in my voice travels across the faded parquet floors, down the dirty carpet hallway to Richard.

"Will do. Bye!" he says loud enough for it to make its way through the single inch of door left open. Flat. Distant. For a fleeting second, I wonder if he knows. The door clicks shut.

I move fast. Turn the shower on. Puffy pink shower cap secured. I have less than 20 minutes to get downtown to Friend of a Farmer to meet my favorite new "friend" for breakfast. Brett texted me an hour ago asking if I could make it work. As if I would miss the chance.

The overcast sky makes the restaurant feel cozier, like rain could start any second and trap everyone inside. The idea of being trapped with Brett doesn't scare me, which is unusual for me.

He stands the moment I walk in. It's only been six hours since he kissed me outside the revolving door at my apartment, and yet he looks at me like it's been weeks. His eyes travel my body head to toe. My hair is pulled into a tight low bun, no time for theatrics. I let my dress do the talking: a neon orange splatter-print DVF wrap, bold and unapologetic. Blue ankle-strap sandals. Bangles stacked in every shade of citrus. Orange is his favorite color. I learned that somewhere between midnight confessions and our ridiculous this-or-that texting game.

Before I even sit down, Brett's talking. Fast. Too fast. I only grasp fragments. What I do catch is that the business deal is happening. In China. His visa has to be rushed. He has 72 hours. He's got to pack. The trip will last two weeks. My brain scrambles to assemble all the details. Trying to determine what it means . . . for us.

He stops mid-sentence when he sees my face.

"Sorry. Let's start over," Brett exhales. "Mike called this morning, basically right after I dropped you off. He's in Brazil. The deal is in its final stages. He needs me in Beijing by the morning of the fifth to finish due diligence. I have to tell the investors whether to buy the company or not. It's all happening."

"The fifth?" I interrupt. "As in July 5th?"

He nods.

"That's four days from now," I confirm. "That's before I leave."

"I know. Crazy," he says, grinning, "but good. All good things."

He skips words when he's excited, like grammar can't keep up with ambition. I am proud of him. I really am. But the news hits like a punch to the ribs. Brett's leaving. Then, I'm leaving. Whatever this is—this life-altering, impossible thing—has an expiration date.

It doesn't feel like "all good things" to me.

The rest of breakfast is pleasant but blurred. I order the restaurant's signature dish: apple pancakes, fluffy and golden. Brett gets black coffee and an omelet with everything, which I now recognize as his standard order. I'm careful with my words. I don't want to sound like a complication. I'm married, for goodness' sake. Why would he factor me into any decision about China?

"Do you have to rush back?" he asks softly. "Or can you hang with me today? I could really use your help."

"I have some time." I smile.

We spend hours zigzagging downtown, stopping at visa offices, luggage shops, and electronics stores. Brett buys a sleek carry-on and a new dopp kit. He holds my hand the entire time. A boyfriend move.

"You know what?" he says, as we wait in line somewhere bureaucratic and fluorescent. "My friends loved you."

"They did?" I feign surprise, but I know I was on my A-game. I'm extra charming when I'm riding this high.

"Of course, they did," Brett insists. "I should tell you, though, they know you're married."

"What?" I stop walking. "You told them? Then, why did you make me take my wedding rings off?"

"I didn't tell them," he says, laughing. "They pieced it together when you didn't stay the night."

He glances down at my left hand. I follow his eyes. Bare. A cold rush floods my chest. I never put them back on.

I dart into the elevator in my building and jab the number 7 button three times, fully aware it doesn't make the car move any faster, but somehow, I'm convinced it helps. I am terrified Richard has beaten me home. I have no logical explanation prepared for why my wedding rings would be off, hidden in the secret pocket of my evening bag.

The doors open. The apartment is dark. I made it home first. Relief crashes over me. I rush to the chest of drawers where I've stored my bags, each shelf lined with lavender drawer liners I picked up from TJ Maxx to mask the dorm-room smell. My fingers tremble as I reach into the black faille interior of the brushed gold Chanel.

Metal meets skin. They're there. Safe. I slide them back on and check the time. 5:15 p.m. Where is he? My phone buzzes. It's Richard.

Where are you? You see the address above, right?

Double shit. In the chaos of going back to Brett's apartment, what was likely our last hurrah before China and Miami and lease endings, I completely forgot I'm supposed to meet Richard and his former boss for drinks Uptown.

Charles, the man who made New York possible the first time around, is the hiring partner who carved out a spot for Richard on his team. His wife is impossibly chic and perfect. Their children are polished and polite. They're nothing short of Kennedy-esque. And here I am. Lipstick smeared. Hair undone. Dress damp with sweat. Skin carrying the faint trace of another man.

Get it together, Morgan. I press a cold washcloth to my face, then my neck, then anywhere that still feels flushed. As if I can wipe away the intensity of what just happened. Impossible. It's burned into me.

The closeness. The abandon. The way I told Brett yes without hesitation. Even with protection, it felt daring. I had never surrendered that way before. Not even in the safety of marriage. Not even when I was on the pill. It shocks me. And yet . . . I wasn't afraid.

For as long as I can remember, the fear of pregnancy has been a shadow trailing every decision. In the South, it was practically Scripture: one mistake could ruin your life. The warning echoed loudly. I have never wanted Richard's baby. So even inside marriage, the fear never left me. Layers of protection. Always. But with Brett, something shifted. At the very moment when I felt him throb inside me, suspended there, catching his breath after, I thought, I wouldn't mind having this man's baby. If that doesn't define crazy, I don't know what does.

July 1, 2009, 6ish—Upper East Side, NYC

I rush out of my apartment and grab a taxi to Paola's, but traffic is a disaster, so I hop out of the cab and walk. With every step, I feel a blister forming on my heel. Before leaving the apartment, I changed into something I thought Richard would approve of.

Over the last year, he's made it abundantly clear that most of my outfits are, in his opinion, too loud. Too accessorized. Too colorful. Too revealing. Even when they aren't. I'll admit I've pushed a boundary or two, but it's rarely into anything truly risqué. My devotion to turtlenecks and architectural vintage silhouettes runs too deep. Over-pleated. Over-puffed. Overthought. Bandage dresses have never been my lane.

Last year at his company's Christmas party, Richard found the perfect way to humiliate me. He does it privately of course, as to not tarnish his image. On the way out of the apartment, I asked for his approval of my outfit. He tells me it's fine.

"You look cute, like a snow bunny," he said. It was almost nice. Sweet. And kind of true. I was wearing a strapless pink satin dress with a sweetheart neckline. Nude hosiery. Ivory quilted slingbacks with black patent leather toes. To cover my shoulders, I draped an off-white bunny stole around them. A bit of cleavage remained; I do have boobs after all, but it was only a peek. You really had to get in there and look to see it.

Walking into the party, inside a museum downtown, armored with Richard's approval, relaxed me. I wasn't so concerned about getting scolded. I settled into the scene. I should have known better.

Moments after receiving a compliment from his male colleague, I was pulled to the side. Richard's grip was firm on my arm. I knew his look well. Disapproval. Anger. Once out of earshot from the crowd, he said, "That dress. It's ridiculous. Too much cleavage. Too short."

I wanted to fight back. To ask him why he approved it in the first place. But I didn't. I cowered. I apologized. I excused myself to the restroom, shoved my chest down as far and as flat as it would go, working against nature. I shimmied the stole all the way to the front to reduce exposure. And I slithered out, much smaller than I entered.

When I finally arrive at Paola's, I rush toward the table.

"Hello!" I greet them. "I'm so sorry I'm late! I completely spaced and thought I was meeting Richard at the apartment and coming together. My fault entirely."

"No need to apologize," Charles says, standing to greet me. "Gave Richard and me time for boring shop talk. Nice to see you, Morgan." He takes my hand and asks what I want to drink, pointing out that I can't go wrong with a red. "They're all fantastic Italians."

Richard stands, following Charles's lead. The restaurant is bustling, filled with locals. They're identified by age, by timeless style originating the phrase itself, and by demeanor, a comfort level almost as if they're dining at home. There is nothing luxe about the place, short of its reputation, longevity, and occasional celebrity clientele. It boasts simple wooden tables covered in paper toppers, wine glasses with rims slightly too thick, and basic black and white octagon tiles.

Charles couldn't care less about any of that. He lives a beautiful life, but at his core, he's a loyalist. I imagine he and his wife, Charlotte, have been coming here for ages to exchange stories about their days—his work in law, hers with charities and children. Perhaps, they decide if they will spend the three-day holiday weekend at Rye Country Club or take a quick flight to Bermuda. They probably discuss their kids' private school applications, lacrosse matches, and riding classes. All the while, they touch each other softly, the way couples do—when they stay in love. I lean over to give Richard a quick obligatory hug for looks. It's forced. I pray it doesn't look as unnatural as it feels.

But Charles is too observant. He studies people. Learns how they tick quickly. It's possible he senses Richard's irritation as much as I do. In this particular case, it's obvious. The disappointment of my tardiness sits on Richard's face like a watermark. And the dress. Not landing.

I bought it in Bangkok at the night market, one of our rituals after long factory days with Greer and Addy. Dusk to dawn, vendors everywhere, trinkets and textiles and ice-cold Singha beers for less than a dollar. The dress is bright red, yes, but modest. High neck. Structured box pleats. Feminine puff sleeves. I belted it to create a waist, but the volume still dominates. There's zero bodycon appeal here. And it sits just above the knee. I thought he'd approve. Apparently not.

When Richard excuses himself to the restroom, I turn to Charles.

"How's Charlotte?" I ask. "The kids? What's new this summer?"

He answers quickly. Too quickly. Then, he leans toward me, close enough that I smell his aftershave.

"You won't do anything to hurt him, right?" Charles asks.

The words freeze me. Where is this coming from? We haven't spoken to Charles in years. He hasn't witnessed the erosion.

I force a laugh. "How would I ever hurt him, Charles?" I ask.

He studies me.

"I just know you can," he says quietly. "I suspect you know, too."

Before I can respond, Richard returns. The moment evaporates. Charles checks his watch. Time to take his town car back to Rye. It feels unmistakable that he orchestrated that sliver of alone time. As he leaves, something settles over me. For the first time since Brett walked over to me at Bemelmans, it occurs to me that Richard might actually care if I vanish. And that realization complicates everything.

July 3, 2009, 1 p.m.—My Temporary Apartment, Midtown

Greer calls. Her voice is breathless, anxious. "I have news," she says. Another baby is on the way. Hers.

I hear myself squeal, bright, perfectly pitched. Congratulations tumble out of my mouth in all the right places. But my face burns red, and tears prick my eyes before I can stop them. Their lives are moving forward in the most beautiful, tangible way. New life. New chapters. Expanding families. And mine feels like it's collapsing in on itself.

I am having an affair. The man I'm falling for is leaving for China the day after tomorrow. I lie and say my mom is beeping in before my sobs swallow me whole. When I hang up, the only person I want to talk to is Brett. This is girlfriend territory. Not "married chick" territory. I text Brett anyway. He replies almost instantly.

Yes! You never have to ask to call me, my perfect girl.

My perfect girl. A recent evolution. A promotion from married chick. He answers on the first ring. A stadium roars in the background. I know he's at his last Yankees game before flying to China. He invited me to join him, but a day game in the Bronx is too risky. Impossible to explain. After a quick hello, I just blurt it out.

"Greer's pregnant!"

The tears come hard this time. Sniffles. Uneven breath. It's not just about the baby. It's what it represents. Time is moving forward. Lives cementing. The one bright, stable part of Dallas is shifting into something new. It won't disappear. But it won't be the same. Brett doesn't tell me I'm overreacting. He doesn't minimize it. I can hear him moving, the crowd noise dulling, like he's stepping away from his seat to focus on me.

"I can get back to The City by three," he says. "Can I see you?"

I swallow and say, "I'm meeting Richard for sushi at 15 East. Maybe, I can slip downtown before? Cooper Square Hotel bar?"

"Perfect," he says. "Three o'clock." A pause. "Everything is going to be okay, Morgan. You'll see. I can't wait to see you."

"You, too. Have fun at the game. Go Yankees," I manage to say, forcing brightness back into my voice before we hang up.

One last meeting. Then, Brett goes to China. And I go to Dallas.

Chapter 10

THE GOODBYE

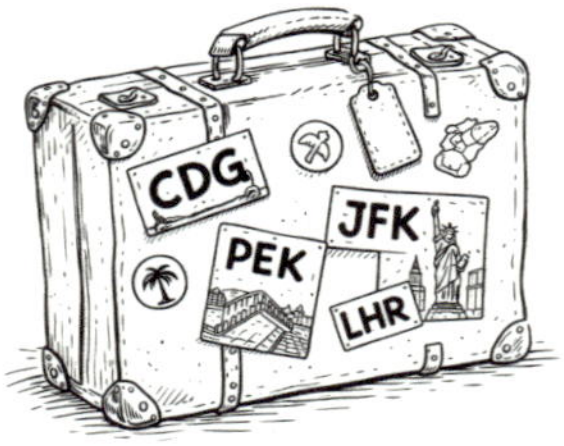

FALL 2007
10 a.m.—Doctor's Office
Dallas, Texas

I am 27 years old when my psychiatrist says, flatly, "You have bipolar." There is nothing warm about her delivery. No cushioning. No softening the language. Just fact. She is dry. Clinical. Always dresses in some variation of the same outfit. Ill-fitting black polyester trousers and an earth-toned sweater, pilled heavily at both elbows. The fabric is worn down where it has rubbed against her clipboard. The cheap particle-board kind with the silver clamp that holds intake forms in place.

I'm not opposed to a uniform. I admire consistency. But this isn't that. It feels like resignation. A quiet giving up. Color would suit her. Something gentle. Something hopeful. A reminder that the room she sits in every day is filled with people searching for relief from invisible illnesses that fracture lives and abduct identities for weeks or months at a time. I ask her how she could possibly know for sure. Bipolar, really?

I've only been seeing her for a few months. My care is now stacked—30 minutes with my psychiatrist, the one licensed to prescribe meds, and 60 minutes with my therapist. They work in tandem, extracting different fragments of me each week. It feels mechanical and disjointed—30 minutes to discuss medication and 60 minutes to unpack a life. If you ask me, it's a broken system.

My psychiatrist does her best to explain her testing process with me. Not at all what I expect. At times, some of the testing feels only marginally more sophisticated than a *Cosmopolitan* mood quiz—same self-reporting, just higher stakes and fewer glossy ads.

There isn't a scan, blood test, or definitive result, no tidy printout to announce: this is it. It's still largely clinical. A series of structured questions. Long interviews. Standardized assessments in "check a box" formats, refined over time—mood inventories, clinical signs, patterns pulled together over multiple sessions. She listens as much as she measures.

She walks me through it: the diagnostic markers, the patterns in my speech, the way my thoughts sometimes outrun themselves. The mood cycles. The impulsivity. The stretches of depression followed by bursts of energy that don't quite line up with normal joy.

She looks for duration. Intensity. Whether the highs disrupt sleep, distort judgment, start to feel less like enthusiasm and more like acceleration without brakes. She compares it against my baseline—who I am when I'm steady, assuming I've ever been.

But the real giveaway, she says, is my body's reaction to serotonin medications without a mood stabilizer. When my previous doctor in New York adjusted my antidepressant dosage to fight my depression, years earlier, I tipped into mania almost immediately. Shopping sprees. No sleep. Grand ideas. A sense that I could solve everything. Textbook.

July 4, 2009, 5:30 a.m.—My Temporary Apartment, NYC

Usually, I leap out of bed on the Fourth; pop on something aggressively red, white, and blue; and play "What a Wonderful World" while brushing my teeth, already tasting barbecue and imagining fireworks in the air. Today, I can't. Celebration feels dishonest.

Yesterday afternoon at The Cooper with Brett felt heavy. Not dramatic. Just weighted. Like the air had thickened and neither of us wanted to name it. I tried to keep things light. Tried not to let my sadness settle over the table like a damp cocktail napkin.

The Cooper is cool in that deliberate downtown way: sleek lines, tonal grays, furniture that looks sculpted rather than placed. The outdoor terrace is framed in tall green bamboo, uplighting casting everything in a flattering glow. Candles flicker even before dusk because the surrounding buildings swallow the sun early.

Brett and I sat outside. It wasn't late, but it felt like twilight. We couldn't stop touching each other. Not overtly. Not like the newlywed couple from *National Lampoon's European Vacation*, about to "pork" at the table. Not the kind of touching that makes strangers stare. Just constant, gentle contact. Fingers laced. His thumb brushing circles into the inside of my wrist. My knee pressed against his. Arms hooked together like we were anchoring each other. Like we had forever.

Which was the cruelest part. Because what we were actually doing yesterday was saying goodbye.

Richard will sleep for a couple more hours. We didn't stay out late. I just wake earlier than he does. Always have. But this summer, the gap feels extreme.

For years, I've referred to my stretches of little or no sleep as "power-through" moments. I spin them into productivity. Deadlines. Creative bursts. I tell people I'm finishing something important. Or I disappear entirely and let them assume I'm resting. It started in college, freshman year. It's remarkable how easily symptoms can be rebranded as personality traits—driven, high-energy, low-maintenance, quirky. The rebranding camouflages my manic moments and makes other people more comfortable. So, of course, I lean into what eases people, what reroutes their questions.

I grab an orange Vitaminwater and step onto the apartment's

balcony. The air is cooler than expected. Overcast. It matches the way I feel. My BlackBerry device sits in the pocket of my fuzzy pink robe. Wishful thinking that Brett will text.

I've technically been alone a lot this summer, especially at the beginning, but since mid-June, there hasn't been a single quiet stretch long enough to process what's actually happening. Not outwardly. Internally.

My therapist in Dallas has been pushing cognitive therapy. The whole "observe the thought, let it float down the river" exercise. It feels absurd when she says it. Stupid even. As if suicidal ideation can simply drift away on a current if I squint at it differently.

Not that I've been actively dwelling on suicide since I got here. I've been too elevated. Too fast. Too bright. It's hard to sink when you're hovering. Still, I know I need to try harder. Sleep more. Drink less alcohol. Stop eating Toblerone for breakfast and only a few slices of turkey meat for dinner. My medication might not be enough help on its own right now, and I'm certainly not helping the chemistry.

My therapist's fear is being realized. The ebbs and flows. The speed. The weight changes. The way my voice accelerates when I talk. The recklessness. The moral lines blurring. What am I supposed to do now? Go back to Dallas? Back to Richard? Am I about to crash so hard I can't resurface? Will I need supervision?

It doesn't take a rocket scientist to know Richard won't understand. I don't blame him. I didn't officially "have bipolar" when we married. So, in his mind, maybe this isn't part of the deal. Not his burden.

I also hide my symptoms well. Too well. Richard has little to no understanding of any defined symptoms of bipolar disorder. He's never researched it. I'm not even sure he believes it's real. And he's certainly not alone in that. Mental illness feels like the cancer of the '80s, whispered about and vaguely shameful. Like in *Terms of Endearment*, everyone is unsure how to speak its name.

And then there's Aaron, Richard's childhood best friend, who loudly insists mental illness is a crutch and a weakness. I know that narrative seeps into Richard's thinking when he's trying to "fix" me with some cure-all like camping. Camping, of all things, is my personal version of kryptonite. Richard's preference is to ignore it entirely. Honestly, his disregard makes it easier to disappear. It certainly made my escape to New York seamless.

After years of missteps and wrong medications and questionable doctors, I felt relief. Immense relief when I received a proper diagnosis. A name. A map. A path forward, however complicated. Richard felt humiliation. Concerned about optics, he asked me not to tell anyone.

I told the people who mattered, the ones who needed to know. But part of me wanted to shout it from the rooftops. If I finally had a map, maybe someone else needed one, too. I thought of all those suffering in silence or acting out without understanding.

The road ahead is long and winding. But at least now, I know in what direction I'm walking. My thoughts are interrupted by the vibration in my robe pocket. Brett's calling. I tug the sliding door shut so Richard can't hear and answer, "Well, this is a surprise."

"I don't think I can leave without seeing you again," Brett says. "My car service is on the way. I could swing by en route to Newark."

I glance toward the bedroom. "Swinging by here, with my husband in the next room, might not be our smartest move," I warn him with a laugh, but my voice is shaky with nerves. "Pick me up at 29th and Madison. I'll grab breakfast sandwiches."

I change quickly, white tank, kelly green running shorts, pink pom-pom socks, sneakers. No time to dig for something cuter. Hair into a messy high pony. A sweep of bronzer. Gloss. Big black sunglasses to hide un-mascaraed eyes. I leave a note for Richard by the sink:

Went for a morning walk. Be back soon. Happy 4th.

The "Happy 4th" is habit. I love this holiday. Something about celebrating the beauty of our flawed nation validates my own shortcomings. It honors something bold and unfinished, that has made mistakes and carried contradictions, yet still insists on becoming better.

My crossbody bag holds keys, a credit card, and nothing else. I slip out silently. The city feels paused. Trash cans are freshly emptied. Pigeons squawk louder than traffic. I stop at a Farmers Deli for egg, bacon, and cheese sandwiches and stand on the corner sipping my Diet Coke.

A grey town car pulls up. The door opens. It's Brett. I fall into his arms without thinking, small, almost childlike.

"Little Morgan," he teases, noting the absence of heels.

"You didn't give me time to plan a proper farewell outfit," I say, grinning. "So, this is what you get. You know . . . you're starting to become the boy who cried goodbye."

His laugh. That laugh. I'm going to miss it.

He's wearing a soft white henley, a grey Ralph Lauren sweatshirt looped over his shoulders, dark jeans, Nikes. Effortless. It's the kind of sweatshirt I'd steal if we were a real couple. I know better than to romanticize him into something mythic. Brett has flaws. I've seen flashes of them already. Impatience. Ego. A restlessness that mirrors my own. A real life with him wouldn't be some glossy montage. It would be messy. Highs and lows. My mood swings ricocheting off his. Fights that burn hot and apologies that take their time. Tears. Doubt. Two strong personalities colliding in a small kitchen at midnight.

But it would be real. "Your hot breakfast, sir," I say, passing him the white paper bag, grease already revealing itself from the bottom.

"Would you like to go on a date to the entrance of the Lincoln Tunnel?" he asks.

"I thought you'd never ask," I reply, sliding into the car. The driver pulls away. There's no way I'm eating now. I don't want his last image of me to be me inhaling melted cheese and bacon grease.

Brett takes my hand. Talks about how he's lived in New York nearly 15 years and can't believe he finally meets someone like me just as he's about to leave. We joke about the obstacles that would exist even if he weren't boarding a plane. But the humor fades. What I've been feeling for 24 hours, the heaviness, settles visibly onto him. Between packing and logistics, he hadn't had time to sit with it. Now he does. We reach the Lincoln Tunnel far too quickly.

"Ride the whole way with me," he says suddenly. "Please. The car can bring you back. I'm not ready to let you out of my sight."

I'm not ready either. And I'm past worrying about the lie I'll tell if Richard asks.

"Okay," I say softly.

Brett doesn't twist my arm. He pulls me into him instead. My back rests against his chest. His chin at my temple. Like we're on a couch on an ordinary night. And that's when it hits me, the ordinary things we will never have—takeout on rainy Sundays, grocery runs, Christmas shopping, meeting parents, shared calendars, shared mornings. I start mourning the nevers.

"Will we stay in touch?" I ask carefully. "No pressure. I just . . . I don't know what happens next."

"And you think I do?" he says gently. "I've never done anything like this. Especially not with a married chick." A small smile.

The car pulls up to Continental curbside check-in. The driver unloads Brett's matching Tumi luggage. Of course, he has matching luggage. He doesn't do anything half way. In the backseat, before he opens the door, Brett cups my face in both hands and rests his nose against mine. We close our eyes. The kiss is slow. Familiar. His head tilts left, mine right. Seamless. The first kiss in the rain, replayed.

He steps out. I stay inside. I don't know why. Maybe because walking him in would make it final. Maybe because I can't cross that threshold without a passport, literal or otherwise. I roll down the tinted window and watch him walk toward the doors. He turns once more. A smile, masking sadness. The automatic doors slide closed behind him.

He's gone.

Chapter 11
THE SURPRISE CALLER

JULY 4, 2009
Morning—Back of a Town Car
New York City

On the ride back from Newark, I demolish the breakfast sandwich. It's no longer hot, but it's salty and rich, comfort in its most basic form. I eat it too fast, barely chewing. Crumbs gather at the corners of my mouth, and bits of English muffin wedge in my teeth. The smell of egg fills the car. Thank God I waited until Brett was gone to eat. I couldn't bear his last image of me to be this one. It's feral, grieving, inhaling bacon and cheese like it might plug the hole he just left behind.

"I'm so sorry," I tell the driver, mortified as the scent lingers. He nods politely in the rearview mirror.

When I finish, I wipe my hands on a napkin and stare out the window. American flags flap halfheartedly in the morning air.

I call my mom. She answers on the second ring, bright and relieved. I can hear it immediately; she's been worried. She always knows when something is off. She's not wrong to be worried. I've been avoiding her. Not because I don't want to talk to her, but because I do. Desperately. I want to spill everything—the affair, the mania, the fear, the unraveling. I want her to tell me it's going to be okay. But I know she has no ability to stamp it with a guarantee.

She has told me time and again, since I was 5 years old, that there is nothing I could ever do to stop her from loving me. There's no problem too big for us to solve together. I've always wanted to believe that completely. With her, I mostly do. With my dad, I rarely did.

They got pregnant with me just a few months after their wedding. My dad has said, more times than I can count, that he "wasn't ready to be a dad." When he welcomed a new baby into his life, my brother, who is 27 years my junior, my dad casually announced to me, "Morgie, when you're 28, the last thing you want to do is stay home with a baby. At 52, it's wonderful!"

Did he forget he was talking to his first "baby" in that scenario? On its own, it's harmless enough. Honest, even. But layered with my dad's other comments and behaviors over the years of my childhood, it shaped something inside me. I grew up believing I had to earn his love. Be pretty. Make all As. Be Homecoming Queen. Date well. Impress people. Represent properly. At times, I told myself I was imagining the pressure, that parents love their children unconditionally. That's the rule. But conditions were often spelled out for me.

"You will love Becky and let her into your life, or no college," my dad warned me. I was 16 when my dad left my mom for Becky, his secretary. I was 18 when he married Becky, and he insisted I welcome her with open arms. But I knew too much.

I knew about the wedding anniversary cards Becky mailed to my mother at our house, mocking their sham marriage. I knew the tone she used when she referenced my father like he was already hers; the way she married another man to make my father jealous; and the way she claimed her miscarriage was a sign that my father and her should be together, after almost a decade of their hidden affair. I knew of my mother's humiliation. And of my own.

I knew about the letters Becky sent to local businesses, signed with my father's legal stamp, instructing them to deny charges to our family accounts at the dry cleaner, at the gas station, and even at the local diner. She let shop owners tell me to my face that the account was not open for me to use, as if I was laundering money, not church dresses, and dry-cleaning other people's clothes on their tab in exchange for cash. Becky never confronted me directly. She let the town do it for her . . . with my father's approval. Likely with his direction, but it's easier to blame the outsider. Fair or unfair, I don't want to believe my own father, capable of extending endless empathy to anyone sitting across from him, somehow couldn't find it for his own daughter.

These aren't catastrophic traumas. No one died. No one starved. But these memories burrowed. And now, sitting in the back of a town car on the Fourth of July, smelling faintly of egg and regret, I have to face the irony. There are no children in my situation. But I am the adulteress now. Just like Becky. The self-loathing settles in, slow and certain, with nowhere else to go.

Time softens things. It brings perspective. Humility. A kind of mercy. But it doesn't erase the echo. Who's the tramp now?

I press the phone tighter to my ear and let my mom chatter about fireworks, a trip to the lake and white potato salad, never yellow. I respond in the right places and laugh when expected. I don't tell her anything real. Not yet. But I need her voice. Even if it's just a temporary distraction.

"Where are you by the way?" my mom asks. "It sounds like you're in a wind tunnel."

Shoot. I should have rolled up the window. I do it quickly.

"I was crossing the street," I reply. "It must have been the wind." There is no reason for me to be in a taxi this early on a holiday.

But telling her where I really am would open a door I'm not prepared to walk through. So, I pivot. Back to our plans for the day. I tell her about the rooftop party Richard and I are supposed to attend tonight at Bill and Edward's, one of our favorite couples. They've just finished a massive home renovation and can't wait to show it off.

"It'll be fun," I say. "I love their friends. And the view of the fireworks from up there will be incredible."

A distraction, mostly. From my impending spiral.

"Boo," Mom says gently, using the nickname she's had for me since I was little. "Are you sure you're alright? You just don't sound like you."

"I'm sure," I lie. "I think I'm just not ready for the summer to end. I love it here. I wish I didn't have to go back to Dallas. You're the only one who really knows how I feel about that place, you know?"

Though that's not entirely true anymore. Brett knows. He knows how heavy Dallas feels to me. How small. How suffocating. He knows I'm dreading it almost as much as I dreaded watching him walk through those airport doors this morning.

As the town car nears the Lincoln Tunnel, I rush to end the conversation with Mom. I know the call will drop underground, and that will lead to follow-up questions. We never hang up without multiple rounds of "I love you," but I compress them into seconds.

"Happy Fourth!" I chirp, clicking off just as the driver rolls forward to pay the toll.

I ask the driver to drop me off at the same corner where he picked me up. For all the driver knows, that's my building. Richard has only texted once since I crossed state lines with another man. Not to ask where I am. Just to ask when I'll be back because "he's hungry."

I tell him I'm close and need to change before breakfast. I can't risk him offering to meet me on the sidewalk while I'm still climbing out of this car. When I step onto the pavement, I thank the driver and shut the door carefully. The city is beginning to stir now. Coffee runs. Early joggers. Strollers with alert babies inside.

My phone vibrates in my bag. I assume it's Richard again. At the next crosswalk, waiting for the light, I dig through my bag to see what he needs. But it's not Richard.

A smile spreads across my face before I can stop it. It's Brett.

Hi, perfect girl. Made it through security. In the lounge and boarding soon. I hope you have a great Fourth!

I read it twice.

If there is anything that can lift my mood, short of adjusting my meds, Richard boarding a train, or Brett reappearing, it's the whimsy of a Fourth of July hair accessory. This year, I have options. For day: a metallic spray of red, white, and blue stars that bob with every step. For night: a headband wired with tiny patriotic lights shaped like fireworks.

There will be no restraint on a holiday. And frankly, I couldn't care less whether Richard approves. We will be with my kind of people tonight. So, I'm going big.

I choose a blue-and-red striped vintage '80s dress with dramatic puff sleeves and a fitted waist, unapologetically theatrical. It once had a matching sash, but that's probably hiding in my fashion closet in Dallas, which is really just a dark storage unit I rent in our building, so I don't "clutter" our shared closet.

Instead, I cinch the dress with one of my mother's old belts, a red rope twisted into an infinity knot with a hidden Velcro closure. It's one of my favorites. It feels like armor and inheritance at the same time. For an emotional and literal lift, I slide into my silver stacked heels, the Chanel pair I wore the night I met Brett. That detail doesn't escape me.

When Richard asks how he looks, I answer "Fine!" without turning around. The silence that follows tells me he noticed. I sigh and apologize, twice. I blame it on not feeling well, due to a migraine threatening to bloom behind my eyes. I swallow two Excedrin in front of him as evidence.

"It's actually great," I say more sincerely when I finally look. Richard's wearing red Bonobos and a white oxford, sleeves rolled. I smile.

There are still moments, brief ones, when I don't feel anger toward him, or perhaps worse, complacency. Sometimes, I can remember the version of us before everything became clinical. Before my diagnosis had to be spoken out loud. Before our marriage felt like a negotiation of symptoms and optics. I remember our fun weekend getaway to Prague, while we were living in London. Our Sundays, spent at the Duvall's ranch, trail riding on four-wheelers. Our shared loved of margaritas and ceviche happy hours alfresco in Dallas. For a split second, standing there in my patriotic excess beside his crisp simplicity, Richard and I almost look like a normal couple heading to a rooftop party.

Almost.

It's a gorgeous day, thick summer heat nowhere in sight, so I ask if we can walk. Bill and Edward's apartment in Chelsea is only about a mile away, an easy stroll. Richard agrees.

About 20 blocks later, after walking a mix of long east-west stretches and shorter turns downtown, we've barely spoken. Just logistics. We remember to stop at the wine shop around the corner to grab a couple of bottles: one as a housewarming gift, one to contribute to the party.

The store is lovely. It has rows of unusual labels, soft lighting, and that faint mineral smell of cork and dust. It even has one of those instant chilling machines, so we're not limited to the tiny refrigerated section. I let Richard choose.

Lately, I prefer that he make the small decisions like where we eat, what we do, which wine to bring, and how to spend our last few days in New York. I don't want to argue. I don't care enough about these moments, nor can I focus long enough to fight for one place over another. So, I nod. I smile. I agree easily to whatever Richard suggests. It isn't peace exactly. It's closer to absence. I feel emotionally void, present in body, but somewhere slightly outside myself, watching us walk down the sidewalk like a couple in a scene of a movie I no longer feel invested in and that I don't want to watch anymore.

Bill and Edward are the more-the-merrier type of couple, the kind who would rather squeeze 10 extra people into a room than risk someone feeling left out. I'm grateful, especially when I hear that my friend Rebecca is included in the celebration today. We vaguely knew each other in college, but we reconnected years later at Fashion Week, colliding at the entrance to the Diane von Furstenberg show. Since then, Rebecca has been a steady beam of light. Human sunshine. Warm, flattering, forgiving. I could use some of her sunshine tonight.

The couple's apartment is wall-to-wall people, 80% men in their late 30s, maybe early 40s, who are polished and put together. They are impeccably dressed with sharp tailoring and fearless patterns. I assume most of them are gay. And while stereotypes are usually lazy and wrong, the "dumb blonde" trope comes to mind. I believe that assuming a man is gay because he dresses impeccably is high praise.

The space is too packed for a proper tour, but Richard and I squeeze through anyway. We listen as Bill and Edward recount the ordeal of combining two separate units, refinishing original hardwoods, debating Mission versus Shaker cabinetry styles, and landing on maple. They proudly show us their his-and-his sinks.

"A game-changer," Bill says. "No more fighting for space at night." He bumps Edward's elbow endearingly.

That actually does sound divine. Sharing a sink with Richard has never felt romantic. It feels territorial and mechanical. We are so out of sync that even brushing our teeth can feel like a negotiation. Maybe I leave the toothpaste cap loose. Maybe he hates that. Maybe he hates me.

Richard beams at their renovation. He lingers in the walk-in closets, admiring the symmetry and order. We had separate closets once in our last apartment. Not now. I know he misses the clean division. My half is organized, but it's in a Carrie Bradshaw way, curated chaos. It's not the Container Store fantasy Richard prefers.

I glance at him. He looks genuinely happy. Jolly, even. There is nothing obviously monstrous about him. Is it all me? Did I bring out the critical, controlling, shaming parts of Richard? It's possible. I'm a pusher. I've pushed a bigger life on him than he wanted. His dream was to be a college professor. Summers in Greece, running the study abroad program, with a slew of students, hanging on his every pompous word as he introduces them to the depths of Greek mythology.

But also, I've seen him speak to his parents and my mom the same way he speaks to me, with the same clipped tone and the same subtle superiority. So, maybe it isn't entirely my fault. Still, I've cheated. And when my affair eventually surfaces, because secrets like this don't dissolve, they detonate, I will be the villain, the adulteress, the "whore," and the one who ruined everything.

Richard will be the victim, the blindsided husband. The story will be clean and simple for everyone else. And yet, somehow, that feels easier to live with than this secrecy. I think I can survive being cast as the antagonist. Because somewhere beneath the noise, I will know the truth. He wanted out, too.

He may never admit it, not to friends, not to family, and maybe not even to himself, but I will know. Since my diagnosis, our relationship has only deteriorated. If I'm honest, I can't think of one thing Richard truly likes about me anymore, except maybe the image of our shiny exterior. He likes the narrative of college sweethearts who made it, as if we're the perfect, glossy couple out of a storybook.

What a joke.

After the apartment tour, I cannot pour myself a glass of wine fast enough. My small-talk game is officially in the toilet. I need liquid assistance. My focus is shot. Everyone's voices blend together like the collective sound of Grand Central. It's a miracle I made it through

Bill and Edward's renovation walkthrough at all. My interior design background carried me, the vocabulary, the right questions, and the appearance of engagement. I do love this stuff—floor plans, cabinet debates, and the subtle politics of finishes. But the internal vibrations are too distracting today. For years, I've made the same tired joke: I majored in interior design, but now, I design clothes for the interior side of our bodies. Cue Chandler Bing: ba-dum bum.

We have an hour before the fireworks start, but the crowd migrates upstairs early, drinks in hand. The rooftop is stunning, with a 360-degree skyline view, featuring the Hudson River stretching wide and expectant beneath the darkening sky. Built-in yellow brick planters overflow with boxwoods and small flowering trees. Teak chairs and low tables create little pockets of intimacy, though tonight, most of them are shoved together to make room for the crowd.

It's already packed. Rebecca is here. I can see her above the crowd, the advantage of her height. Relief floods me when I spot her. I beeline toward her. Her greeting is warm and enveloping. She carries the conversation effortlessly at first, which is a gift because my brain is scrambled.

When it becomes my turn to answer questions instead of asking them, I pivot to discussing Jet Set Lingerie. Richard isn't within earshot, so I won't get the side-eye that says why are you talking about this again? It feels like the safest subject with Rebecca.

She has always been supportive, so I let myself open up, cautiously. I tell her about Maidenform's interest in our company and the Saks meeting around the corner. I recount the QVC presentation at their Fort Knox-style campus in Pennsylvania with the metal detectors, the rehearsed pitches, and the surreal feeling of selling underwear under fluorescent lights to a panel of strangers. I tell her about casually bumping into Richard Simmons in his signature short shorts and colorful workout tank. It's not bragging. It's more of a confession. The last 18 months have been brutal with the economic fallout and fear. We need something big to shift the tide.

I don't tell Rebecca about Greer being pregnant. That's not my news to share. But we talk about Addy's baby on the way and how it will change things. In beautiful ways. In complicated ones, too.

The sky deepens into navy. The rooftop crowd swells. It's person-to-person now. Warm skin, perfume, cologne, condensation from plastic cups. I haven't seen Richard in a while, but I doubt he's looking for me either.

And here, physically wedged between bodies, I don't have to shrink myself on purpose. There's no space to twirl. No room to be animated or exuberant or "too much," as I've been told. I am quite literally contained. In my box.

While Rebecca updates me on the chaos and glamour of her own fashion-world orbit, I feel my phone vibrate deep inside my clutch. Not a text. Not an email. It's a call. Balancing my plastic cup of chardonnay between my teeth, I wedge open my bag with one hand and dig for the phone with the other. It's an odd time for a call. I want to be sure everything is okay. Fireworks will start any second.

My heart stops. It's Brett. But how?

Did the plane not take off? Is he still in New York? My pulse jumps into my throat. I have to answer. I pull the cup from my mouth and mumble to Rebecca that I need to take this call. I push through the crowd, apologizing, sidestepping, and squeezing past bodies. The phone is still ringing in my hand. Second ring. Third. Please don't hang up.

I need to find a quiet place. Behind the elevator shaft, there's a shadowed hallway, barely wide enough for one person. It will do.

"Hello?" I answer cautiously, bracing for a mistake. A pocket dial.

"Hi, perfect girl!" Brett says. "I just landed. Walking to immigration. Apparently, they're taking temperatures before letting us through, but I couldn't wait to hear your voice."

For a second, I can't breathe. He landed in China. He's calling me from the other side of the world . . . on what must be an outrageously expensive roaming phone plan. He's giving me live updates. We've blown past casual into relationship territory.

"Hi!" I lower my voice. "I can't believe you're calling."

I glance over my shoulder. The rooftop is flooded with laughter and anticipation. No one is paying attention to me.

"I just couldn't help myself," he says. "Fourteen hours without hearing your little Southern drawl was a long time."

I've never thought of myself as having an accent, but I know it isn't true. In Texas, it's subtle. In Manhattan, it's a glowing marquee.

"I'm thrilled," I manage. "Just . . . surprised."

"I know you're skeptical," he says, warmer now. "But this, whatever this is, it's not over."

My heart feels like it's hovering somewhere outside my body.

"I'm almost at the checkpoint," he continues. "I have no idea how I'm getting to my hotel without speaking a word of Mandarin, but can I call you tomorrow?"

"Yes! Yes, of course," I reply. The words stumble out. I want to sound composed. I want to sound ecstatic. I feel both and neither. "Text me your email. I'll send you a time. I'm not sure how texting works internationally."

"Perfect," he agrees. "I'll do that. Miss you."

"Miss you, too," I say instantly, too loudly, before remembering where I am. We hang up. For a second, I stay there in the shadow of the elevator shaft, staring at the dark screen in my hand.

Just as the first fireworks burst over the Hudson, I step back into the crowd. The skyline ignites in red and gold and green and blue. The rooftop erupts in cheers. And for the first time all day, I feel something bright and uncomplicated. Nothing can dim me in this moment. Not Richard, not the diagnosis, not even the looming return to Dallas.

I am lit from the inside.

Chapter 12

THE MIAMI VICE

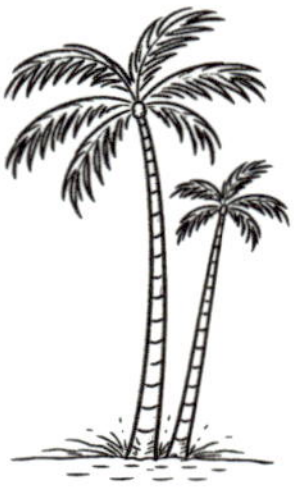

JULY 4, 2009
Near Midnight—My Temporary Apartment
Midtown, New York City

The second Richard and I get back from Bill and Edward's party, I pull out my computer. Richard is already in the bottom bunk with his nose buried in a book. I tell him quietly that I need to respond to some design questions from our Thailand factory and don't want the glow of my laptop disturbing him. He nods without looking up. I slip into the den.

I'm curled on the couch in my cotton pajamas. They're cheap Wal-Mart ones, white with tiny black polka dots, threadbare, and comfortable. I've already decided they won't be coming back to Dallas with me. Some things are easier to abandon than pack.

I open my Hotmail account and search for the old Gmail invite that I never used. I scroll and scroll, annoyed at the archaeological dig that is my inbox. Six pages deep, I find it.

Create new account. A fresh address. For one person only.

I giggle as I type: morganisperfect@gmail.com.

Nothing could be further from the truth. The irony is so sharp it's funny, almost tragic. And yet, Brett sees something in me. Or maybe, he sees the version of me I know exists beneath the static. The kind, generous, curious version of me. The one who laughs easily. The one who loves deeply. He manages to look past the manic volatility and focus on the good. There is good in me. I know there is. Somewhere.

God made me. God loves me. Even if I don't feel Him as clearly right now, even if I imagine Him watching this summer unfold with disappointment, my faith is steady enough to believe He is still near.

The password box blinks at me, calling me to respond.

Summer 1998—My Hometown, Murray, Kentucky

Light spills in from matching stained-glass windows, illuminating the double rows of people in obedient bands of jewel tones. Whether they like it or not, they're shining. Their Sunday bests imply they do.

Just off to the side, the mahogany baptismal font gleams with understated self-importance, its pristine surface seems less like a vessel for water and more like a place where sins come to be respectfully acknowledged . . . and then gently reupholstered. The backs of gray-haired men in navy sport coats with gold-crested buttons, pleated khakis, white Brooks Brothers shirts, and polished wingtips dominate the view, followed by grandmothers with perfectly preserved hair, lacquered into place like time never touched them.

I'm 17 years old, perfectly postured in the pew, wearing an ivory crepe drop-waist dress with delicate pleats, a French brand I found on sale at Off Fifth in Nashville. My long blonde hair is sun-streaked, and I'm tanned from the summer sun. I'm leaving for The University of Alabama in a week.

After the church service, couples line up to wish me well.

"Show them Kentucky girls are best, now," someone encourages.

"We'll be waiting to hear about the Dean's List and which top sorority you pick!" another promises.

They mean it kindly. Encouragingly. But the expectations feel heavy. No one considers that I might fail. That I might spiral. That I might not make the cut. They see the perfect small-town girl I've always been. With my parents' messy divorce still fresh, being "perfect" is convenient. It redirects the gossip. It tempers the narrative. I'm their only child. I can't add to the drama. I can only distract with good reports. So I do all the right things. I get into a great sorority. I make the Dean's List. I have cute fraternity dates on football Saturdays.

But threaded through all of it are the shadows: The weeks I don't get out of bed. The classes I skip. The emails I ignore. The manic bursts that follow, staying up all night to "fix" everything at once. Rewriting papers in a frenzy. Reorganizing closets. Making impossible promises. Hiding in my closet with the lights off, not answering my friends when they knock to see if I'm alive.

Those are the pieces no one in those pews ever wants to see or hear about. The secret evidence that I am not, in fact, perfect. I have carried those fragments for years, protecting the façade.

July 4, 2009, Late Night—My Temporary Apartment, NYC

I send my first email to Brett:

Hi B!

Thought you might get a kick out of this email address. I created it just for us, just for you. :) I hope you made it to your hotel okay . . . and that you're having sweet dreams (of me). Talk soon!

Your perfect girl

Already anticipating his response, I add the new Gmail account to my BlackBerry so I can check it from anywhere. Discreet. Portable. Private. If I need to delete it, I can. That's what I tell myself.

I tiptoe into the kitchen and eat a few saltines in the dark, leaning over the sink so crumbs won't betray me in the morning. It's the first thing I've eaten since that frantic breakfast sandwich in the back of the town car. My stomach growls.

I open the fridge and find its crown jewel, the last wedge of

Laughing Cow cheese. I spread it carefully across two more crackers and sprinkle a little salt and pepper on top. Midnight delicacy. Dinner, technically.

My mom may be conflicted and worried I'm not eating enough but also secretly pleased I look "trim." It's that complicated maternal pride that lives somewhere between protection and projection. I close the fridge carefully and head back to the bedroom. Richard is already asleep, book resting on his chest. His breathing is steady, unbothered.

I climb into my own bunk and pull the thin comforter over my shoulders. The room is still. I let my eyes close and invite the only thing that feels uncomplicated right now, the possibility of dreaming about Brett. About walking down a Greenwich Village street, his arm wrapped around me so tightly that his hand folds all the way across my collarbone, resting just beneath my chin.

His signature move. I fall asleep trying to feel that weight again.

July 5, 2009, Early Morning—My Temporary Apartment, NYC

I hit the streets, BlackBerry in hand, forcing myself not to check my new email account until I'm safely outside the apartment. Today is going to be a doozy. It's packing day.

I am wildly unprepared, physically and emotionally. My summer of escape passed in a blink. Tomorrow, I'll hand over the apartment keys, still dangling from that hideous lanyard I never bothered to replace with something charming. Tomorrow night, Richard and I will board a flight back to Dallas together. And just like the last time I had to leave New York, I am operating in full denial.

Last time, I left with a moving truck and big plans. This time, I'm leaving with just three suitcases, and far more secrets than I brought. The logistics are manageable. The leaving is not. I don't feel like I'm going home. I feel like I'm leaving it. Or maybe, it's already left me.

New York didn't just house me this summer. It held me. It distracted me. It expanded me. It gave me permission to be looser with the edges. Dallas feels like a contraction. And then, there's Brett.

Can a person you've known for less than three weeks feel like home? Can someone who exists mostly in stolen hours and secret emails feel steadier than the life you've built for years? The thought lodges in my throat as I walk. Maybe, home isn't geography. Maybe, it's recognition.

And for the first time in a long time, someone recognizes me for who I really am, not who I have forced myself to be.

The day is dreary, a soft gray that flattens everything, but it can't dull my affection for this city. I see New York through rose-colored glasses even when she smells like trash, even when a rat darts across my path, even when everything costs three times what it should and I absolutely cannot afford it. She's magic to me.

I'm underdressed for the cold. It's barely 60 degrees, but I head north anyway, resisting the urge to check my phone. My fingers sting. I wish I drank coffee. Sitting on a bench in Bryant Park with something warm in my hands while reading a flirty email from Brett sounds lovely. I duck into Starbucks and order a hot Passion Tea with milk. Tart and creamy. Balanced.

It takes me back to days in London, the first time I ever added milk to tea, or rather, tea to milk. I'm a milk-first girl, which I learned is a controversial declaration at The Ritz on Piccadilly during high tea. The waitress interrogated me gently, as if the order revealed something about my character. Who knew milk hierarchy mattered so much?

London was one of the better chapters of my marriage to Richard. Looking back, it makes sense. Richard was studying law abroad for a semester. He was busy and absorbed. I had endless alone time. I wandered Bloomsbury. Climbed Primrose Hill. Drifted through tiny boutiques and down Marylebone streets, staring at Georgian façades. I dreamed up businesses. Explored design districts. I felt expansive.

In many ways, it was my first escape. Richard was there physically, but I allowed myself more room to be me. And he seemed too distracted to police it. In London, I wasn't manic. I wasn't depressed. I was centered. It lasted for a good bit, until a weekend getaway to the City of Lights.

Fall 2003—Paris, France

Stepping off the train in Paris, almost six years since my first visit, feels both impossibly long and not long at all. I'm no longer 17 and wide-eyed in quite the same way; I arrive this time with my husband, the term still new enough to say it, and feel a small, private flicker of disbelief. The city doesn't seem surprised by either of us.

Richard and I begin, as everyone should, with a dinner that goes on too long in the best way, tucked into a hidden spot along the Seine on the Left Bank, all low light and clinking glasses, too much wine, too many baguettes, the kind of excess that feels like permission rather than indulgence. It's a form of self-medication for me. The next morning, we wander without direction, finding ourselves in Montmartre, where I sit for a portrait that renders me less as a woman and more as a mildly concerned monkey. We laugh, because what else is there to do.

There's a boat ride, of course. The river does what it does, carrying everything gently forward while the city performs itself along the edges. It is, on paper, all exactly as it should be. And still, somewhere just beneath the surface, I feel a small shift, a rearranging I don't know how to name.

Instead, I fixate on something simpler, more manageable: a visit to a proper French *pharmacie*. Richard kindly obliges, even though he has been rather disappointed in the lack of sex in our marriage. Still, I am determined, oddly focused, rather, to fill a basket with the shop's superior creams and treatments, the kind that make our expensive American versions feel like overcompensating imposters. The labels my high school French teacher raved about all four years. It feels like a small, controllable victory, something I can take home, something that promises, however falsely, to keep everything just as it is.

After 10 minutes into collecting creams and serums, struggling through my rusty French as I stroll through aisles of simple, yet elegant packaging, the ground gives way. My mind begins to race, not excitedly, but chaotically. The letters on the labels blur. My own hands feel foreign. I bend my wrists sharply, wanting them to break off. The same elegant paper boxes are now suddenly abrasive. Unbearable. I can't touch them for a second longer. I have to leave. I have to get out.

"Are you okay?" Richard asks.

He rests his hand on my shoulder, a sign of concern. I jerk away.

"Don't touch me. You're making my skin crawl," I whisper sharply, scrambling to put away the items in my basket, but making a mess of it all. "Please just get us a taxi."

It's not him. My skin is crawling all on its own. I'm 22 and newly married. What is happening to me? And how can Richard possibly help? He really knows so little about me and what really goes on inside my brain.

London has been a dream. Such a high. I should have known a crash was en route. It's a common trend now, one I wish would politely move to the "Out List."

Richard is only 23. His bride, the one who vowed everything to him, is recoiling from his touch. I can't imagine how it feels, the confusion and the hurt. Neither of us are equipped for this. A brick is laid in the wall forming between us.

Back at the hotel, it deepens. I beg Richard to draw the curtains, seeking total darkness. I murmur something about a migraine to quiet him. My body shivers with restless energy until sleep finally overtakes me, wrapped tight in an itchy hotel blanket.

When I wake, Richard's eyes are drilling into me. He's not angry, but determined. Vigilant.

"As soon as we get back to Dallas," he declares, "you're going to see a new doctor, someone who can fix this."

July 5, 2009, 7 a.m.—New York City | 8 p.m.—Beijing

I round the corner of Bryant Park and find an empty bench tucked behind the library, facing the carousel. A gold plaque reads:

Have a seat.

Close your eyes.

Think of someone you love.

I sit. I close my eyes. Brett's face appears instantly. The wood is cold against the backs of my bare legs. Running shorts were a poor choice. Too late now. I open my BlackBerry and pull up my new email account, waiting for it to sync. One new message. From him.

This is perfect. The perfect email address for my perfect girl . . . I'm safe and sound in my new hotel. It's in the Diplomat District, on the 14th floor. I'm trying to adjust to the 13-hour time difference, but it's not going so great. Luckily, I had a few fun dreams about you! I'm going to work out and get some food. Work starts tomorrow. Any chance we can talk today, I mean tonight for me? Your day? I think you go back to Dallas tomorrow, right?

Yours, Brett

I respond quickly.

I can talk now. Xx M

Minutes later, my phone rings.

"Hey, sexy," Brett says.

The word makes me unsteady every time. No one has ever called me "sexy" before. He's talking fast. Faster than usual. Excited. Animated. For a split second, a dangerous thought crosses my mind.

Are we both manic? Stop. Bite your tongue, Morgan. One unstable person is complicated enough. Two would be catastrophic. I push the thought away.

Brett tells me about Beijing, the language barrier, the taxi fiasco, the way even hotel names are pronounced differently. It took four taxis before one understood Kempinski, (or rather ky-bin-si-gee). I hang on every detail. He makes it sound adventurous instead of terrifying. I laugh with him. I wish I had been there.

I don't have much to report. I've only been sleeping and walking, but I tell him I'll spend the day packing and watching the Wimbledon final. Andy Roddick versus Roger Federer. An American hasn't won since '99. He perks up at the sports reference.

With the time difference working against us, we decide to start emailing "fun facts" back and forth. There's still so much we don't know about each other and so much I want to uncover. Before we hang up, Brett wishes me luck packing. He wishes me luck going back to Dallas. He tells me everything will eventually work out. My brain knows he can't possibly know that. But my heart believes he means it. And somehow, from more than 6,000 miles away, that's enough.

I walk back toward the apartment with a strange lightness in my step. Maybe, my life will work out after all. Even if tomorrow, I'm flying back to Dallas.

Packing takes almost no time at all. Intentionally, I brought mostly old pajamas, worn sheets, and cheap towels, things I wouldn't mind abandoning. I toss them into the trash without ceremony. It feels symbolic, even if it isn't.

I fold everything else neatly, laying clothes flat inside my suitcases, layering handbags and shoes between them, each tucked carefully into its dust bag. My travel outfit stays ironed and waiting in the closet.

Toiletries I won't need in the morning are sealed and zipped away.

I'm finished before the second set of Wimbledon really gets going. Roddick takes it.

"Go USA," I say softly to no one in particular.

Richard watches the match from the other couch. We don't sit together. We don't reach for each other. Snuggling feels foreign now, if it was ever truly ours. I try to remember a time when sitting side by side with Richard felt natural. I honestly cannot imagine not touching Brett if we were in the same room. An email from Brett pings in with happy face emojis and a celebratory *Yay, Andy!*

I smile at the screen. I message him to get some sleep. It's already 11 p.m. in Beijing, and he has a massive day of due diligence tomorrow with the team. He ignores my suggestion. More flirty messages trickle in.

The match stretches on for nearly four hours and 20 minutes. It's one of the longest Wimbledon finals ever. Brett stays awake for most of it, commenting in bursts, but during the final set, his emails stop. He's asleep, I assume. And then, Roddick loses.

Now, I have to get ready for one last dinner in Manhattan. Richard and I stay in the neighborhood. The restaurant is fine but not memorable. The food tastes like nothing. Conversation barely registers. The entire meal passes in a haze.

Tomorrow, we leave. I can feel New York slipping from my grip.

July 6, 2009—NYC to Dallas

I usually love airports. Busy departure boards. The click of heels on polished floors. The quiet promise that something new is about to begin. But as the taxi pulls up to the terminal, all I feel is dread.

The check-in back to Dallas is uneventful. I don't have to reshuffle my bags to meet the airline's weight limits. A true miracle. It sets a calmer tone than other travel days Richard and I have shared.

I recall the infamous 86-pound suitcase. We were Aspen bound last February on a couples' trip with Greer, Rhett, Addy, and Sam to the Duvall's gorgeous new vacation home. I was allowed 70-pound luggage with my Continental status, which meant redistributing 16 extra pounds into my carry-on and tote in the middle of the curbside check-in line. I managed it, of course, like a pro, but in the flurry, I bent down to repack and gave the curb a brief, unintended view of my backside. My dress was flowy, comfortable for travel and light enough for the hot Dallas air that rolled in far before asked. The wind simply caught my hemline.

Richard wasn't wrong to point it out. It was revealing, accidental but revealing, nonetheless. A normal husband might have laughed, tugged the hem down playfully, and whispered something mischievous. Instead, what followed was a full lecture in the lounge, delivered in a low, tight voice as the bartender hand-dried glasses three feet away.

I remember thinking even then, it doesn't have to feel this way. Now, sitting on the plane, I let my mind drift. What would travel be like with Brett? Champagne roadies in the back of a car service to the airport. Fingers laced together during check-in. He would insist on carrying my bags. He'd push for first-class upgrades just because it felt celebratory. If a flight were delayed, he'd turn it into an adventure instead of an inconvenience. He wouldn't pout. He would live in the moment and somehow coax me into doing the same.

Less managing. Less bracing. Less walking on eggshells. More laughing. More ease. I don't know if I'd even be good at that kind of spontaneity. I'm wired for contingency plans and emotional weather reports.

But God, it would be refreshing to try.

July 7, 2009, Morning—Our Apartment, Dallas

I wake to a life that feels like it might be slipping back into "normal," whatever my new normal is. I'm back in our semi-temporary apartment, this one a cookie-cutter "luxury" unit, after moving out of the gorgeous Providence Group property we'd been in before. That one felt like a gift. A perk of Richard working for Greer's father-in-law's company. It was comped, impressive, and out of our budget. This one just feels . . . fine.

I unpack my three mismatched TJ Maxx suitcases, each one collected on sale over the years. I wonder if I'll ever own a coordinated, grown-up set of luggage, the kind that glides instead of wobbles.

I pull on a simple kelly green sundress, left behind in my Dallas closet. It's one I didn't deem worthy of New York.

I eat a granola bar for breakfast. I roll the empty suitcases down to my storage unit, the wheels clacking against the concrete. On the walk back, it hits me for the first time: I have nowhere to go.

When I left in early spring, we still had our Jet Set Lingerie office with its pink walls and the inspiration hallway. Lined with movie posters, from *9 to 5* to *View from the Top* to *Troop Beverly Hills*, it was our little shrine to ambitious women with big hair and bigger dreams. Now, it's gone. No office. No desk. No place to show up to work.

I assume we'll work from Greer's house, but I don't want to presume. Rhett might get tired of us taking over, though, I'm fairly certain she prefers her beautiful home to this below average apartment. Plus, Richard is already irritated by how much time I spend with the Twins. He'll hate Greer being here. This morning, on his way out the door, he already expressed discontent of our Miami trip in two days.

Why am I here? Why couldn't I figure out how to keep the apartment in New York?

Norm, my little Brussels Griffon, is the only thing I was excited to come home to, and he's still with Richard's parents until after Miami.

My mind drifts. I wonder if Brett likes dogs.

It's been at least five minutes since I checked my email. I refresh again. It's a reflex now. A twitch. One new message. It's short.

Can you talk?

The reply flies out of me.

Yes!

Brett calls immediately. The excitement in his voice makes me feel less self-conscious about the excitement in mine. Today, we talk about childhood homes.

I tell him I grew up on Olive Street in the same tiny town, but in two different houses, until I left for college. He tells me he has only lived in two homes, too, though his parents have since moved into a "grown-up" house on a golf course, but he's never actually lived there.

I tell him my mother set the table every single day with the good china, even on random Tuesdays. He laughs and says his family didn't even have furniture in their formal dining room while growing up.

God, for someone who's spent more than a decade in New York, he's so normal in the best way. Yes, he appreciates beautiful things. But he doesn't expect them. He works for them. He's comfortable without them. He's scrappy. Like me.

Greer beeps in. I know I need to answer her. We have to figure out the next couple of days before Miami. It's already 11 p.m. in Beijing and 9 a.m. here in Dallas. Brett should be sleeping. He has another massive day ahead, and it sounds like the deal is accelerating.

"Have the best day, perfect girl," he says.

"Sweet dreams, my Brett."

"Only of you," he replies.

And we hang up. I stare at the phone for a second longer than necessary. Back to normal. But nothing feels normal anymore.

The next few days move quickly.

Greer decides we should work from her house, so we set up in the small office just off her kitchen. It's intimate but decorated to a T.

Two matching built-in desks, a shared printer, samples tucked neatly into custom cabinets. The wallpaper is a soft, expensive blue, chosen at the design center with her mother-in-law's help. Even the desk chairs match, upholstered in a muted ikat that feels both tailored and feminine. It's beautiful. Effortlessly elegant.

No more packing orders ourselves. No more tissue paper and shipping labels and late-night runs to FedEx. We moved fulfillment to a family friend's center back in Kentucky, slightly expensive per pick-and-pack, but necessary. Strategic. Forward-thinking. Babies are coming. The business has to evolve if it's going to survive. It was the right call. Still, it feels odd not to physically touch what we're building.

The only moment that feels uncomfortable is the one I had been quietly dreading, as I explain that Richard and I will be staying at a different hotel in Miami. The trip starts tomorrow.

Greer, Addy, their husbands, and two other college couple-friends of theirs are all staying at The Delano, a perfect choice. The Twins and I stayed there for Addy's bachelorette party a few years ago. It has soaring Art Deco ceilings, gauzy white curtains dividing the lobby into romantic little alcoves, and candlelight flickering everywhere.

Richard didn't want to stay there. He said he wants space, not as in square footage, as in away from those people. I didn't argue.

If I'm honest, I want space, too, but for entirely different reasons. I want privacy and time to message Brett. I want late-night phone calls without thin hotel walls and shared elevators and accidental run-ins during email checks.

I let Richard's preference become the explanation. But I know it's more complicated than "space." He has never fully articulated what unsettles him about the Duvalls or their circle, but I suspect it's rooted in something deeper, something tender. He grew up with very little. His parents didn't go to college. No country clubs. No generational wealth. Just above food stamps really.

Richard pulled himself up from nothing. It's impressive. But there is a chip that lives on his shoulder. Country clubs infuriate him. Ivy League pedigrees irritate him. He'll casually remind anyone who will listen that his law school was "harder than Harvard because Harvard doesn't give grades." Passed-down wealth seems to provoke something sharp inside him. Instead of dismissing it, he absorbs it. And it curdles. I've hidden this before, from Greer specifically.

Once, Greer saw a text flash across my phone, something biting about Rhett and his "friends." It was Richard asking me to invent an excuse so we wouldn't have to attend a dinner. I covered for him and said it was taken out of context. She knew it wasn't. She was gracious enough not to press.

Today, when the hotel question came up, I chose a different lie. I said we were staying at The Mondrian because it was half the price of The Delano. I framed it as a budgeting choice, my own financial concerns. Realistically, after a summer of careless purchases, the lower cost was also necessary. Though not a choice I would have made.

It was an easy out. And I took it. Greer was incredibly kind. Her only disappointment was that we might have less time together. That sweetness made it worse. Secretly, I wish it were just us girls. A celebration without husbands, hierarchy, insecurity, and the politics of success and status. I think they might wish that, too. But our work lives and our marriages are braided together now.

July 11, 2009, 3 p.m.—South Beach, Miami

Our flight lands after theirs. By the time Richard and I drop our bags at The Mondrian, on the opposite side of the peninsula, and make our way to The Delano, everyone is already in the pool.

Sunlit. Loud. Happy.

One of the Twins' college roommates, Annie, has made matching airbrushed T-shirts for everyone. They're ridiculous and perfect. It's the kind of thing that looks best when you're already inside the joke. I feel like I'm arriving late to something that's already formed without me. It's probably in my head, but I've always felt slightly peripheral around the Lehigh crew. They have never been anything but warm, inclusive, and easy. Still, I'm an outlier.

My hair is bigger and blonder. My dresses are brighter. My accessories are louder. Greer and Addy and I get mistaken for triplets all the time, but somehow, it works for them. Twins can carry more. Everything is cuter in pairs.

Richard and I claim a crisp white chaise and slip into the pool with our cocktails. With two sober husbands and two pregnant women, the vibe is surprisingly restrained, buttoned-up, and responsible.

I, on the other hand, feel three sheets to the wind, whether I've had one drink or five these days. For a fleeting moment, I convince myself the mania might be tapering off. Maybe, it had simply been Manhattan. Maybe, I had just absorbed the city's tempo, borrowed her urgency, her sleeplessness, and her appetite for more. I let myself believe I had caught a case of the city. But Miami proves otherwise. The buzz didn't fade when the skyline changed. It followed me.

It's still early in Beijing, but Brett is awake and emailing more than ever. I'm in and out of the pool, pretending to towel off, pretending to check something, pretending to need the restroom. When the Twins ask where I keep disappearing to, I blame it on drinking too much water on the plane. Damn their observant pregnant soberness.

As long as he's emailing, I'm responding. Thankfully, Richard doesn't seem to notice. It's fine. It's all fine.

Brett writes that he's going to the Great Wall in the morning and wants to call me from the top. Of course, I want to talk to him from the Great Wall. I decide I'll slip away during dinner and blame it on my mom calling. The Twins won't question that. My mom and I talk all the time. She's my constant.

I actually laugh to myself imagining that Richard might be less irritated if he knew it was another man instead of my mother.

The tropical air meets me before the door does—thick, salted, a little sugared with perfume and heat. The restaurant hums at a frequency just above conversation, a constant rise and fall of laughter. The atmosphere glows in a shade of red and hot pink. Glassware catches it, skin softens under it, and even the ice in the cocktails seems to hold the color for a moment before giving it back.

Every table is full, pressed close together, candlelit, and topped with tropical florals. It's a little cheesy, but it works in the space. Waiters move with ease, threading through the narrow spaces like a maze they solved eons ago.

I'm loopy from a full day in the sun. I'm talking too fast and too loud, but I'm detached from the words themselves. They're outrunning my thoughts. At one point, Richard places his hand on my knee. He squeezes hard. Forefinger and thumb imprinting my leg. It's the signal.

Stop.

He's done it before. The pressure is sharp enough to bruise. And I bruise easily now because of one of my meds. But tonight, for the first time, I don't stop talking. I'm done shrinking.

If Brett isn't real and this implodes and I end up back in Murray, Kentucky, living under my mother's roof, which is the last place I ever want to land, then so be it. But I will not be silenced with a knee squeeze again, even if I probably do need to shut up.

I slide my clutch next to my left thigh so I can feel the vibration through the silk of my pink Tracy Feith dress. When I slipped it on earlier, I thought about how much I wanted Brett to see it.

The phone buzzes. I check discreetly. It's him.

I mouth "my mom" to the table and slip toward the entrance, pushing through the restaurant doors and out onto the sidewalk.

"Holy shit!" Brett says, breathless. "I'm on the Great Wall, and all I'm thinking is I wish you were here."

"Goals," I say and laugh softly. "Tell me everything. Is it really that great?" I add a funny tone to it.

Brett gives me every detail in rapid-fire. He's in a crowded section now but says Mutianyu is the better part. That's where he wants to take me. We'll stay at the Commune. He says it like it's already decided and inevitable. And I follow him there in my mind. As if I'm not leaning against a restaurant wall in Miami while my husband and closest friends sit 10 feet away inside. Of course, I'll be there with him. That makes more sense than anything else right now. I don't properly calculate how long we've been talking, but I feel the tug to go back in.

"Brett," I start, wanting to call him "Love" or "Baby" or something that makes him mine, but I don't. "I want to hear more, but I should get back to dinner. Everyone will wonder. I told them it was my mom."

"Of course," he says warmly. "Go have fun. We'll talk tomorrow. Your tomorrow," he clarifies. "I miss you."

"Miss you t—"

"Morgan, I'm serious about you visiting. We'll make it happen."

Standing there in the humid Miami night, I believe him.

July 12, 2009, 10 a.m.—South Beach, Miami

Last night, no one said anything at dinner about how long I'd been gone while I was talking to Brett. Not a raised eyebrow. Not a sideways glance. But today, by the pool, the questions begin to surface.

We're back at The Delano. The sun is already sharp; the sea of white loungers is almost blinding. Brett and I are still in a full, feverish back-and-forth. Emails in short bursts. Quick replies. It's addictive.

Richard is stretched out on a chaise and reading. Aloof. Greer and Addy float in the pool, cooling their bellies, glowing in that effortless way pregnant women sometimes do. Radiant. They look so beautiful and so anchored in their lives.

When I leave the pool for the fifth time to check my phone, Greer climbs out behind me, water dripping. Concern written across her face.

"Everything okay?" She asks. "Who're you emailing so much?"

The irony is that my extended family is genuinely in the middle of some weird drama back home. I use it to my advantage. I reference the call from my mom last night, layering in just enough details to make it believable. Greer nods. She buys it. Or at least, she chooses to.

I walk a few feet away and resume typing a message to Brett, describing the way my swimsuit ties at the hip, the color of the water, the heat on my shoulders. I give him visuals.

Later, Richard looks up from his book. "Want to play Kadima?"

It catches me off guard. Kadima is our thing. We've played on every beach we've visited together—Mykonos, Menorca, St. Vincent, and the Grenadines. We always pack the paddles. It's one of the few rituals that still feels like us. I'm surprised he asked. Naturally, I say yes.

I set my phone face down on the chaise, tucking the device under a towel, out of the direct sun. I pick up the wooden paddles. Richard and I walk across the hot sand toward the shoreline. The ball pops back and forth between us. An easy rhythm that almost calms me. Sun in our eyes. Salt in the air. For a moment, it feels simple. Almost happy.

We play Kadima for nearly an hour. We don't talk much, and we don't need to. For that stretch of time, it feels uncomplicated. When we walk back toward the pool, I actually feel excited for dinner. I'm ready to shower, get dressed up, and celebrate my favorite Twins, my best friends. Turning 30 feels big, joyful, and worth honoring.

And then, the mood shifts.

The second Richard and I reach the pool deck, the group's energy changes. Almost theatrically. The eight of them climb out of the water at once, each announcing a different reason they suddenly need to leave.

"I'm exhausted. I need a nap," Addy says, rubbing her tiny bump.

"I booked us facials," Annie adds, glancing at Claire, the other college roommate.

"Couples' massage," Greer announces, squeezing Rhett's hand.

The others follow like a chorus, with smiles, nods, and quick explanations but no real eye contact. It's not even three in the afternoon.

"Okay. No problem," I say, forcing brightness into my voice. "We'll head back to our hotel and get ready. Can't wait for tonight!"

Wrapped in thick white Delano towels, they offer quick, damp hugs and scatter. Richard and I stand there for a second. He looks as stunned as I feel. We brush it off and pack up swiftly. The ride back to The Mondrian is under 20 minutes, but my phone buzzes three times. Brett. I can't answer. I shoot off an email before Richard notices.

Can't talk. Can you call back in 15? Why are you awake??

I peel off my wet bikini in the bathroom, wringing it out carefully and hanging it over the towel bar, straight and neat. From the other room, I ask Richard if he minds if I take a walk to grab a Diet Coke.

"The minibar only has Pepsi," I plead lightly.

He barely looks up from his book. "That's fine."

Perfect. I slip into my terrycloth tunic and white patent medallion sandals and head downstairs. I can't call Brett; the international charges would be obscene. So, I have to wait for him to call me back.

Please don't fall asleep. I'm dying to hear his voice.

The lobby is bright white with harsh black accents. Club music pulses through the space. Suddenly, all I want is Sinatra and Palm Beach rattan. My bell-sleeve mod tunic feels conservative in a hotel built for bodies and spectacle. I pass beneath the dramatic black spiral staircase and step outside by the pool. The swimsuits here are barely garments, more like rubber bands artfully arranged. Biscayne Bay stretches out, calm and blue. After a chilly New York summer, the heat feels exhilarating. I close my eyes. Let the breeze hit my face.

My phone rings.

"It's really you!" Brett's voice is warm and unmistakably slurred.

"Well, hi there," I tease gently. "Sounds like someone had a big night." I can almost smell the alcohol through the line.

"So sorry," he apologizes. "Long day. Went out with some guys from KKR. We had a grand time. It'd be so much grander if you were here, of course. I wish you were here . . ." He's stepping all over his words. It's sweet but a little irritating.

"Slow it down, mister," I say. "You sound . . . well, drunk. Four or five sheets to the wind perhaps. But go on, please, I love hearing how much you miss me."

He laughs softly. "Oh Morgan, I miss you so much. I'm sorry I kept calling," he pauses, "But something happened."

His tone shifts. It's the first time I've heard worry in his voice. My stomach drops.

"What happened?" I ask. My mind goes to dark places.

"I called earlier," he says. "I thought it was you, but it wasn't."

"What do you mean? You dialed the wrong number?" I ask, laughing, picturing his tipsy fingers fumbling with country codes.

"No," he says quietly. "I called you. And Greer answered."

The sound of her name catches me off guard. Sudden, disorienting. I almost want to laugh again, to make it small. Maybe, it's nothing. Maybe, it's everything.

Chapter 13
THE DENIAL

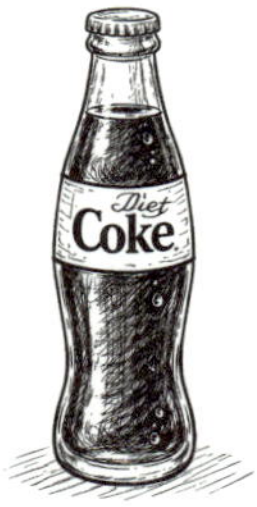

JULY 12, 2009
Late afternoon—South Beach, Miami

The humid air forces me to sweep my hair into a top knot. A sheen of sweat forms on the back of my neck. I can feel my pulse everywhere—wrists, throat, behind my knees. It's too present, too loud, like my body has turned the volume up without asking me. My palm sweats, clenching the phone.

"What did you even say? I'm sure everything is fine. She didn't even mention it." I try to laugh it off. If I keep moving, keep smiling, surely it will stay light. Maybe it doesn't have to become some big thing.

I crack open one of the two Diet Cokes I bought at the shop near the hotel. It's shockingly cold; the carbonation, sharp and aggressive. Condensation drips from the can onto my feet. Brett's voice derails the pleasure of my first sip.

"Morgan," he says. His voice stiffens. Clearer. "It didn't go well. God, you sound so much alike. I thought it was you."

"Okay," I say slowly. "So, what did you say?"

"I opened with 'hey, sexy,'" he explains. "And when she reacted, I realized it wasn't you. I panicked. I made up some random guy's name."

My stomach tightens. He's saved in my phone as "Elizabeth." I cannot, for the life of me, remember why I chose that name. At the time, it must have felt clever. Logical. Protective. Now, it feels absurd.

Why did Greer answer my phone in the first place? Did she hear it buzzing on the chaise near the pool? Was she conveniently walking past my chair, and she just grabbed it automatically? It's something she would do without thinking. But why didn't she say anything to me about it?

"What part didn't you get right?" I ask carefully.

"She said something about Elizabeth. Asked if this was Elizabeth," Brett says with a groan. "My head was spinning from drinking this insane Chinese liquor, Moutai. Apparently, it's some rite of passage when you arrive here as an expat." He starts rambling.

"Baby," I interrupt gently, "I love your drunken cultural commentary. But I need to know how you ended the call with Greer."

He pauses. "Aww. You called me baby. I love it," he gushes.

This guy is so easily distracted. Heat rises into my cheeks. The word slipped out without thought. It felt natural. Comfortable. I'm not even panicking anymore. Greer answered my phone. So what? If she gave it any weight, she'll bring it up at dinner. We'll laugh it off.

"You are, right?" I say softly, confirming the "baby" part.

"Yes," he says. "And you're mine. But, Morgan," Brett continues, "I think we've been outed." There's something in his tone, not dread exactly. Something with less heaviness. Almost relief. It's not because he wants my life to implode. I don't believe there's a cruel bone in Brett's body. But I suspect his tolerance for secrecy expired weeks ago.

"I really don't think we have anything to worry about," I insist. "How could she possibly connect the dots? Please don't spiral over this. Greer would have said something. We've been friends too long."

As I say it, I hear the flaw in that logic. Nearly three decades of friendship hasn't stopped me from lying so far. But Greer is pregnant. And turning 30. And renovating a house. She's building a future. She does not have the bandwidth for my madness.

"I guess you could be right . . . " he says, but he sounds deflated. Disappointed, almost. "Can I be brutally honest?" he asks.

"Isn't that kind of our thing?" I tease. "Or do you usually win girls over with unemployment stories and tales of your man-whoring days?"

"Ouch," he laughs. I can picture the grin on his face, that heavy five o'clock shadow, the tired eyes, and the boyish charm.

"Yes, honesty is our thing," he says more seriously. "I was relieved when I thought the truth was finally out."

My breath catches.

"I mean, it made me sick to think I couldn't be there, next to you, if it blew up," he goes on. "But Morgan, in case I haven't made it clear." He pauses and then leans into a *Jerry Maguire* movie reference. "You had me at 'I'm married.'"

I exhale slowly. He says it like a joke. But it isn't one.

Time gets away from me. I rush back to the hotel room, knowing a frustrated person is waiting. Only made worse by my damp, unfixed hair and lack of makeup. "I know. I know. I have to hurry," I frantically blurt out as I enter. "I couldn't find Diet Coke anywhere near the hotel." It was a lie, but I'm hoping it will grant me some understanding.

"Just remember these are *your* friends," Richard remarks.

It isn't what he says; it's the way he says it. The way he says everything—tinged with condescension. It's interesting how they are my friends, yet without them, the career he got to step into wouldn't exist. It wouldn't exist for him anyway. They wouldn't know he existed. Of course, he is qualified for it, but that is beside the point.

"I'll be ready in 10," I quip, making it a point to be ready in nine.

Richard and I don't say a word to each other on the walk to the elevator. I'm oddly focused on how confusing the carpet is. Hotels never seem to get this part right. I get that a print won't show dirt like a simple solid will, but why do hospitality designers consistently choose the most hideous rug patterns in the entire free world? I just don't get it.

Richard and I arrive with everyone else. I haven't had a drink in hours, but I still feel drunk. Or unmoored. Maybe both.

Are the Twins acting strange? Or am I sunburned, exhausted, and running on fumes? Did I sleep last night? I try to reconstruct it. We came back from dinner. Emails with Brett. Sudoku, maybe? A bath? Did I actually fall asleep? There are gaps. So many gaps this summer.

We sit. I'm across the table and two seats down from Greer and Addy, the birthday girls, but far enough away to feel exiled. The table stretches endlessly, like one of those childhood slip-and-slides, and I'm sliding toward the grass-stripped, muddy end, alone.

I order champagne when the waiter comes. Then, I excuse myself to the restroom. I don't need to go, and Brett is asleep in Beijing, but my body is bubbling from the inside. I don't belong here. I'm not sure where I belong anymore, but it's not here. These people are so good. Kind. Stable. Building families. Moving forward. Salt of the earth. I'm not. My path feels jagged and fractured.

When I return, a steak is in front of me. When did I order that? I consider correcting the waiter. Maybe, it's a mistake, but I can't remember what I ordered. I just smile and say thank you. I love rare steak, but I'm deeply unsettled by how the food got here so quickly and by how time seems to be slipping through cracks I can't see. How long was I gone?

"Boo, are you okay?" Greer calls from what feels like another zip code.

Is my face giving something away?

"Of course, birthday girl!" I chirp. "Are you having fun?"

Before she can answer, sparklers erupt. Waitstaff swarm with towering desserts, flames crackling. We sing. For a moment, I see us as we were: disco naps, Diet Cokes, peddling panties to celebrities in nightclub bathrooms, guerrilla marketing in sequins, Olive Street birthdays in Florence Eiseman dresses, our mothers filming us on VHS, Virginia Slims 120's balanced between their fingers. The '80s. Carefree.

Easy.

But now, I'm here in body only. My mind is elsewhere. My spirit is a mess. I try to pull myself back into alignment, but I can't find the girl everyone needs me to be. She's transformed into a pink balloon, filled with helium, floating higher and higher.

Everything feels like déjà vu, except it's happening in real time. Greer and Addy see it. Of course they do. No one knows me more deeply than they do. They know I love them. And because they know me, they can feel the drift. I think Greer has felt it for months. The hardest part is knowing that, at some point, they'll pull back, too. Not out of cruelty. Out of survival.

The check comes. Richard, "crocodile arms" as my dad often refers to him, pins his elbows close. His arms suddenly shorten. Quickly, he conveniently steps away for a bathroom break. Rhett swoops in to cover it all, always the most generous.

"No dancing?" I ask lightly.

"Pippy, we're just so tired." Addy says. They don't physically gesture to their pregnant bellies, but the implication is there.

"Of course," I say. "Totally understand. It's your night."

It is their night. But I'm not fully in it. Goodnight hugs begin. Addy holds me longer than usual, heavy and intentional. Greer's embrace is similar, reluctant and nervous. I pull back slightly, search her eyes. They flash towards the floor.

"I'll see you for brunch tomorrow though, right?" I confirm. "At The Mondrian? By the pool? Then, we can head to the airport together. I think we're on the same flight."

In unison, almost rehearsed: "Sure thing, Pip. See you tomorrow. Love you."

"Love you, too," I say. "See you tomorrow."

They never show up.

Chapter 14

THE CONFESSION, PART I

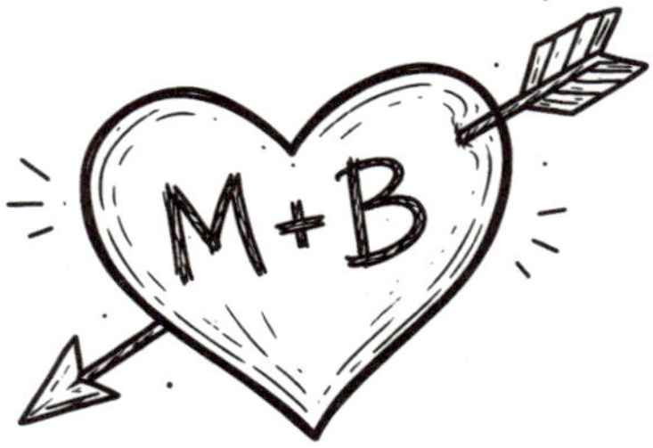

JULY 14, 2009
9 a.m.—Our Apartment
Dallas, Texas

A loud knock jolts me awake. For a second, I don't know where I am. I'm still wearing the top I wore on the flight home from Miami yesterday. No pants. Those are crumpled on the floor beside the bed, tangled with my shoes and purse, like I dropped everything mid-step. The room is too bright. Thin slats of light cut through the blinds.

I'm alone. Richard left early for Baltimore to check on a project. I don't remember him saying goodbye. Maybe he did. Maybe, I mumbled something from under the covers. It has to be at least 9 a.m. It's unlike me to sleep this late. Even when I've barely slept, I've still been awake before dawn. But I can't remember going to bed.

I know we got back from the airport late. I know I was exhausted. But the stretch between baggage claim and crawling into this bed is a blank strip of film. The flight is hazy, too. Did I drink? Yesterday, at the pool, I had one piña colada. I remember feeling puffy in my bathing suit. I don't think I ate the rest of the day.

I still can't make sense of why Greer and Addy never showed up for brunch. It was the one piece of the weekend I had pictured clearly ahead of our arrival. Poolside food. A surprise birthday dessert with singing. Virgin drinks for them with silly umbrellas and garnishes.

I know they're pregnant. I know they're tired. I know South Beach at noon isn't exactly nesting energy. But they didn't come. They didn't even invite me to join them wherever they went instead. I half-expected to bump into them at the airport lounge, to linger, laugh, and compare notes on the weekend. But we never crossed paths. They must have changed their flights.

I'm trying, truly, to be a supportive friend. I'm trying to be thrilled about the babies. And I am happy for them, somewhere inside me. But I'm scared. It's not the babies. It's what they represent. Change.

For six years, Greer and Addy have been my exit ramp. My cover. My joy. My shield. They've been the reason I could step out from under Richard's thumb without it being a fight. They've been the distraction when my moods get dark. They're the proof that I am still alive inside. And soon, they'll be mothers. Their world will narrow in the most meaningful way. I'll move from best friend to Aunt Morgan. I don't know how to do that.

I think of my grandmother. The last long conversation she and I had was in her formal living room in Kentucky, sitting on the cane-back sofa she found in Palm Beach and surrounded by chinoiserie screens and delicate porcelain birds she'd collected over decades.

She mentioned my closeness with the Twins. Out of nowhere. She wasn't critical. Just observant. Wise in that subtle way older women are. She said that friendships as intense as ours might not be the best thing for marriage. She didn't know that they were the only reason my marriage has survived this long. They were my coconspirators in PG rebellion. Without their guardrails, I've gone to NC-17 in record time.

But it's all been with Brett. Every cell in my body is magnetized toward him. If I imagine the future, he's there. I have no map for how. No logistics. No plan. Just certainty.

Yes, my behavior has been outlandish. Much of it has been fueled by mania. Now, I know that intellectually. I can name it, categorize it, and reduce it to something clinical and temporary. But knowing it hasn't stopped me. If anything, it has given me language to excuse it—to call it a phase, a surge, or something passing through me rather than something I am choosing.

And still, I crossed a line I once believed impossible to cross. Not by accident. Not in confusion. But with a kind of clarity that felt, at the time, like truth. That's the part I don't know what to do with.

Because even now, I can feel the distortion in it, the heightened color, the urgency, the way everything narrows until only one thing matters. I can see how my mania sharpens desire into something that feels like destiny. How it edits out consequence. How it turns risk into something almost revered.

And I'm aware of all of that. I am. But I'm also aware that I wanted it. That I still do. That I'm grateful for it. Who the hell is grateful for mania? Perhaps someone not in her right mind.

There is actually a part of me that wonders if Brett is even real? Or did I conjure him in some heightened, shimmering state? Perhaps I'm mad. But if he is real, I believe that if Greer and Addy met him, it would click. They would see it, too.

They would see how Brett looks at me. How he doesn't try to shrink me. How he doesn't press on my knee under the table to quiet me. How he doesn't box me in when my highs or lows show up. They would understand. So why can't I tell them? Why can't I let them in?

Another knock.

"Pippy, are you in there? It's me."

Greer.

My stomach drops like I've missed a stair in the dark. Why would she come here? I don't want her to know I'm still in bed.

I scramble, grab my pants from the floor, shimmy them on, put a toothbrush in my mouth, spit mint foam, and panic. The fact that I didn't see her yesterday suddenly feels like an advantage. My day-old outfit passes as "already up," an odd silver lining.

I open the door in the middle of saying "Sorry!"

"Hey, Pip," Greer begins. "We need to talk."

Her voice is flat. Not angry. But serious in a way we rarely are with each other. We've survived hospitals and divorces and funerals with inappropriate jokes and Diet Coke to wash them down. We've always found the funny seam in the darkest fabric. That's how we've stayed standing. But not today.

She leads me to the bedroom, grabbing two Diet Cokes from the fridge on the way like muscle memory. To anyone else, it might look strange, skipping the couch and heading straight for the bed, but this is how we've always done it. Cross-legged on top of covers. Carbonation between us. Truth in the air.

We sit facing each other. I'm vibrating from the inside. She starts.

"Yesterday, when you and Richard were on the beach, I heard your phone ring," Greer explains. "I answered it."

The air leaves my lungs. So, Brett was right. I was in denial.

"Elizabeth popped up as the caller," she continues. "With everything going on with your family, I thought you'd want to take the call. I was going to come find you. But it wasn't your cousin. Pip, who is Keith?"

Keith? Part of me wants to laugh. Brett, drunk in China, inventing an alter ego. Why is that the name that came to his mind?

"It wasn't Keith," I say carefully. "It was Brett . . . the guy from Bemelmans. He was just calling from China."

The word just lands like a lead balloon. Greer doesn't buy it.

"Morg," she starts, "I know it's more than just a call. More than just a kiss. I found the emails."

My skin goes hot. "You read my emails?" I ask, stunned.

"I forwarded them to myself," she confesses.

The ceiling fan ticks above us. Cool air glides down my back while my insides combust. I should be furious. But I know us. We've never had boundaries. Not really. We've always been three halves of the same brain. If it were Addy, she would've done the same thing. In her way, it isn't betrayal; it's intervention.

"Addy and I are worried about you," Greer continues. "You're not yourself. It's like you're in and out. Are you taking your meds?"

I am taking them. Every single one. Lamictal. Zoloft. Seroquel. I haven't missed a dose. But I also haven't slept. I've barely eaten. I've been floating for weeks. Still, that's not what I'm stuck on. I'm stuck on Greer reading the words that were only ever meant for Brett and me.

"Why didn't you just talk to me?" I ask.

"Richard was right there," her tone easy. There's kindness in her voice, but it's anchored by a certainty that makes it clear she doesn't regret what she's done.

And there it is. The entanglement. Husbands. Bosses. Best friends. Business partners. It's not just my secret. It's a web.

"You're going to destroy your marriage," she says with volition, fresh blonde curls framing her tan face, her eyes glossing over with tears she can hardly hold in place.

My marriage is already ash. I want to say out loud, but I don't. To protect her. It's too sharp, and in this moment, she seems like the more breakable of the two of us, even though I know she's here for me, bracing me against a fall I won't quite admit is coming.

"What do you even know about him?" she presses. "Is he really in China? What is he promising you? How is it enough to walk away from almost 10 years?"

The questions stack so fast I can't catch one to answer. And underneath all of them is the real one: How could you risk us? Because this isn't only about Richard, it's about the three of us—the version of a life we built. It's the rhythm we've had since we were girls in smocked dresses at scavenger hunts and matching pleated skirts at tennis team matches.

Greer doesn't stop. Her concern is real. It's love. But it's built on something incomplete. She doesn't have what she needs to understand this, and I'm the one who kept it from her.

"Morgan, you love Richard," she says. "He's all you've wanted."

But he isn't. Richard is what I chose when I didn't know how to choose myself.

"You can't do this," she goes on. "It will change everything. Our relationship. The business. Where would you even go? Back to Murray? In with your mom? How would you pay for anything?"

It's seven years too late to confess that I wanted to run out the back of the church on my wedding day. Seven years too late to admit I married out of fear of not knowing what came next. Seven years too late to claim confusion without it sounding like mental illness. She will think it's the bipolar disorder talking. Maybe it is. Maybe it isn't. Maybe it's both. I don't trust myself enough to know what's up and what's down right now. But I know, with a clarity that feels almost dangerous, that I would lose everything to be free of this life as it is now.

And I cheated. That part is undeniable. I didn't leave my marriage bravely. Self-loathing washes over me, like a tidal wave that doesn't arrive all at once. It gathers first, a strange pull. Then, it rises, impossibly tall, blocking out everything else, until it hits. It isn't just water; it's a force, taking my footing instantly, folding me into it, and spinning me in a direction I can't navigate.

I could have done this cleanly. I could have told Richard the truth before stepping over the line. I could have packed my bags and taken the shame back to Kentucky, like a grown woman. Instead, I lit a match. In my overwhelmed state, I fold. I say more things I don't mean.

"I messed up," I whisper. "I don't know what I was thinking."

A tear slips down my cheek before I can stop it. It's the first one I've cried since she told me she was pregnant. She looks scared, not angry, but actually scared. There's a stillness to her, the kind that comes not from control but from not knowing what to do next. Even the way she holds herself, with her hand instinctively resting on her belly and her shoulders drawn in just a touch, looks as if she's trying to make sense of something that doesn't fit. And in that moment, I realize something sharp and true: Greer isn't fighting for my marriage; she's fighting for the version of our lives that makes sense to her, for the safety of what's familiar.

"You have to tell Richard," she says. "If you don't, I think Rhett will."

The floor tilts. It feels like I'm on the Perfection game board of the '80s. The pieces will start flying soon.

Rhett? Richard's boss? This is bigger than my heart. It's corporate, and it's clear that my emails were shared with the crew.

"I need a minute," I say. "Richard is still on a plane."

"Then call Brett first," she suggests. "End it. And call Richard next."

End it. The words feel like a physical blow.

"I haven't told Rhett everything," she adds quickly. "But he's worried about your health. He thinks Richard needs to know how serious this is."

My health. Not my happiness. My health. I nod, obediently.

"Okay," I say, and my voice trembles at the idea of saying goodbye to Brett. "I'll call him first. Then Richard."

It's the script of a responsible woman who fixes her mistakes.

"Can I meet you after?" I add too lightly. "At our favorite diner?" Seems a shame not to take her out for lunch in her darling dress, a sunny shade of yellow, ironically joyful for the heaviness in this room, on this bed, now sprinkled with tears.

A look of shock washes over Greer's face. I said it too casually. Am I just supposed to break my own heart, blow up my marriage, and then meet her for a tuna melt? Even I hear how unhinged I sound. The truth is, I don't know if I'm strong enough to do what she's asking.

I know I'm not going to end it with Brett. Not in five minutes. Not today. Not tomorrow. Not because Greer sat cross-legged on my bed with a Diet Coke in her hand and fear in her eyes.

But I had to get out of the conversation before I agreed to more things I don't mean, before I let shame or guilt start drafting my life for me.

Richard can wait. Rhett can tick like a moral time bomb. Right now, I have an important Skype date to prepare for.

I move fast, almost mechanically. In a bathroom of maple cabinets I would never pick with granite countertops that scream basic, I apply concealer, bronzer, blush, mascara, and lip gloss. My toiletry bag is still half-packed, nothing "Morganized," as the Twins would tease. No tidy display. No curated calm. Just urgency.

I yank the blinds up with more force than the cheap cords deserve. They groan in protest and the light floods in harsh but workable. I position myself on the sofa where the oil painting of Petros the Pelican hangs behind me. It's from my study abroad in Greece when I was a different version of myself. My mom had the painting framed, as a reminder of who I was before everything got so tangled.

I log into my brand-new Skype account. It's 10:30 a.m. here and 11:30 p.m. in China. The ringtone bursts through my speakers, tinny, clubby, cartoonish, like Mickey Mouse Clubhouse for adults. It's Brett. Unreasonable butterflies flutter inside me. I click "answer."

There he is. Not a selfie. Not a memory. In real time. Breathing. Blinking. A little rumpled. In a white V-neck with a small bolognese sauce stain just below the neckline. Messy hair. Sleep still clinging to his face.

"Hi, perfect girl," he says. "Sorry about the bedhead. I set an alarm for you. Been asleep for a couple hours. Crazy day here. I think we're closing the deal. And . . . " The longest pause. "They asked me to stay. To help run the company."

The words hang in the air. Stay. In Beijing. Permanently, maybe? I can't take it on yet. My mind is already too full of thoughts, coming in like overcaffeinated interns—insistent, urgent, and completely gone if I don't let them speak the second they arrive.

"Okay, we will revisit that, but first," I say, "Greer knows."

Brett's face shifts instantly. He looks relieved in a way that feels unexamined, like he's been willing this outcome without considering its weight.

He sighs. "I knew it. There was no way she bought the Keith bit."

"Where did Keith even come from?" I laugh despite myself.

"Old colleague. I panicked," he explains.

I don't know why the name tickled me. I can't recall ever having met a Keith. It felt both oddly specific and completely invented. I'm guessing Greer didn't know a Keith either, which probably only made it more suspicious. Would a John or a Bryan have slipped by more easily?

Seeing Brett, even on screen, drapes everything in a sense of calm. The looming confrontation with Richard. The Rhett ultimatum. The possibility of my life imploding. For a moment, the chaos blurs at the edges. He studies my face.

"What happens now?" he asks. "How did Richard take it?"

"I haven't told Richard yet," I admit sheepishly. "He left this morning. Greer came over. They all know. Rhett apparently plans to tell Richard if I don't."

I lace it with sarcasm, but underneath it is something else. Unburdening. The fantasy of someone else dealing with the disaster of my own life for me.

"Morgan," Brett says carefully, "what's the plan? I agree with Rhett. Tell Richard. You want to, right? You want the truth out."

The truth. Such a clean word for such a messy thing. Brett knows about my bipolar diagnosis. The medications. The sleeplessness. But he doesn't know how much I've protected Richard. How I've curated the image of us. How deeply I believe in marriage, even after crossing the line. My faith still whispers about vows and covenants and sacred promises. Even as I sit here, camera on, talking to another man.

"Yes," I say slowly. "I mean, no, I don't want to have to do this. But yes. I'll tell Richard."

I'm not afraid of the shame that will follow my truth, not really. Or the blame. It's already formed. I suppose I'm a little afraid of Richard, but even that feels distant and dulled. His opinion of me fractured a year and a half ago, the moment I said bipolar disorder out loud, repeating my diagnosis back to him.

What unsettles me is something else entirely.

The older version of me, the one I haven't fully outrun but just buried, the one who understands consequences, and the one who still believes in lines you don't cross—she's still inside me somewhere, tucked away for now, but intact. And I can feel her waiting.

What will she do when it all arrives: the rumors, the chatter, the catty names spoken just loud enough to be heard? Will she resurface all at once, horrified and ready to crush the new me? Or will she disappear, eclipsed by this version that feels so untouchable?

I don't know which would be worse. Because right now, I feel almost immune to it, as if I could stand in the middle of it all and not flinch. But I have the distinct sense that she would. And I'm not sure I'll survive becoming her again—or losing her entirely.

Brett exhales at my affirmation. He's reassured.

And then he says it plainly: "I told the investors I'd stay. But only after I go back and see about things. My apartment. And most importantly . . . a girl, you."

There it is. Even if everything ahead is a dumpster fire, and it will be, this part feels hopeful. Not manic glitter. Not fantasy projection. He didn't hesitate. He factored me in.

With or without Brett, I know I can't stay in my marriage to Richard. But knowing Brett is real, that this isn't just some chemical mirage born of sleepless nights and Manhattan lights, sends a current of calm through me.

For the first time all morning, I don't feel cornered.

It's almost noon. The sun is directly overhead, but you can't tell from the cloud cover. I light a candle, Jo Malone's Pomegranate Noir, foolishly hoping it might overpower what's about to be said. The smell of the burned-out match lingers in a thin ribbon, curling upward, carrying finality with it, like a small ending you can smell.

Richard landed in Baltimore 30 minutes ago. I don't text first. No warning. I just call.

He answers on the second ring. His voice is flat and uninterested, like I'm interrupting an event on his calendar I'm supposed to know about.

"Hey, can we talk?" I ask, code for this won't be pleasant.

He sighs, saying I need to make it fast. He has meetings. His tone makes my resolve wobble. I'm thinking too fast. I'm feeling too little about things I should feel deeply about. Be quick, Morgan. Do this.

"Richard, I crossed a line this summer," I say, diving in before I lose my nerve. "I met someone. And I crossed a line. Emotionally."

That part is true. I am falling in love with Brett from 6,000 miles away, through screens and time zones and insomnia.

"What do you mean?" Richard asks. "Morgan, what did you do?"

The way he says my name makes it feel diminished. Clinical.

My courage fizzles. I tell him about inappropriately long conversations, texts, emails, and the first "almost kiss." And then I stop. I let silence imply that was the end. I omit the the Skype calls. The planning. The "see about a girl." The future tense. The thought of explaining how this could happen, filling in all the holes from years of omission, exhausts me. I stop. I brace myself for Richard's interrogation. It doesn't come. Just three questions.

"Is that it?"

"Yes," I lie easily.

"Is it over?"

"Yes," I say. "He moved to China." It's a convenient truth wrapped around a much bigger lie.

"Who else knows?"

Of course, that's the one thing that matters most to Richard. Reputation. Optics. Control of the narrative. I tell him Greer knows. I don't elaborate. I don't confess that the entire Miami crew probably dissected my instability poolside while he and I were on the beach.

He exhales. Short. Tight. "I have to get to my meetings," he says. "We'll talk more later. But you making a mistake doesn't mean I don't get to go hiking this week. I didn't do this. I'm still going to Aspen."

Music to my ears.

"Definitely," I say quickly. "This is my doing. You deserve to go."

And I mean that part. Because his trip to Aspen buys me time. Thursday to Monday. Time to think. Time to choose where I will land. Time to get at least a couple ducks in a row. At the moment, the ducks are everywhere. In the road. Under the bed. Running wild. I need a few days to gather them. To pack. To slip out. To avoid the long, drawn-out autopsy of a marriage that has been dying slowly for years.

Should I go to Kentucky? My mom's house perhaps? That'll be a reset no one saw coming.

Richard ends the call with: "We'll talk when I get back."

No yelling. No prodding. No devastation. Only logistics deferred. When the line goes dead, I sit very still. My plan isn't honorable. It's strategic. Defensive. Self-preserving. Selfish. Plain and simple. If he comes home from Aspen and wants to label me as the wife who blew it all up, fine. But I won't be standing in the doorway when he does.

I know that I'm hanging by a single thread here. The main goal is to pacify Rhett and survive the week. Then run.

Before I head out for the afternoon, I send an email to Brett, telling him that I talked to Richard. I didn't get into the details. We can talk about that on our next call tomorrow morning. It's still the middle of the night for him.

But Brett doesn't wait. Minutes after I pressed send, my phone rings. I've just gotten into my car to go meet Greer for lunch.

"Hi!" I answer perkily.

"Hi," he whispers, sleepy talk, "I couldn't wait. How did it go? I'm worried about you. Are you okay?"

I can't lie to him. "Yes, I'm okay," I assure him. "But I couldn't fully go through with it. Over the phone, it felt off. I told Richard that I had an emotional affair over the summer, that you kissed me, but . . . "

"And . . . " Brett pushes.

"And then, he just really didn't ask much more of me, so I didn't give it. I let him think it was over," I admit. After a long silence, I add, "Brett, I really need a minute to figure out what I'm doing. What am I actually going to do?"

It was a rhetorical question; I didn't expect Brett to have a plan for me. I didn't want a "fix." Not from him.

"Richard gets home in two days and then he leaves almost immediately for a hiking trip" I explain. "He'll be gone, and I will figure out what to do and where to go."

"I know where you can go," Brett says, "assuming that you're still in this with me." I can almost hear the corners of his mouth turn up into a small smile.

"Oh, I'm in," I say affirmatively. "Where am I going?" My voice ticks up.

"To see me," he says, no longer sleep whispering.

I laugh. "As much as I want to see you," I say, "China is not on my bingo card just yet."

"Not China," he explains, laughing. "New York! I'm flying back on Friday. I land at 5 p.m. Come and be with me!"

I don't hesitate. "Yes," I agree. It's abrupt. I don't think it through. I don't want to. "I'll be there."

"Are you sure?" he asks. "If so, that's the best news ever, but no pressure."

"I'm sure," I insist.

"Okay then," he says. "I'll look for a ticket for you in the morning, my morning I mean. But, Morgan, Richard needs the full truth."

Oh man, not Brett, too. Everyone is really taking this so seriously. I don't think it's going to be all that bad. I don't think Richard is really going to care half as much as everyone thinks.

"I know, I know." I appease him. "But for now, you get some sleep! Dream of our reunion at the airport on Friday."

I pull into the mostly empty parking lot of one of Dallas's signature strip malls. The sky is dark, the kind of July day where the air feels suffocating. It's still, only the noise of traffic in the distance.

Greer is already inside, waiting in our usual booth. The table is the same as always, ivory laminate, slightly worn at the edges, almost completely hidden beneath oversized laminated menus and an army of condiments. Ketchup. Mustard. Sweetener packets. And then the extras that make this place ours: little bowls of capers, whole pickled pepperoncini, and a lineup of Texas hot sauces in every shade of red and green.

She looks up when I walk in. Her eyes are tired. A little sad. But she is still so beautiful. Her pregnancy isn't showing yet, not in any noticeable way, but there's something already luminous about her. Warmer. A glow that has nothing to do with makeup or lighting. It's subtle, but it's there.

"Boo," she says gently, "how did it go? Are you okay?" Her voice isn't accusatory. It's careful. Protective.

I slide into the booth across from her and start at the beginning. It's clear that she doesn't fully believe that he is in China, but I assure her he is. It's nice to be able to not lie about that detail.

When I move on to the call with Richard, something in me gives way. The tears just start. No warning. No dramatic build. They fall steadily. I don't try to stop them. I'm sure she thinks that I'm crying over Richard, over what happened on our call. But that's not it.

It's not about Richard. Not really. It's exhaustion. It's the fatigue of pretending. Of managing perceptions. Of carrying secrets in every room I walk into. My body feels like it has reached capacity. And crying feels like relief. Greer reaches across the table without hesitation, her hand warm over mine.

"Greer," I manage through the tears, "I couldn't tell Richard everything over the phone. I will. I promise. But I need a little time. Until he gets back on Wednesday. Can you give me that?"

There's no pause.

"Of course," she says immediately. "Anything you need. I promise Rhett doesn't know everything I heard or read. I won't tell him until you're ready. I promise," she reiterates.

I believe her. I trust her. Greer has always been on my side.

She has supported me since we were 6 and 7 years old, when Raymond, the neighborhood bully, tried to knock my tree house down and she stood at the bottom of the ladder like a tiny, furious bodyguard. Through scraped knees and sleepovers and whispered secrets under covers with flashlights, she and Addy have always had my back. Even now. Even when they don't agree with me. Even when they're scared.

In this sticky strip mall diner, with hot sauce bottles between us and the sky threatening rain, I feel it clearly: Whatever comes next, I am not alone.

Chapter 15

THE CONFESSION, PART II

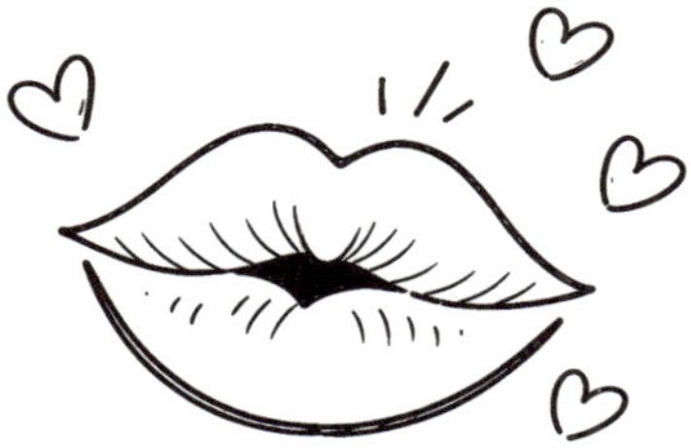

JULY 14, 2009
Afternoon—Shopping
Dallas, Texas

The day feels slightly out of focus, like I'm moving through a thin layer of haze. Pornkiat, our Thai manufacturing partner, asked Greer and me to do some comp shopping to determine if there is an opportunity to offload his overstock to American liquidators. So, we start at TJ Maxx, clipboards in hand, scanning for price points and patterns. On most days, we love the "Teej," the possibility of it. The oddball treasures. The thrill of spotting something designer buried between the ordinary. Not today.

I push through racks of tiny, clear plastic hangers that clack together like impatient teeth. Bra straps are knotted around each other. Sizes are scrambled. The lace looks tired beneath the unforgiving fluorescent lights. There's no romance here, no curated seduction, just markdown stickers and mismatched sets. You don't come here for beauty. You come here for numbers. For margins. For reality.

Greer moves beside me, flipping tags with steady focus. I can see the fatigue in her, too. But hers is sacred. She's first-trimester tired. Cell-dividing tired. Her body is silently constructing a human being from scratch. And then, there's the other layer of exhaustion she's carrying, the emotional weight of me, her manic best friend whose life is teetering toward something explosive.

I'm not just tired; I'm hollowed out. For the first time since my official bipolar diagnosis, I fear this might be more than a phase or a high that will eventually level out. I'm afraid that I may have pushed myself toward an edge I don't fully understand, and worse, might not be able to step back from.

I call my mom on the drive home. I need a dose of Mona.

Greer has an early dinner with Rhett, so we cut our comp shopping short. Neither of us says it, but we both know. She needs her husband's arms. And I need solitude.

Mom answers on the second ring, bright and warm as ever. Instant comfort. I've always known how lucky I am to have her, but today, it feels essential. Like oxygen. Her excitement at hearing from me gives me a lift, a small, steadying surge of energy.

I tell her nothing. Not about Greer reading my emails with Brett. Not about Richard. Not about my Friday plans. Not about the tectonic plates shifting under my life.

Today, her intuition guides her to softness instead of questions. She's gentle. She doesn't pry. What a gift. To be loved by someone who demands nothing in return. No timeline. No explanation. No ultimatum.

We talk about family: my grandfather's recent health scare, my cousin's diabetes tests, and some bizarre legal drama swirling around extended relatives. It's been a strange year for our family tree. We even laugh a little about how refreshing it is that, for once, the drama isn't centered around us. During the worst years of my parents' divorce, Mom and I used to joke that we were the black sheep branch of the family tree, sticking out in a grove of snow-white Southern Baptists.

The joke stings a little now. Because I know I'm about to add another chapter to that broken branch. Another story for the pews. Another whisper. But not today. Today, I keep it locked up.

It feels nice to talk about something other than my own brewing storm. It's nice to just be a daughter catching up with her mom. This time, I don't rush our drawn-out goodbye with three rounds of "I love you" and one "Oh, wait, did I tell you . . . ?" And, finally, the last "Okay, really, bye."

I hang up just as I pull into my parking spot. The apartment is stale when I open the door. No Richard. No Norm. For the first time since I woke up, I am alone.

The thought of solitude makes my shoulders drop. Not in defeat. In relief. Tonight, I'll eat cereal for dinner. I'll have Honey Bunches of Oats first, straight from the box like an appetizer, and then Fiber One sprinkled over Activia yogurt for the main course. An epic solo feast. I'll put on reruns of *Sex and the City* and let myself drift back to Manhattan in my mind. If my eyes cooperate, if the words stop jittering on the page, maybe, I'll read a few chapters of *The Widow Clicquot* and imagine bold women building empires from nothing.

But first, I will check my email. Brett usually writes to me first thing in the morning, his time, telling me some silly fact about himself. Yesterday, it was deeper. He wrote about the Catholic Church, growing up in it and eventually leaving it, during the scandal. I was comforted when, in the end, he confirmed the importance of his faith.

I loved that part.

But it struck me; we've never gone deep on the subject of religion. Sure, I've alluded to my Christian upbringing, but my actions of late reflect none of it. Are we really aligned? Am I even aligned with myself right now?

My faith in God hasn't wavered. But it's distant. I'm not angry about having bipolar. To me, it's no different than diabetes, a condition to manage, not a moral failing. But that's not always how "the church" treats it. Mental illness is often a hushed topic. Tucked away. Reserved for the poor, the unstable, or the spiritually weak. No one hides diabetes. Richard would never have asked me to keep stories of my insulin deficiencies a secret.

But bipolar? That silence he requested, it was the final crack that sent me running from Dallas. I've dropped my basket this hard before, in a totally different way, and survived. I think I can do it again.

The apartment is pitch-black. I must have closed the blinds after my Skype call this morning. I drop my Goyard tote onto the floor. It spills slightly open, packed too full. Laptop, manila folders, overstuffed wallet, loose makeup pouches, Band-Aids, bobby pins. The straps are worn. The bottom is dusted with saltine crumbs and lip gloss smears.

My tote is a mirror of me. Still cute on the outside. A little chipped. Chaos inside.

I kick off my sandals and pull out my laptop. I can't wait another second. What will Brett's email hold today?

Meg Ryan in the '90s rom-com pops into my mind—her anxious, hopeful look while she waited for her computer to announce: "You've got mail!"

There he is.

Subject line: *NYC Visit*

For half a second, panic flashes. What if he's canceling? Chill out, Morgan. He already asked for your Continental number. He is a follow-through kind of guy. Still, I brace myself as I click. Relief floods me immediately. He's booked my ticket. First class. Upgraded with his frequent flyer miles. We will land within 15 minutes of each other at Newark airport. Same terminal, most likely.

Every detail is mapped. Every move is deliberate. He is in this.

Then, paragraph two stops me cold. He invited his parents. They are coming to the city to see him before he returns to Beijing. And to meet me. He adds: *Assuming that's okay with you.*

Wow.

Under normal circumstances, I would be floating. But these are not normal circumstances. I am manic. And I am married. He is moving to Asia in two weeks. How could this possibly work? Before my doubt can grow teeth, I reply:

Wow, B. That is some big news. But what the heck? Count me in. :)

Should I leave my wedding rings at home? J/K! Talk tonight your time? Not long before I see your face now. Zhù nǐ jīntiān gōngzuò yúkuài.

Your Perfect Girl,

M

I Googled how to write "have a good day at work" in Mandarin pinyin. He explained pinyin to me yesterday. It's Mandarin in our alphabet, not characters. It's entertaining to learn about his new world.

I close the laptop and shuffle to the pantry. I pour some cereal into a bowl. Then more. Then the other box. As if the cardboard somehow understands that, after tomorrow, I may not be here to finish it. I eat standing at the counter, in the dark apartment, with the sound of my neighbors' feet on the concrete outside, my only soundtrack.

Tomorrow, everything changes. Tonight, it's just me, cereal, Carrie Bradshaw, and the girls.

July 15, 2009, 7 a.m.—Our Apartment, Dallas

I wake to the sound of Skype ringing from my computer. It's infinitely kinder than an alarm clock. I'm still in yesterday's clothes, but this time, I'm on the couch. Two cereal bowls sit in front of me on the glass coffee table, the flakes swollen and lifeless in cloudy milk. The TV is on, a paused image glowing faintly into the dim room.

Another round of Skype rings. I scramble up, disoriented. The computer rings again, and I answer without checking a mirror. The camera flicks on. Instant regret.

"Morning!" Brett beams. "I see someone was sleeping hard."

"Hi," I croak, my first word cracking out of a dry throat.

"I'm sorry to call so early," he apologizes, "but I've got a work dinner in half an hour and didn't want to miss you."

"No, no, I'm glad you called," I insist. "Just wish I had 30 seconds to look cuter."

"You always look cute to me," he says easily. "I might like this best, though. I love being the first person to see you wake up."

I laugh. "That's generous," I say. "I can see what I look like, too."

He grins wider. "Hey . . . I hope it was okay that I asked my parents to come before we talked about it," he says, a bit sheepish now. "When I told them I'm moving to China long-term, they wanted time with me while I'm back. I thought, what better time than when they could meet you, too?"

How is he so unfazed by the chaos of my life? Honestly, how am I?

"I'm flattered," I tell him. "And I'm a little nervous. My life is . . . messy right now."

"I know," he says carefully. "But this might be our only window for a while. I want them to meet you. Morgan, we'll work this out. Eventually."

Eventually. I cling to that belief. When I'm talking to Brett, everything feels solvable. With Greer, the room is crowded with consequences: divorce, broken trust, and endings. When I'm alone, I swing back to affirmations: I can change my life. I can survive this. On the phone with Richard, I retreat into myself, hard and shelled, surviving by denial.

How do I deny Brett's offer? He wants me to meet his parents. He's building me into his future plans with no guarantees about how that future even begins. It's what girls are taught to want.

"Well," I say lightly, "I guess I'll see you in Newark then. I'll wear my meet-the-parents best. It's been about 10 years since I did that dance, but I think I remember the steps."

We flirt a little longer before he has to leave for dinner. Peking duck at one of Beijing's most famous spots. He says he can't wait to take me there. I believe him. We hang up feeling buoyant. It's the last time we'll speak before our planes land within minutes of each other, inside the same New Jersey terminal where we kissed goodbye, outside of it, just weeks ago.

Richard gets home this afternoon. No time for a call tonight. Tomorrow, Brett will already be in the air to America when I wake.

My body is here. My mind is already at that airport gate. I picture weaving through Newark's crowd, rolling suitcases bumping into ankles, scanning faces until I see Brett. His pace quickening. His arms wrapping tight around me like it's been years instead of weeks. His hands on my face. The way he looks at me, not like I'm fragile or failing, but like I'm the person he's been waiting for.

The lift. My feet leaving the ground. The pause. The kiss. Passionate. Effortless. Certain.

My BlackBerry buzzes and shatters the scene. A text from Richard.

Sorry I didn't call last night. Needed some space. Going straight to the office when I land. See you tonight.

I hadn't noticed we didn't speak last night. There was a time when we checked in constantly, for no reason except that we wanted to. That ended some time ago. Mutually.

See you tonight. Let me know if I can pick up anything for your trip. I know you're heading out early tomorrow.

Of course I want to make sure his trip runs smoothly. It's better for everyone. And in this case, it makes my trip to NYC easier to sort out. I still haven't figured out how I'm pitching it to him, but that feels like a tomorrow problem. Telling Greer—that's today's real hurdle.

I put on Simon and Garfunkel's "The Only Living Boy in New York" and let it play through my laptop speakers. With a strange brightness rising under my skin, I pull outfits from my closet. A few dresses. Beautiful lingerie. I slide my carry-on out from the back shelf, roll everything carefully, place it inside, then tuck the suitcase back where it belongs.

There's one perfect, parent-approved dinner look missing. It's hanging in Greer's closet. I'll find a casual way to borrow it.

In the shower, steam rising, curtain drawn, "Bridge Over Troubled Water" starts to play.

When you're down and out . . .

In the dim steam, something colder creeps in. This isn't impulsive anymore. It's planned. Mapped out. Timed. I'm about to take off my wedding rings, hide them in a drawer, and board a plane to meet another man's parents as his girlfriend. And I don't even feel that guilty.

It unsettles me. The ick isn't the affair. The ick is the familiarity. The realization that somewhere along the way, my actions mirror my father's. The cheating, yes. But more than that, it's knowing that I would do it all over again for this result. There is no repentance in that.

Summer 1990—My Hometown, Murray, Kentucky

I'm 9, almost 10 years old. It's Sunday, deep into a Southern summer, sharing the space with mosquitos and humidity. After church, we take separate cars to the country club. Mom and I need one for meeting friends at the pool, and Dad for golfing with his favorite foursome. Dad pitched the two-car idea, framing it as thoughtful, in case he adds an extra nine holes with the guys.

My dad knows my mom doesn't want to be stuck at the club, so of course, she agrees to his plan. Before we leave the house, she reminds him that we made family dinner plans to join the Pickens at their home, post pool and golf, implying he can't be too late.

Miraculously, he arrives shortly after us. Right on time.

It's a magical summer night. Lightning bugs fill the sky as I play with friends in their sprawling backyard, overlooking a massive wheat field. The Pickenses' house is nestled at the back of a cul-de-sac in one of the most popular family neighborhoods in Murray, one packed with kids. Quite the opposite, of ours. My family lives right in town on Olive Street, just off Main, and not far from our town's quaint court square. All the homes in our area of town are old and charming, but it isn't this. This neighborhood has a vibe. Spotlight Tag and Kick the Can games run rampant on nights like this.

Sunkissed and chlorine-logged from all day in the pool, followed by running all over the neighborhood, all the kids land in the home's upstairs TV room after dinner, while our parents play Rook. At some point, the men retire to Dr. Pickens's man cave to catch SportsCenter. My mom comes upstairs around 9:30 or 10 p.m. to tell me it's time to head home. We're all exhausted.

I say goodbye to the crew. Mom and I go downstairs to tell dad we're ready to go. Dr. Pickens meets us at the top of the stairs of the basement. Before Mom can ask, he covers for Dad. Something about my dad's back hurting, and that he left to go home a little while ago.

I can tell Dr. Pickens's excuse stirred a rage inside my Mom, but I'm not sure why at the time. She hurries me to the car. In minutes, we're on our way home. Or, so, I thought. Her aggressive driving is out of character. Her silence is a dead giveaway that something is off. For the first time in my entire life, I feel scared in her presence.

When we get to the corner of Main and 16th, she turns left. Home is straight. I don't ask any questions. I grip the bottom of my seat to give my idle hands something to do other than peel back the layers of my fingernails. Suddenly, I have a sense of where we're going, though, I don't want to believe it. I thought our family was healed. I thought we survived the brink of divorce last year. I thought dad stopped cheating. I thought our family of three was spared. But I'm just a kid. What do I know?

Mom pulls into the parking lot of a small apartment building. In all my life living in Murray, I've never noticed it before. It's just off Murray State's campus, across the street from the building where my dad teaches one of his two real estate law classes, an add-on task to his law practice. For a moment, I feel relieved. Perhaps, he stopped by to pick up papers to grade.

The apartment building looks run down, more like a roadside motel. It's two stories with doors on the outside and one shared staircase in the middle. My dad's new car, a silver Pontiac Grand Prix STE, is parked underneath the only streetlight in the middle of the lot. My mom pulls in beside it, right behind another car, stamped with a bumper sticker I've seen before: "If you're rich, I'm single." It's Becky's car.

I can feel the heat from her anger. Dad isn't here for work. I know that much. Mom gets out of the car and slams the door. I follow her instinctively. I'm not sure what else to do. I feel myself shaking and realize I am sobbing. She takes my hand. She feels like a stranger, a person who I've never met. My mom is only 35, but in this moment, something in her face hardens into age. Her color rises quickly, starting at her chest, climbing her neck, settling high in her cheeks in a flush that looks feverish. Her mouth presses into a line too firm to be natural. Her eyes don't dart or flash, they fixate, on a single door.

Hand in sweaty hand, we walk up the second-rate staircase, stepping over a stray cat at some point. Somehow, Mom knows exactly where she is going, walks right up to one of the apartment doors. The welcome mat is cheesy, a silly pun that I don't get, with paw prints on it. She bangs on the door. Two full rounds of beating.

Hot tears roll down my face. I wipe the snot away. No one comes to the door. One more round of beating. No one says a thing on the other side, but Mom and I can hear scuffling inside, as if dad's car isn't already proof.

"I know you're in there, Mark!" Mom shouts. "You're a coward for not answering the door!" No doubt everyone in the complex hears the entire interaction.

She storms off, pulling me behind her. We get back in the car, heading home. She hasn't cried up until this point, but as she watches me put my seatbelt on, her body convulses with sobs. I know it isn't because of my dad. It's because of me. In an instant, she's back in her right mind. She is my mom again. The guilt of bringing me along is too much for her.

"It's okay, Mom," I say. "I'm okay. It's not your fault."

She does her best to calm down and drive us home safely. She takes Main Street, past the Hungry Bear, the best pancake spot in town, past the Dairy Queen, known for its signature chili dogs. She handles the car far less aggressively than on the way to that hellhole. We're home in less than 10 minutes.

About 20 minutes after that, my dad pulls into our driveway, a full circle drive that wraps around the back of the house. It's easy to spot someone coming in at night because the car lights shine through the front windows of the house first and travel all the way around to the back. I rush upstairs, with a half-eaten orange sherbet push-up pop in hand, to change into my pajamas and avoid the aftermath that is surely coming.

I hear Dad come in the back door, just off the kitchen. The storm door slams behind him. My father's anger doesn't arrive all at once—it builds, visible before it's spoken. His ears flush first, a deep, unmistakable red that spreads outward, as if the heat has nowhere else to go. It's a stark contrast to his silver hair. His jaw tightens, working slightly, like he's holding something back and failing. His hands betray him. They don't rest. Shaky.

Rage is something I've rarely seen in him, if ever, before. For all his marital shortcomings, Dad is super even-keeled with me; he's not the yelling kind. Calm. Steady. Absent sometimes sure, golf always calling, but also kind. Everyone loves my dad. My mother included. If she didn't, then she wouldn't be so mad or so hurt right now. She doesn't embarrass easily. Her reaction has nothing to do with that. She sincerely wants their marriage to work. But Becky, her cat claws, are deep into my dad. Becky is only 23. But to 9-year-old me, she seems just as grown up as my parents.

Trying to decipher the maturity difference of a 37-year-old married man and a 23-year-old single girl, when your main focus in life is which Lisa Frank Trapper Keeper you're going to get when school starts back in three weeks, is an impossible task.

Almost 20 years after that night, I know that 23-year-olds actually know zilch. Becky was a just kid. Still becoming. Trying to find her footing, following her heart, without the life experience to fully grasp the ripple effect of it all. It doesn't erase the pain. But it softens the edges. She didn't set out to shatter our family. She was a young woman in lust, making adult decisions without the tools to understand their weight.

My dad's anger was misguided at the time. Obviously, my mother shouldn't have brought me along to confront him at Becky's apartment. But surely, he could see that none of it would have happened without his actions. He took no responsibility for his behavior.

As I think back on this, for the first time, I realize that may have been his cruelest act. Maybe, this is where I choose differently. Maybe, this is how I stop repeating the story.

If I'm honest, I'm sure my mother wasn't perfect in their marriage. No one is. It takes two people to fracture something sacred. I know that now in a way I couldn't understand as a child. Marriages are layered and complicated and rarely one-sided.

But this part of my story is mine to own. Whatever is broken between Richard and me, whatever rules or silences or shames built the distance, I chose the weak exit. I didn't sit across from him and tell the whole truth when it first started cracking. I stepped outside of it.

No matter how justified I've felt, no matter how lonely, no matter how unseen. I took the bad guy's way out. And maybe, the only way to be different from my father is not in avoiding the mistake, but in how I handle the aftermath. Own it. Say it plainly. Stand in it. As soon as Richard is back from Aspen, I will tell him everything. Not the edited version. Not the diluted one. Not the half-confession. All of it.

I don't know what that will cost me. My marriage, certainly. My reputation, probably. Maybe even most of the relationships I'm clinging to. But still, I will face it.

July 15, 2009, 1 p.m.—Our Favorite Diner, Dallas

At lunch with Greer, I muster the courage to tell her about my trip to New York. I feel like I might share the actual reason at this point, but I worry opening the Pandora's box of my situation will make its way to Rhett and wreck my entire plan, so I hold off.

I tell her I'm going back to New York for an event, while Richard's in Aspen, to get away and clear my head. I tell her I found a cheap room in the Flat Iron, one we've stayed in before for the COTERIE wholesale market, safe and easy. When she asks if I really need this, I remind her that New York is my happy place, and I confess that Dallas is not. Unsure if she's buying my story, I choose to believe that she is. At some point, she stops asking me questions. We move on.

We head back to Greer's house, so I can find the dress I was hoping to borrow in the back of her newly renovated closet. Rhett nailed their home addition. They officially live in a grown-up house now, matching their beautiful grown-up life.

When Greer comes back into her bedroom from a call she needed to make, she finds me trying on the dress, likely catching the puppy love grin on my face, reflecting back at her in the full-length mirror.

She stops dead and asks, "Morgan, are you really going to New York by yourself?"

"Yes, Boo," I reply. "Brett really is in China." I know what she's really asking.

I got an email from Brett before he went to sleep, detailing the plans. WD-50, Wylie Dufresne's Michelin Star restaurant, for our first meal. The meet-the-parents dinner.

Greer's colorful Milly dress, a 1960s retro fit and happy print, is spot on. While riding high on the anticipation of it all, I completely miss my phone ringing.

"Pippy, your phone," she tells me, picking up my BlackBerry from the end of her bed, dressed in a fresh new Frette duvet cover as part of the renovation. She glances at the caller. She holds it out in my direction and, in a disturbing tone, states, "It's Richard."

On the other end is an angry man-toddler, who is upset that Rhett thinks he shouldn't go on this hiking trip. I listen, in silence, trying not to show emotion on my side of the phone. It's surprisingly easy. I don't actually feel anything associated with what he is lecturing me about.

"Why is Rhett telling me my marriage is in crisis mode, Morgan?" Richard asks. "Does he know something I don't? Do you have more to tell me? Where are you right now?"

I don't know which one of his questions to answer first. Looking down at the floor, nervously picking the skin off my lips, I dart my eyes to Greer. She's noteably not surprised by his call.

I start with the last question. "I'm at Greer's," I tell him.

"I just got to the office," Richard explains. "Rhett says you and I need to talk. Meet me at Starbucks in 10." It wasn't a question.

Well, if Rhett thinks so . . . I guess I have no choice.

I take off Greer's dress, quickly roll it up, and tuck it inside my purse. I rush to change back into the clothes I put on that morning, an ivory puff sleeve button-down shirt piped in whimsy black trim with a grosgrain ribbon necktie. As I slide my skirt back up, I realize it's the same skirt I wore to breakfast with Brett. I think I'll keep it forever.

I arrive at Starbucks' just as Richard pulls into the next parking spot over. He taps on the passenger window mouthing for me to unlock it. I guess this means we aren't going inside to order a tasty treat.

I unlock the door, and he slides in through the small crack. I didn't park well and got way too close to the white line, per usual, leaving little room to open the door all the way. Richard manages to squeeze through, but I swear I sense a laugh. My driving skills or lack thereof are a common joke among our friend group.

Once he locks in on my eyes though, any sign of a laugh, smile, or general kindness ends. Should I feel scared?

I don't. Despondency perhaps? A few of my doctors over the years have used this word . . .

"Why does Rhett think you and I are in crisis mode, Morgan?" Richard asks before uttering a simple hello. "Why does he think I shouldn't go hiking this weekend? What are you not telling me?" He keeps going, with zero breaks in his questioning for me to actually answer.

"Are you lying to me?" he demands. "What did you do? Is there more to your story? How much more? Is this guy actually even in China? Did you cheat on me? Did you sleep with him? Did you . . . " Richard is still going strong, getting louder, sharper with each question, but I interrupt him.

It's time. This is it. I take one more deep breath. Let's give him what he wants.

"Yes, Richard," I confess. "Of course, I slept with him."

Chapter 16
PRETTY LITTLE PILLS

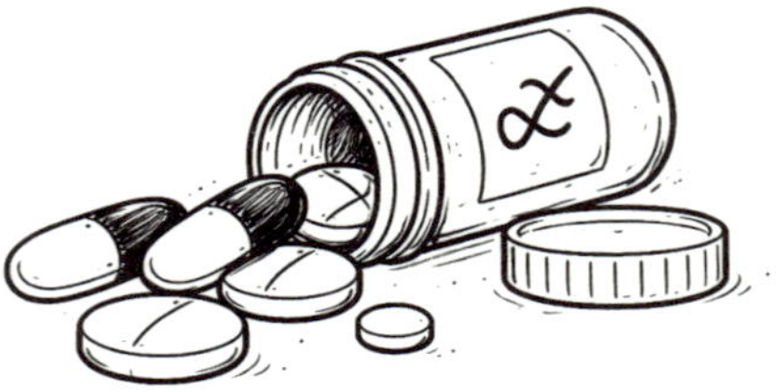

JULY 15, 2009
2 p.m.—My Car
Dallas, Texas

After 30 seconds of silence thick enough to choke on, something snaps. The questions come like gunfire. No space between them, no air for me to breathe. Richard barrels ahead, each question more explicit than the last, more invasive, more determined to hurt as much as to understand. He leans forward, forearms pressing into his knees, closing the distance without realizing it. His demanding questions for details keep coming:

"Did he wear a . . . ?"

"How many . . . ?"

"Did he . . . ?"

"Did you . . . ?"

"Was it good for you?"

Finally, a crack, not in Richard's volume, but in his rhythm. Less precise, like it slipped out before he could shape it. The questions stop.

My body jerks like I might throw up. But it isn't nausea from food; it's from truth. The truth rises fast and violent, demanding to come out.

And I let it. I answer Richard, one question after another in quick honest blows, never breaking the eye contact he commanded from the start:

"Yes."

"A lot of times."

"Yes."

"Yes."

"Every time."

My final answer detonates. I know it as soon as it leaves me. It cuts. I didn't mean to be cruel. But it's true. And it fell out of my mouth at the speed of it all. My voice surprises me. Calm. Even. There's no trembling. No bargaining. Richard asked. I answered.

Somewhere deep down, a softer version of me recognizes how brutal this must feel for him. But I don't pull back. I don't edit. The part of me that has been hiding and swallowing and reshaping truth for years is done doing that. The release I feel is overwhelming.

Richard's anger is real. But beneath it, I see something else. Humiliation. It's there in the way he holds himself too rigidly, like posture might keep everything else from slipping. His shoulders square, but not naturally. Forced, as if he's trying to occupy more space than he feels entitled to. There's a flush that creeps in, covering every inch of his cheeks, like rosacea, a color he can't control. It betrays him even as the rest of him tries not to.

I didn't just betray him privately. I cracked the image and the carefully managed story of who we were: The happy couple. It's the narrative Richard cares most about. How it looks. I get it. I've lived it. Honestly, I'm the one who's been protecting our image more than anyone. I built it.

But I can't do it. Not anymore.

There's something almost procedural about our exchange. Neither of us is crying. Neither of us sounds heartbroken. It's as if we're dissecting a body that has already died. If someone neutral were watching us in this car, they might find it strange that this conversation is happening at all because Rhett insisted it should. That I gave Richard a half-truth first, and he accepted it. That he only pushed harder when someone else told him he needed to.

If Richard truly wanted to save our marriage, wouldn't he

have canceled Aspen? Suggested counseling? Demanded we hole up somewhere and fight for it? Maybe, he didn't ask because he didn't want to know. Maybe, he didn't ask because he didn't want to cancel his hiking trip. I can relate. My reason for not telling him is because I didn't want to cancel New York. There's bitter symmetry in it. Perhaps the only thing we've remained aligned on is protecting our exits.

I know, without a doubt, Richard would rather be wandering the aisles of REI right now, stocking up on dehydrated meals and high-performance hiking socks, than sitting here in my car absorbing the anatomy of my betrayal. Richard and I . . . we've been hiking in different directions for years now. I've just been doing it in heels.

I can't help but wonder, if the tables were turned, would I be furious? Would I feel betrayed? Or would I feel . . . relieved? Would I demand every detail the way Richard just did? Would I want to know the mechanics of it all? Or would I cling to ignorance as a shield?

I think there was a version of me, years ago, that it absolutely would have shattered.

Back in 2004, when Richard and I were living in a beautiful floor-through apartment on 61st Street, he came home late. I didn't think too much of it until he said, "I need to tell you something."

His tone made my stomach drop. With his long days, late nights at the firm, and dinners entertaining clients alongside polished colleagues and chic, self-possessed women—infidelity had crossed my mind more than once. I'd always brushed it off as immaturity, my own FOMO, or maybe even some lingering narrative about my own daddy issues.

But hearing him like that, I couldn't help but wonder if I was dismissing it too quickly or recognizing something I didn't want to name?

Richard and I weren't having sex often by any couple's standards, but especially for a couple in our early 20s. I fibbed about our sex life to friends, even my close ones. The truth embarrassed me. I felt defective. Delinquent. Ugly. Unworthy of touch. Trapped by the lack of desire to touch him. Richard would occasionally voice frustration, but not aggressively. Over time, I leaned into the assumption that maybe he didn't want me either. It was a tidy solution to my own indifference.

We stood beneath the apartment's high ceilings in the candlelit glow from a fireplace full of ivory pillar candles, camouflaging the lack of logs, while he struggled to begin.

"I don't know how to say this. I'm ashamed," he confessed.

"Of what?" I asked, bracing. My palms got clammy. My throat dry.

That old, familiar feeling slipped in—the one from childhood, when my name was called from the other room and I could hear it in the tone before I knew the reason. The slow walk toward the formal living room. The way the apricot faille wingback always felt a little too hard, too upright. The pause before my mom began talking, suspended with possibility. I never knew which version it would be—something I'd done, something my parents had done, or a lesson disguised as concern that left us all feeling uncomfortable.

Richard continued, "Lately, after work, I've started going to strip clubs. For lap dances."

Of all the possibilities circling around my brain, this wasn't one. Richard having a fling with an intelligent, chic lawyer at the firm who reads *The New York Times* front to back and loves rhetoric? Sure. My brain could get there. But lap dances from unsanitary strippers, spinning on germ-filled poles? The sting surprised me.

"Like with guys from work?" I asked. "Do you feel pressured to fit in or something?"

Richard shook his head. For a second, I thought he might cry.

"No," he answered. "I've been going by myself. It started out of curiosity and then . . . "

I raised my hand to stop him. Diana Ross style. I didn't want the rest. But he continued anyway.

He went on about his loneliness, circling it like it was something I should have already seen. He said I'm distant. Untouchable. That word hit harder than the rest. Mostly, because I knew it was true. When I felt depressed, I retreated, inward. Hiding.

Richard continued explaining his physical curiosity in broad terms, almost theoretical at first. Like it wasn't about anyone in particular, just the idea of wanting more, something exciting. And then, more plainly, he told me that I don't satisfy it. There was no cruelty in the way he said it. That was almost worse.

He said he feels detached from me. That I'm not really here anymore. That I'm like a version of myself—recognizable but hollowed out. An empty shell.

He kept talking and talking, like if he just explained it clearly enough, it would all make sense to me. Said that he just wanted to feel something. Anything. Even if only on the surface. Even if it was with someone who didn't matter.

But underneath all of it was the steady implication: I drove him there. Straight to the poles, and not the voting kind.

Truthfully, he wasn't wrong about my withdrawal. Or any of it really. I was detached—from him, from myself, from almost everything at that point. But Richard's loneliness didn't erase the ick of what he did.

Going to a strip club alone. No bachelor party crew. Before sunset. The image formed instantly. Lonely men in business casual, laptop bags slung over shoulders, searching for something transactional and fleeting. It felt desperate. Sad.

More than anything, I was shocked he told me. Why confess? Why place that image in my head? Why make it real? Was there actually more to tell?

"Promise me you won't tell Greer and Addy," he demanded.

Weird, he went there first.

"You don't need to worry about that," I told him. And I meant it. I didn't want to share it. I didn't want to know it myself. I needed distance from it.

I walked into the bedroom for space and put on *The Notebook*. We'd bought it on DVD a few days ago. It was dark and cold in the room. I pulled the duvet back and let my hands slide under the cool side of the pillow. The film's peaceful opening scene filled the room with a warm orange glow, mirroring the sunrise reflecting on the lake outside Allie's window. I decided to let someone else's epic love story fill the room for a while.

Back then, a little part of me shattered inside. My depression swooped in hard and fast. The meds from my NYC doctors missed the marks. I built walls around myself. Honestly, Richard didn't have a chance.

What hurt then feels obvious now. Of course, he was lonely. I was, too. Lonely and confused and lost. And now, oddly, all I wish is that he had properly cheated all those years ago, so then, this whole thing could be a cat's game of Tic-Tac-Toe.

Though, I know that's not really how it works.

"Let's see what an absolute cliché you are, Morgan," Richard says, his tone turning angrier than before I answered all his questions. "What is he some big deal fashion exec?"

"Actually, no," I spit out. "He's an unemployed accountant from Ohio."

The response is like lighting a match to gasoline. Something in Richard gives way the moment Brett becomes a real person, not some faceless fantasy, not some reckless fling. He is no longer a caricature of a man, but a normal, competent person.

If I had cheated with some arrogant cliché, a flashy villain, maybe Richard could reduce it to a joke. Maybe he could frame me as foolish, blinded by ego, and taken in by someone obviously beneath him. He could roll his eyes and call it predictable.

The idea that I chose someone grounded, someone without theatrics, spins Richard out. It means this isn't about rebellion or chaos. It means I had found something real. And that reality unleashes something feral in Richard. The anger doesn't flare, it bleeds out of him.

To Richard, it isn't just about sex anymore. It isn't even about betrayal in the physical sense. It is about comparison. About replacement. About the possibility that someone else offered me something he either couldn't or wouldn't.

"You fucking slut," he accuses, his voice flat. "All these years, all these things I've done for you, given you, and this is what I get!? You are an embarrassment. I hope you're ready to be penniless, homeless, and alone. You'll get nothing from me. I'm going to tell EVERYONE what you've done, knock you down from that goddamn pedestal people put you on." His voice raises with every slur.

To survive the moment, I leave it. Not physically, I'm still in the car, still pinned under the weight of Richard's anger, but mentally, I'm gone.

Brett's face floods my mind. His effortless curls that refuse to be tamed. The white shirt, never overly pressed, one button too low. The ripped jeans. His strong hands. His contagious smile. I want nothing more than to be wrapped in his arms. Out of this suffocating car. Out of Dallas. Out of this version of my life. Free.

My tears come suddenly, violently. Not graceful. They spill over before I can stop them. Richard keeps spewing words like knives at me.

He's right though. I was never meant to be on that pedestal. It was built by expectation, by image, by playing a role too long. The perfect girl. The good wife. The college sweetheart who made it work.

But that's not why I'm crying. I'm not crying because I'm afraid of losing my place on the pedestal. I'm not crying because the church ladies will whisper. I'm not even crying because Richard is calling me horrible names. I'm crying because, somewhere along the way, I have become someone I barely recognize.

I don't know how to unwind myself without hurting everyone. I can feel the ground shifting beneath me, and there is no version of the future that doesn't cost something enormous. I know, deep down, that even if Brett disappears from my life tomorrow, my marriage will still be broken.

Because I'm finally, fully exposed. The tears aren't shame. They're grief. For the life I thought I was building. For the version of me that tried so hard to be good. For the fact that freedom and destruction are arriving hand in hand.

"Get out of the driver's seat," Richard snaps. "I'm driving home. The last thing I need is you hysterically crying and driving off the road. Everyone would blame me. You'd be the victim then, not me."

Victim. That's where his mind goes. Not, our marriage is falling apart. Not, we need help.

I push the car door open and step out. July wraps around me like wet wool. The air is unmoving. My tears mix instantly with sweat dripping, mascara trailing, salt stinging my lips. My body won't stop shaking, just a deep, internal quake I can't stop.

I've never believed Richard would physically hurt me. The way he squeezes my knee and tightly grips my arm is about control, not violence. But tonight, his behavior feels different. Not necessarily dangerous, but volatile, like something brittle has finally snapped.

I don't want to get back in the car with him. I don't want to go back to our apartment. I don't want to sit in any space with him. But I walk around the car anyway, submissively, and I slide into the passenger seat. Click the seatbelt. Fold into myself. Small. Silent. Trying to take up less oxygen.

Richard pulls out of the parking lot without looking at me. In all the times he's been "fed up," this time feels final. And a small, shameful ounce of relief moves through me.

He's done, too. There's something clarifying about mutual surrender. Then, he says it.

"Call your mom right now," he insists. "Tell her what you've done. Tell her every terrible detail. Tell her to come get you immediately, or you'll have nowhere to sleep tomorrow."

His cruelty is precise. He knows exactly where to strike. Honestly, I find it fair, and his words are not surprising at all.

My mother is the one person who loves me without terms. Of course, Richard wants to make me confess to her in real time, to force the humiliation out loud.

I would choose Brett again. I would do it all again. I know that. Even now, with the wreckage unfolding in real time, I know I would. And I know, without question, that my mom will always have my back. She has proven it over and over. Fierce loyalty. Unwavering love. But the thought of telling her like this, with Richard in the driver's seat, listening, correcting, interjecting, makes my skin crawl.

I'm not afraid of Mom's judgment. I'm afraid that her feelings will be hurt. I'm afraid that she will somehow blame herself for my silence, for my inability to open up to her. I should have told her before now. I should have told her when I called on the drive back from Newark. Before secrets calcified. Before other people were involved. Before this became a spectacle. Maybe it would have saved me.

I press and hold the #2 key on my BlackBerry. Memory dial. Mom's landline. She should be home. Cordless phones are always scattered everywhere. Kitchen counter, bathroom sink, patio table, like a trail of breadcrumbs. One is always within reach.

She answers on the second ring. "Hi, Boo! What's up?" she asks, always making sure I know my call is wanted.

Richard thinks this phone call will shatter me. He doesn't understand that she is my foundation. I open my mouth. Nothing. No words. Just loud, unfiltered, guttural sobs that surprise even me. Not the silent, controlled tears I've been leaking since yesterday. This is different. This is body-deep, animalistic crying.

I cried like this when Greer moved to London, but that was temporary. She was back in five months. Plus, no one saw it.

I cried like this when I was 8 years old, and my dad told me he was in love with Becky and might leave us. Though, my tears turned out to be premature because my mom and dad stayed together another eight years before he left for good.

But it's the same cry. The kind that feels like the floor just disappeared from underneath you. There's something about betrayal and departure that hooks into the child version of me.

"Morgan?" my mom asks. Her voice tightens immediately. No more pep. Just alert. "Honey, what's wrong?"

I can feel Richard beside me. Silent now. Waiting.

"I messed up," I finally choke out. "I messed up really badly."

There's no sharp inhale. No immediate interrogation. Only her routine breathing on the other end.

"Okay," she says gently. "Start wherever you can."

Not, what did you do? Not, how could you? Just. Start.

I glance at Richard. He's listening for shame. He loses patience with my inability to speak and yanks the phone from my hands. The motion is fast. Sharp. Forceful enough to make my breath hitch. He's never been a physically imposing man. He tells people he's 5-foot-11, but I've stood next to him in bare feet enough times to know that's a generous estimate. His build is average, a little soft around the edges. Not out of shape, just undefined.

Richard could never scoop me up effortlessly the way Brett does, spinning me and making me feel weightless and wanted. But in this moment, Richard feels enormous. My failure inflates him. Fills the space. He looms over me like some distorted version of a genie, swollen with power, but instead of granting wishes or cracking jokes, he spits fury.

I slide lower into the passenger seat, pressing into the perforated leather, wishing I could dissolve into it. Vanish. Evaporate.

"Mona," he barks into the phone, "come get your daughter. You need to get here as fast as you can."

I hear my mother's voice faintly, trying to interject, but he plows over it.

"Morgan, tell her," he demands. "Tell her what you've done."

He thrusts the phone back toward me. It slips for a second. My fingers fumble before catching it. I bring it to my ear, hand shaking.

"Mom . . ." I begin. My voice is wrecked. "I . . ."

"Boo," she says, steady and calm, cutting through the chaos in the car. "Are you safe right now?"

"Yes," I whisper. "I'm safe."

Richard exhales sharply beside me, angry at the direction this is going.

"I made a mess," I continue, trying to breathe through the sobs. "I cheated. I had an affair."

It's out. Silence on the other end for a second. She's processing.

"Okay," she says, her words measured. "We will figure this out." No yelling. No panic. Just a unified "we."

Richard huffs in frustration. "You don't understand, Mona," he says, interrupting again. "It wasn't just emotional. She . . . "

My mom cuts him off, politely but firmly.

"Richard," she says, in a cool voice now. Controlled. "I will talk to my daughter. You don't need to narrate." The shift is subtle but powerful.

For the first time since Richard and I left the Starbucks parking lot, the power dynamic changes.

I'm still shaking. Still ashamed. Still responsible for what I've done. But I'm not alone in this seat anymore. Richard wanted a spectacle. What he got was a mother.

I feel like a dog. No, it's worse. I'm like a mutt with her master's hand clamped around her snout, nose shoved into a mess she made, forced to inhale the evidence until shame becomes obedience.

That's what this feels like. Not accountability. Forced submission. When I'm with Richard, my default is obedience. It's efficient. It costs less energy than pushing back. Less conflict. Less escalation.

But something strange happens when I'm away from him. With distance, his voice, that flat, disappointed monotone, fades from my head. It's almost hypnotic when I'm around him, as his disapproval seeps into everything I do. When I'm gone long enough, his voice quiets in my mind. I remember what my own thoughts sound like. I become someone I can tolerate again. Not perfect. Not manic-free. Not saintly. Just . . . me.

I'm not "the Morgan he signed up for." As if there was a pristine, perfectly calibrated wife he was promised and then somehow swapped out. I'm not even sure the girl he references ever existed. Maybe she was 19 and masking her true self. Maybe she was manic and sparkling. Maybe she was just trying very hard to be lovable.

I have spent years chasing her.

Therapy. Medication. Dosage adjustments. New doctors. Journaling. Faith counseling. Lifestyle changes. Sleep hygiene. Food tracking. Mood charts. I've made every attempt to sand down the edges and return to the version of myself Richard believes he married.

Trying to "be" her. Trying to earn back approval. Trying to fit into a silhouette that shrinks every time I almost reach it. At some point, it stopped being about managing bipolar disorder. It became about managing Richard's comfort. And I am exhausted. Not from being ill. From feigning wellness.

Several months before our wedding, I went on birth control. My gynecologist recommended starting six months ahead of time so my body could "adjust," and so I could manipulate the dosing schedule to avoid having my period during the wedding or honeymoon. If I'm honest, that manipulation felt like the real reason. Southern brides and pristine are practically synonyms. God forbid one of us bleed beneath a white, poofy veil.

Birth control and I didn't jive. Or at least, that's what I told myself.

Looking back, I'm not sure that was entirely true. Many bipolar symptoms surface in your early 20s. The timing aligned. But the pill was an easy villain. The hormones got blamed for everything—the mood swings, the crying spells, the self-harm thoughts, the insomnia, the disappearing sex drive.

After Richard and I returned to Dallas from his semester abroad and after my Parisian spell, he pressed me to get things "sorted out." I made the promise that I would, so as soon as we got back, I started seeing a new doctor, a man. I wasn't thrilled about seeing a male gynecologist, but the appointment took months to secure, and Richard was being insufferable.

At the appointment, I listed my symptoms carefully: depression, erratic sleep, intrusive thoughts, anxiety. Somewhere in the middle, almost as an aside, I mentioned that I have no real sex drive.

Out of my entire list, which included suicidal ideation, and emotional volatility, my doctor exclusively latched onto my lack of sex drive. He prescribed testosterone on the spot. To "balance" me out. Nothing for the depression. Nothing for the lack of sleep. Nothing for the despair. My libido took center stage.

I'll never forget that doctor. Slender. A Texas tan. Slightly longer hair than the conservative male doctors I grew up around. Mid-to-late 40s, easily more than double my age at the time.

While my bottom hung on for dear life at the end of the paper-covered exam table, my legs spread open, my socked feet awkwardly resting in metal stirrups in the utmost vulnerable position, he began explaining how to apply the testosterone cream he prescribed. I assumed the exam was over.

It wasn't.

He stayed there between my legs, talking about a "magic cream," the cure-all that would fix my sex drive and my sadness in one convenient swipe. Then, without warning, his verbal instructions became a physical demonstration.

He didn't announce what he was about to do. He didn't ask permission. He simply spread his fingers and touched me, stroking, demonstrating, telling me this is where I should apply the cream each night, rubbing it in "until it fully absorbs."

"Or," he added with a casual, off-putting chuckle, "you could let your husband do this part."

My body tensed. He saw the disgust register on my face. He pulled his hand away quickly, peeled off his gloves, and his demeanor.

"We're done here," he said sharply. "You can get your prescription on the way out."

I failed his unspoken test. My discomfort was the problem, not his actions. I walked out in a daze.

In my gut, I knew what the doctor had said and done wasn't just off-color joking. It was wrong. A physician should never use authority that way. But I was 22. Scared and unsure of myself. Who was I to accuse a doctor? Perhaps I misunderstood. Maybe his behavior was normal, and I was the perverted one for thinking otherwise.

So, I did nothing. I picked up the prescription even though I had no intention of using it. I couldn't go home empty-handed. Richard was desperate for a solution, so I paid the $15 co-pay, took the white paper bag stuffed with instructions, and drove back to our apartment.

Later, when I actually read the cream's instructions, my insides filled with rage. It said to apply the cream to "wrists, lower abdomen, or inner thigh."

Not one mention of genital application. Not one. On top of feeling violated, I now needed to find another doctor.

And starting over in mental health care is its own special version of hell. Every new appointment requires you to unpack your entire psyche like a suitcase dumped onto the floor. Why can't mental health be charted like a broken bone or a past surgery? Why do we have to narrate our worst chapters from scratch every single time?

It doesn't make modern-day sense.

I put the phone back up to my ear, glancing down to see mascara tear stains all down the front of my ivory blouse.

"Mom," I say, struggling to catch my breath, "I slept with someone. It started back in June. Richard wants me out of the apartment immediately. Can you please . . . please come to Dallas and get me? I need you." I can hardly get the words out before Richard takes the phone back.

"Let us know what time you will arrive," he tells my mom. "I'm taking her home to pack a suitcase now."

"Richard!" I can hear Mom's rage through the phone. I know it's not directed at me. I think she's always hated him, but out of respect to me, she's done her best to hide it. Now, all bets are off.

"I'll be there first thing tomorrow morning," Mom says. "But please tell me, do you think she is stable? Is she safe?"

"She's fine," he says and hangs up.

I sense Richard is still talking. Words aimed at me. They hover somewhere near my face and dissolve before reaching my ears. The car is heavy with his voice, sharp, relentless, bouncing off the windows, the dashboard, my skin.

At some point, my body stops absorbing it. It rolls off me, like water off a duck's back.

Along the way, Richard runs out of ammunition. Or maybe he grows tired of firing into the silence. We pull into the garage and walk up the stairs without a word. He would never make a public scene. It allows a temporary reprieve, until the apartment door shuts behind us. The second it closes, I walk straight to our shared closet.

My carry-on is still tucked in the back of the closet, half-packed for New York. Seeing it there makes my chest tighten. God, I wish I could call Brett.

Richard follows me in. Our walk-in closet, usually spacious, lined with neatly hung shirts and color-coded dresses, suddenly feels like a crawl space. The lighting is dimmer. The smell of leather handbags and shoes mixes with lavender sachets, tucked here and there, and the lingering scent of Agent Provocateur from blazers and cocktail dresses yet to be dry-cleaned, for budgeting purposes no less.

"Who knows?" Richard demands. "Who all knows the truth? Was this some big joke between you and the Twins? Hiding it from me all summer while you gallivanted around New York, out until dawn?"

I suppose most happily married women don't frolic through Manhattan without their husbands until sunrise. But then again, I can't recall how happily married feels, so what do I know?

"Greer knows a lot," I say carefully, while starting to fill a duffle bag with the basics: jammies, undies, a few simple day dresses and sandals. "But she's not in on it. No one's ganging up on you. This is all me. I'm the only one to blame."

I hesitate. He steps outside the walk-in and paces up and down the small hallway that connects to our bedroom on the left and the bathroom on the right. His feet leave imprints in the shag-like carpet.

"Is that really what you're worried about?" I ask. "Who knows?"

I shouldn't have said it. I know the rhythm by now. Let him win, and it spends itself faster. Push back, and it escalates. Tonight, I pushed.

"I guess you'll blame your 'disease' for this, won't you?" he says, lifting his hands to mime air quotes, the contempt unmistakable.

The "disease." It's the thing he tolerates publicly and resents privately.

"No," I say, "I won't." My voice is steady now. The tears are gone. I'm strangely calm. Hollow, almost.

He watches me, waiting for the deflection.

"I think I'm probably in a hypomanic state right now," I continue, squeezing my now overpacked duffle between my knees to get the zipper to close. "But that's not the full picture."

The air tightens.

"Maybe mania lowered the barrier when I first met Brett," I explain. "Maybe it compromised my judgment. But it continued because I wanted it to. Bipolar or not."

I swallow, desperately wishing for any kind of liquid. Thinking bourbon would make this easier, while knowing water is the better choice. "I did this," I admit. "No excuses. I'm not blaming anything or anyone."

There's a long pause. "But mania aside," I add, my voice rising despite myself, "I don't regret it. And I'm sorry. I'm sorry I'm not who you thought I was or who you want me to be. I'm sorry I can't be that girl."

Another beat. I hear it come out of me before I can soften it. "Honestly, I don't want to be that girl," I confess. The words echo in the closet, bouncing back at us from the overly textured walls, smaller and harsher each time. That was it. A nail, clean and deliberate, in my own coffin. Richard erupts. It's not subtle. His restraint gives way all at once, like he's been waiting for this moment so he can meet it head-on.

"Oh, you don't?" he comes back, sharper now, louder.

And then it starts.

He doesn't ask anymore—he lists. Repeats. Reframes. Every detail I've already given him comes back, stripped of anything soft, arranged to hit harder. There's a force to it now, a tempo that doesn't leave space for interruption. He's not trying to understand. He's making sure I understand. There's something almost methodical in it—the way he keeps going, keeps pressing, like he's determined to grind it down to something undeniable. Something I can't escape.

This isn't anger looking for answers. This is anger that's found its footing. And now, it wants to make sure I stay exactly where he's put me. I try to let his words float down the theoretical carpet river of our hallway, but my cognitive therapy skills need more advanced practice to observe and release—they keep catching. And they're pulling me down. Further and further.

My madness has slowly killed my marriage for years. The affair was the slaughter.

When Richard tires of listing all the bad things coming my way, he takes a green bottle of Rolling Rock from the fridge, flips on the TV, and crashes on the couch.

He spoke a lot of truth.

I am a mess. A sinner. The outlier now. No longer neatly aligned with Greer and Addy's manicured lives of charity luncheons, ranch weekends, and country club ease. I'm the fracture in the Jet Set Lingerie trio. A disgrace.

Richard will make sure the story travels. Everyone in our circle will know of my brokenness. They'll learn that I'm unstable. That I'm impulsive. That I can't be trusted to hold a life together, much less a marriage.

They'll know that I was distant. Cold, even. That I made myself unavailable in ways that justified what came next. They'll hear about my diagnosis, carefully placed, not cruel, just enough to explain me. To make it all make sense.

They'll learn I'm the kind of woman who stepped outside her marriage without hesitation. Who blurred the lines easily. Who didn't think far enough ahead to understand the consequences.

Some will decide I've always been like this, that it was only a matter of time. A few might grant grace, call it a phase, a breakdown, something temporary. But even that will carry its own kind of distance.

And what won't be said, but will be understood, is that I became someone they wouldn't quite know how to hold onto anymore. Not fully. Not the same way. It all feels like more than one person should be asked to hold. I want to make it stop.

And now, there's Brett. He's planning a new venture in China, stepping into something expansive and promising. A new city. A new title. A future with clean lines stretching ahead of him. He doesn't need this weight. No one does. Not even me.

I walk into the kitchen. Our apartment has an open-concept floor plan—the living room, dining room, and kitchen all bleeding into each other with the same bland laminate floors. Only the bedroom and bathroom are closed off. There is really nowhere to hide here.

Richard is staring at the TV, jaw tight, not even glancing up.

I open the cabinet and take down a Waterford Marquis tumbler, our wedding registry glassware. My mom and I used to laugh about those shipments. Box after box arrived at her house, most of them rattling with shattered pieces because the company couldn't be bothered to wrap them properly. Nine out of 10 were broken before they even reached us. Little crystal omens. Like spending my engagement night at a Super 8.

I pull the pitcher of Crystal Light pink lemonade from the fridge and pour a glass to the very top, meniscus style. I set the pitcher back inside and rest the glass carefully on the island, staring at the speckled, outdated granite.

The island drawers have always been a fight, two oversized junk drawers that refuse to stay organized. I've sorted them a dozen times, but they revert to chaos almost immediately.

I slide open the left one and reach deep into the back, past the

Gorilla Glue and past random screws and receipts and matchbooks from forgettable Dallas restaurants. My fingers close around three prescription bottles.

Klonopin. Full.

My doctor prescribed the medicine to help me sleep. Instead, it makes me jittery and restless. I stopped taking it but kept filling the script each month. They've been collecting in the back of this drawer like spare change. Finding the right cocktail of drugs to stabilize me feels like a lifetime project.

"You know," Richard says suddenly, eyes still fixed on the TV, "your beloved Duvalls? They hate cheaters. They'll take my side."

I don't respond. My mouth has caused enough damage today. Besides, choosing sides feel irrelevant. What does social allegiance matter now? I've spent 28 years being good, and it'll be erased in a single headline. I can't make it quiet fast enough.

I slip all three bottles into the tiny side pocket of my black mini skirt. They bulge awkwardly against the fabric. I pick up my overfilled glass and walk to the bedroom. I close the door. The click hangs in the air.

I sit down in the narrow hallway outside the closet. The contractor-grade carpet scratches against my legs. I stretch them out in front of me, ankles crossed, shoes still on, the same spectator wedges I wore to Gemma, less than a month ago.

For half a second, I'm back in that taxi. Crossing Bowery. Heart racing. About to meet a man who might change everything. But I don't deserve that life. I didn't properly earn it.

The glass sweats in my hand. The pills press against my thigh. All I can think is I need out. Now. Even if it's only for a moment.

I open each pill bottle, lining them up like little toy soldiers.

I pop 15 pills from the first bottle. Down the shoot with a big gulp of tart pink lemonade. Only five calories a serving and all I had been drinking the last few days.

The next 15 pills go down easier. Like my body knows exactly what to do. It's surprising because I have always hated swallowing pills.

Four more gulps.

Half a bottle of pills each, chased by Crystal Light, and I'm done.

Everything narrows.

Then smaller, and smaller.

Then gone.

The curtain closes.

Only darkness is left.

Chapter 17
THE ALLY

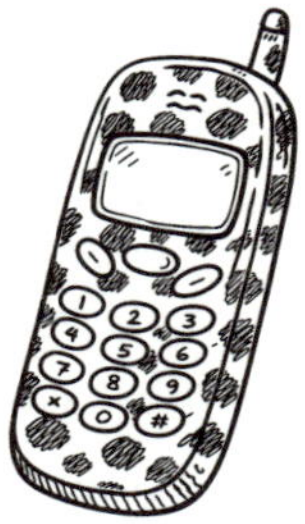

JULY 17, 2009
Afternoon—Legacy Hospital
Dallas, Texas

I wake to voices I know. They're low, almost reverent, like church whispers. One male voice, Richard's. The others sweeter, layered together—my mom, Greer, and Addy. For a second, I think I'm dreaming. My head feels pressurized, like it's been sealed inside a pot about to whistle. My eyelids are impossibly heavy, stitched shut with invisible thread. I pry them open anyway.

The ceiling is wrong. Speckled tiles in a grid. Fluorescent light is dulled to evening dim. A curved metal track suspends baby blue curtains around my bed. Guardrails rise on either side of me, boxing in a narrow twin-size mattress layered with stiff white sheets and a thin polyester blanket in the same institutional blue as the curtains.

Sterile. Everywhere. My right arm throbs. I glance down without lifting my head. Bruises ladder my forearm. A clear tube snakes from my skin to an IV bag hanging on a metal pole. I'm wearing a hospital gown. It's white flannel, dotted with tiny pink and blue flowers and trimmed in darker blue piping. My throat burns. Raw. My nose stings like it's been scrubbed from the inside. No one notices my eyes open. They're absorbed in their hushed conference. One voice is missing.

"Where is Brett?" I whisper.

The words barely make it out. My mouth is desert dry. My lips cling to my teeth, like I've forgotten how saliva works. In an instant, Greer and Addy are at my left side. My mom appears on my right. They move like a rehearsed trio, shushing me gently, wrapping arms around my shoulders, clasping my hands.

"I need to call him," I try. "He has to be wondering where I am."

Why are they shushing me? Why aren't they helping? My head drops back against the pillow. It's too heavy to hold upright. My limbs feel like they are filled with wet sand. The room is hazy, like I'm looking through frosted glass. I can't focus on anything for long.

"No, no, Pip," Greer murmurs, squeezing my hand. "Not right now."

"Morgie, I'm here," my mom says. Her eyes are swollen, glassy with tears, but she forces a steady smile for me. A shadow moves behind her. Richard steps forward.

He looks tired and empty but still composed. Showered. Pressed chinos. Navy half-zip. The uniform of control. He's the only one who appears fresh. My mom, Greer, and Addy look like they've been here for ages. Wrinkled clothes. Smudged mascara. Hair twisted into careless knots.

I have no idea what time it is. Or what day. The light filtering through the narrow hospital window is golden and low. The sun is setting.

"What day is it?" I ask.

"It's late Friday afternoon. You've been out of it for over 24 hours. Have somewhere to be?" Richard quips sarcastically.

I try to rewind. Why am I here? Why am I not in New York? Why does everyone look shaken, like they've just watched something almost irreversible happen?

Everyone except Richard. He doesn't look scared. He looks inconvenienced. Tapped out. His patience seems burned clean through. If emotions were a pie chart, his would be labeled: put out.

And then the flashbacks hit me, in shards. My left palm. Small blue tablets. Each stamped with a "K." The sharp citrus taste of powdered pink lemonade. The pills stacked awkwardly at the back of my tongue, chalky and uncooperative, refusing to go down all at once. My eyes clamp shut.

Fluorescent lights flash in my memory. Rapid, white, blinding. A strobe above me. I'm horizontal. Strapped down. Something hard beneath my back. There are large black streaks running down the front of my ivory blouse. Mascara? Vomit? Both? The image freezes there. Nothing after.

The fog doesn't lift. The weight of it, what I did, what almost happened doesn't settle yet. It's like my brain is buffering, refusing to load the full file. All I can think is that I need to call Brett. Before I can even ask, Richard steps forward and holds out my phone. I stare at it.

"This will be the last time you have access to this for a while," he says evenly.

Even through the haze, I understand the implication. The adulteress doesn't get privileges.

"Pippy," Addy says gently, leaning close. "You need to call Brett. Tell him it's really over. Tell him you're going to work on your marriage. You can do this."

Her eyes are pleading. She wants to rewind the world to before all of this happened.

My mom is already handing me a massive cup of water, packed with crushed ice and a bendy straw. She knows my throat won't cooperate without it. She doesn't look entirely convinced calling Brett is what I should do, but she stays quiet.

Her quiet is out of character. Normally, she would step in. Redirect. Ask questions Richard doesn't want asked. But not now. Even in the haze, I can see it. In the window of my unconsciousness, he had a moment with her. Already framed the situation. Already made it clear, in his way, who's in charge here.

I push myself upright and try to stand. The room spins. Greer grabs my left hand. Addy steadies my waist. I'm embarrassingly weak, leaning into them like a child learning to walk. We shuffle to the far corner of the room, as if distance will somehow manufacture privacy. It won't. The room is too small. I can feel all of them behind me.

I dial from memory. Five rings. Voicemail.

"Leave him a message," Greer whispers. "Then, this can be over. You can start fresh."

She means well. She always does. I swallow. My voice comes out unfamiliar, flat, stripped of color.

"Hey . . . it's me," I say, starting the voice message.

Silence swells. I don't want to say the next words. I don't want to end it. But I am outnumbered. And weak. And dependent. So, I let them feed me the script.

"It's Morgan," I continue. "I'm calling to tell you this is over. I need to work on my marriage. I can't see you anymore. I'm not coming to New York. I'm going to stay married."

The words feel foreign in my mouth. "Goodbye," I finish, void of emotion, as if it's coming from somewhere outside of me.

Tears surge up, hot and immediate, but I swallow them back. I will not give Richard the satisfaction of more hysteria. I lower the phone. The air feels sucked out of the room.

And then, salvation. A nurse steps inside, clipboard in hand. I have never been so grateful for an interruption.

"What on earth are you doing out of bed, Miss Morgan!?" she gasps.

Her voice is warm and booming, wrapped in a syrupy Southern drawl that somehow fills every sterile corner of the room. "Now I'm thrilled to see you've come back to us," she says, "but get yo' bottom back in that bed. It is far too early for you to be standing. You're gonna be foggy for a good long bit." She winks. "You are one lucky girl, you know that? Most people your size wouldn't survive this."

She says it like a victory. Like she personally pulled me back.

It's obvious this nurse has bonded with everyone in my hospital room over the last day. She offers a side hug for my mom, a squeeze of Greer's shoulder, a knowing look at Addy. She moves to my bedside, adjusting monitors, checking my IV, close enough to read the exhaustion etched across my face. She's in her mid-50s, maybe, and the kind of woman who has seen everything and knows when to protect her patient from the world.

"Now friends," she says, turning her back slightly to Richard, addressing only the women, "it's about closing time. Sure, she's been sleeping, but her body needs real rest. Uninterrupted rest. I'm giving you a 15-minute warning, ladies."

Then, after a beat, she adds, "Richard, as her husband, you're allowed to stay." Her tone drops for that last sentence.

Another knock. A doctor this time. Crisp. Efficient. A chart tucked against her chest.

"Good evening, nice to see you're finally awake," she says, not unkindly, but without the nurse's same charisma. "Here are the results of the tests that were requested for you."

The doctor hands me a folder.

"Requested for me?" I ask, my voice genuinely curious, still scratchy from the tubes. I glance inside the folder quickly. "Are these standard tests for suicide attempts?"

It seems unlikely I was the one who requested anything, considering everyone keeps mentioning how long I was unconscious.

"No," she says carefully. "They're not standard in overdose cases. But your husband requested them. For your safety."

The word safety hangs in the air. She glances toward Richard in a way that feels . . . cautious. Richard does not have power of attorney over me. I know that much. There's no world in which he should've been able to authorize any unnecessary testing or treatment without my consent. I open the folder fully. Heavy silver prongs hold a stack of papers in place. Across the top of the first page, in bold type:

LABORATORY RESULTS

My name. The date. A vertical list.

To see every STD under the sun listed so closely beside my own name—to see HIV there, too, negative or not—feels paralyzing. As a child of the '80's, I was taught to fear that disease above all else.

The letters feel enormous. Obscene. Clinical.

Conscious for only a matter of minutes, my mind is still fogged from sedation and survival, and suddenly, I'm staring at words that make me feel contaminated.

"You had all these tests run while I was unconscious?" I ask Richard, louder now. The doctor and my mom both turn toward us.

Richard doesn't hesitate. "I have to take care of myself, too," he says. "You could've given something to me."

He's furious. I understand it. But his fear outpaces our intimacy.

I hand the folder to him, my eyes fixed on the floor. "You're good," I say quietly. "All negative."

I can't bring myself to look at Greer or Addy. Shame floods every inch of me. Like what Brett and I had in New York has been translated into something contaminated with STD testing. Born in sin, how could it possibly be sacred? How could it last?

The doctor clears her throat and announces she's heading out for the evening. My nurse steps forward again, reclaiming the room with her gentle authority. "Alright now," she commands. "It's time for everybody to scoot. She needs sleep."

My mom leans in, kissing my forehead. Greer squeezes my hand. Addy brushes hair off my face. They look wrecked.

I'm grateful for the nurse. For her boundaries. For her insistence that my body needs quiet. But as they gather their things, one thought feels pressing: I need my mom. I need time alone with her. To tell her everything. To apologize.

Greer and Addy pack their things slowly, like leaving requires strategy. There are two rounds of hugs. Maybe three. Wet cheeks pressed together. Fingers gripping tighter than usual, like if they let go too fast, I might disappear again. I tell them what they already know: They have been my lifeline. They've stood beside me in every season, from awkward adolescence, heartbreaks, and business launches to funerals, weddings, and manic summers. I thank them for loving me in the good and in the bad.

When I piece together the timeline of the last 24 hours, the weight of it overwhelms me. Addy's husband drove her, five months pregnant, 13 hours through the night from Knoxville. They only stopped twice. Sam brought his exhausted, nauseous, growing-a-human wife across state lines because I swallowed a handful of pills. Well, a lot of handfuls.

Greer arrived at the hospital at the exact moment the ambulance doors opened. "I thought you were dead," she says, and her voice breaks in half. That sentence alone could undo me.

Their dad fought leukemia for 13 years, more than a decade of hospital corridors and whispered updates and holding hands that kept getting colder. The two of them have already exceeded any reasonable trauma quota for one lifetime. And I added to it.

They rushed to my side while they're both pregnant. While their bodies are busy building miracles. My tears don't stop. They just keep coming. I don't know how to make this up to them. I don't know if I ever will. When they finally step out of the room, I can feel the emotional temperature rise before Richard even speaks. He doesn't address me. He addresses my mother.

"Mona," he begins, "Morgan's life will never be the same again. I won't allow it." His voice is measured, almost professional.

"What if she had died and people thought I did it?" Richard continues. "Do you know how that would've ruined my life? What she's put me through deserves consequences."

Consequences.

"No computer, no phone, no travel," he declares. "She doesn't deserve any of it. She'll have to ask permission for everything, assuming I even let her stay."

He says it like a policy update. Like new terms and conditions. I hear every word. But something strange happens. Richard's words no longer pierce. They hover at the surface and fall away.

It's a bit fascinating really that, when he found me unconscious beside three empty pill bottles, his first instinct was not grief or fear, but reputation management. That someone might think he murdered me. It's such a dark thought it almost tips into absurdity.

He thinks my life will never be the same again. He's right. It won't. But not in the way he means. God saved me. And now, I have to go live the life He spared.

By some divine grace, I am still here. I survived myself. And if I have survived that, I can survive the fallout.

My mom isn't staying at the apartment with Richard. Obviously.

After his little speech, it's clear that this is in everyone's best interest. Another minute with him, and Mom might "spike his Tab with Drano," like Brenda in *Adventures in Babysitting*, an all-time favorite movie of mine. The ridiculousness of that line floats through my head and almost makes me smile. Haven't thought of Tab in a good bit . . .

Mom is staying with Greer and Rhett instead. She insisted she'd take a taxi back to their house, didn't want to burden them or make Greer wait up.

Per hospital policy, Mom walks out with Richard. Before she leaves, she hugs me so tightly my ribs ache. When we pull back, her eyes lock onto mine. She says nothing. Not the million things I know she's thinking. She holds them in, sensing that my guilt meter has already shattered the glass. I can barely hold her gaze. What I did was her worst nightmare. Even the thought of losing her only child is too much to bear, much less the actual possibility.

I wish I hadn't scared her. I wish I weren't manic. I wish the Twin's mom hadn't been forced to show up on her porch with a plane ticket already bought. I wish she hadn't had to drive 120 miles at 90 miles an hour to make that flight. I wish I didn't feel like a bipolar burden.

Letting Mom walk out the door feels wrong. I keep my goodbye to Richard brief.

"I'll come back tomorrow after I stop by the office," he says, like this is a routine check-in.

Fine by me. The longer he stays away, the better. As Mom follows him out, she looks back at me one more time. I mouth, I'll be okay, and force a smile.

The lights stay dim after they leave. The room exhales. So, do I. Without the adrenaline, my body crashes. My eyelids surrender.

It feels like I've only been asleep for a few minutes when I jolt awake. There's a stranger in my room. A nurse I haven't seen before. Younger. Alert. Watching.

"I'm so sorry to startle you," she says gently. "A nurse on duty has to check in every 15 minutes while you're on suicide watch."

"Oh," I say, the words feel heavy. "Okay. When does that end?"

"You have about 48 more hours to go," the nurse confirms. "Has no one explained that to you?"

"Not really. I woke up to a full audience," I say quietly. "And my husband was asking a lot of questions. I'm not sure I understood the answers. Would you mind going over it again?"

"Of course, sweetheart," she offers, pulling a chair close to my bed. "You'll be under mandatory watch for 72 hours total. After that, you'll be transferred to an inpatient psychiatric facility. They're currently checking for open beds that align with your insurance coverage. Once your time here is up, you'll be transported by ambulance to whichever facility has availability. You'll stay there as long as your care team deems necessary."

Each sentence feels like a brick stacking on my chest. Involuntary. Ambulance. As long as they see fit . . .

I start to feel boxed in by the details when there's a knock at the door. My heart jumps. It's irrational, wild, and hoping for something I know is impossible. For a split second, I picture an alternate universe where someone tracked Brett down and told him everything, and he rerouted his flight to sit beside my hospital bed.

"Boo, it's Mom," she says, coming in the room. "I forgot something, so they let me come back up . . . "

Not Brett on a white horse with pink peonies in hand. But exactly who I need.

"Is it possible she can stay . . . just a little longer?" I ask the nurse. My voice sounds small. Desperate.

The nurse checks her watch, then looks at us.

"I'll be back for my next check in about 15 minutes," she says, smiling. "You two don't get into too much trouble before then, okay?" She giggles lightly. I imagine that's how you survive a job like this, small jokes for levity.

"Thank you," my mom says before I can.

And when the door closes again, it's finally just us. As soon as the nurse disappears down the hallway, my mom moves fast. She steps to my bedside, her back to the door like a lookout, and instead of leaning in for a hug, she opens her palm. In it is her faux tortoiseshell-wrapped Nokia cell phone.

"What's Brett's number?" she asks quickly. "I know he's who you really need to talk to. Am I right?"

I nod before I can stop myself. Tears rush in, hot and grateful.

"How do moms always know?" I whisper.

"As long as I am on this earth, I will take care of you," she says, steady and certain. "Your happiness is my priority. Husbands sometimes come and go. But not moms. Certainly not me."

Her left hand squeezes mine.

"Now. Give it to me," she says.

"9 . . . 1 . . . 7 . . . 8 . . . 0 . . ."

Both of her hands fly up in front of my face, the phone still clutched dramatically in her right one.

"Wait. Stop!" she gasps. Her eyes widen. "His phone number is your birthday?"

She looks like she's just cracked a prime time mystery.

"Oh my gosh," I say, mostly to myself. "I never noticed that."

"Well, I came in here feeling bold," she says, lowering her voice conspiratorially, "but this has got to be a sign."

I know that statistically speaking, a New Yorker with a "917" area code having my birthday in their phone number isn't exactly divine intervention. But I let Mom have it. She deserves a win. She types in the rest as I call out the numbers and hands me the phone. My heart pounds. I don't know if Brett will answer an unfamiliar number.

The phone rings and rings and rings once more. The space between each tone stretches like a hem being let out—slow, deliberate, and just a touch longer than it should be. "Hello, this is Brett," he finally answers.

It takes a second for my throat to cooperate. "Hey . . . it's me."

There's an inhale on the other end. "Oh my God," he whispers. "It's you. Are you okay?"

He sounds stunned. Relieved. Afraid. I hear him murmur to someone, possibly his parents, that he needs to step away. The background noise evolves. Less clinking silverware, more distant city hum.

"I'm surprised to hear from you," he says. "I got your message as soon as I landed. It gutted me."

My heart sinks. "I'm so sorry," I say. "A lot has happened. I want to tell you everything, but it sounds like you're at dinner. WD-50? With your parents?"

I can see my plans so clearly: the borrowed Milly dress, the booth, his parents leaning in, amused by my stories, plates arriving with theatrical flourishes, and dry ice curling across the table.

"Of course, you can tell me anything," he says quickly. "I'm at dinner, yes, but all I've wanted is to hear your voice. To make sure you're okay. That voicemail . . . you didn't sound like you. Morgan, what's going on?"

The words lodge in my throat. "Things got really bad," I manage. "After we last talked. Everything came to a head and . . . "

My voice breaks. I can't stop the tears this time.

"Brett," I whisper, "I tried to kill myself."

Silence. Only sounds of city noise filtering faintly through his end. A passing car. A door shutting. He's moved outside. When he speaks, his voice is different. Stripped raw.

"Oh, Morgan . . . " He exhales shakily. "I am so, so sorry."

"It wasn't that I wanted to die," I rush to explain. "Not really. I just couldn't stand being inside my own body anymore. I needed it to stop. I needed out. Any way I could."

There's a long pause.

"I wish I had been there," he says barely above a whisper. "I wish I was there right now." Another breath. "Can I come to you?"

I didn't know how he would take it. Yes, I had told him about having bipolar, the diagnosis, the medications piled on my nightstand. But telling someone you're bipolar, or rather, you have bipolar, is theoretical. It's a story.

This? This is blood and bone. An actual suicide attempt. An ambulance. A 72-hour hold.

In my marriage, mental illness has always felt like something inconvenient. Something to fix. But suicide isn't manageable. It's catastrophic.

When Brett asks again if he can come see me, I explain why he can't. Mandatory hold. Locked doors. Limited visitors. I tell him how grateful I am that he even wants to be here.

"And ignore that voicemail," I add quickly. "That wasn't the real me. I was coached through it."

He doesn't hesitate. "I know."

So, I tell him everything. All the little details of my current situation. How long I have to stay in this hospital. That they're finding me a bed in a psychiatric facility. That I'll be transported by ambulance. That I won't have my phone. And for the first time, I don't feel shame saying it out loud. Not because I'm numb. Not because I'm detached. Because I don't feel judged.

Through the sounds of a Manhattan street, through sirens and muffled traffic, I can feel Brett's empathy. It's physical. Like a weighted blanket settling over my nervous system. Like someone has turned the volume down inside my chest. He isn't trying to fix me. He isn't trying to minimize it. He isn't making it about himself. He's just there.

After 45 minutes, and three exceedingly less gentle reminders from my suicide-watch nurse hovering nearby, Brett says he needs to go back inside to dinner with his parents.

I imagine them sitting at WD-50, confused, watching their son pace the sidewalk with a phone pressed tightly to his ear. I can't take on their confusion, though. Not tonight.

There are so many things I wish were different. The obvious one: that I hadn't swallowed handfulls of pills. The quieter one: that I was there at WD-50 with Brett instead. Wearing the borrowed dress. Meeting his parents. Talking about a future that belonged only to us.

But something stops the fantasy. Even if, someday, I do have the chance to meet Brett's parents, I will be damaged goods.

Not because of my illness, at least not for me. I can say "psychiatric hospital" without flinching, but divorcée? That label somehow feels worse. Who knew that being institutionalized would be easier to admit than failing at marriage?

"Morgan," Brett says gently, "I'm here for you. Whatever you need. I'll be there. Just say the word."

In mania, thoughts lie. They told me those 90 blue pills would rescue me. That they would erase the chaos. What they didn't say was that they could erase everything. Mania shrinks the future down to a pinhole. It removes consequences. It makes the present moment feel like the only moment that will ever exist.

"You are real, aren't you?" I ask him in earnest.

I glance down at my hospital gown, faded, wrinkled, patterned with tiny flowers. My face must be swollen. My nose raw. No makeup. No gloss. Nothing curated. If only I could see myself through Brett's eyes.

"Thank you for being you," I say softly. "I don't know when I can call again. Richard took my phone. This is my mom's. Can I try you tomorrow?"

"I'll answer anytime," he says. "No matter what. And I'll wait for you. However long it takes."

There's a pause. Neither of us knows how to end a conversation like this. Finally, he breaks it.

"I miss you."

"I miss you, too."

I can feel a small smile stretching across my tired, tear-stained face. Two more goodbyes. Then, the line goes silent.

From across the room, where she's been falsely busying herself with a Sudoku book, my mom catches the smile. We lock eyes. Nothing is said, but it's understood. Her instinct, subtle but insistent all week, was spot on. I see her shoulders drop in relief. A small exhale, unmistakable ease.

A sliver of peace, finally finding its way back to both of us, in smoothe unison, like synchronized swimmers surfacing together.

Chapter 18
THE CUCKOO'S NEST, PART I

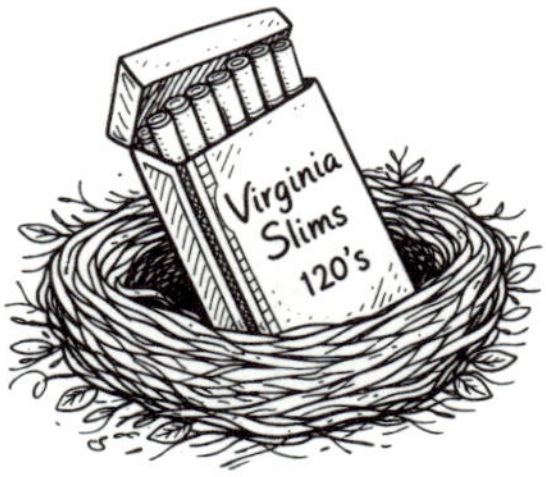

JULY 20, 2009
10 a.m.—Legacy Hospital
Dallas, Texas

Today is the day. After far longer than anyone anticipated on the 11th floor of Legacy Hospital, a bed has finally opened up for me. The paperwork is nearly complete. The ambulance will come soon. I am being transferred.

It's only 10 a.m., but the day already feels worn down at the edges. Since sunrise, no fewer than 10 nurses, doctors, social workers, and case managers have filed in and out of my room asking the same question in slightly different ways:

"Are you sure about East Pines?"

It's not because I have the option of walking out into the world alone; that door is closed. It's because East Pines is a state-run facility. Which is to say: not glossy.

They've shown me the alternatives. Private facilities with soft lighting and landscaped courtyards. Places with websites that look like boutique hotels. The "Canyon Ranch of Crazytown." Serene patios. Yoga studios. Words like holistic and restorative are splashed across their brochures in calming fonts. They also carry seven-star price tags. It seems one week in the "Bipolar Riviera" could cost more than my entire college education.

My mom keeps telling me not to worry about the money. "We'll figure it out," she says. "You don't have to go somewhere like that."

But I do.

The East Pines brochure has a rough matte finish, and the paper is crap quality. It doesn't sell you on hope with filtered photos and spa robes. It's the place you go when there are no other options or when you refuse to pretend there are.

But I am resolute.

When I am released, wherever that lands me, the bills will be mine. I am not sticking Richard with this expense. This will not be another item on his list of grievances against me. And I'm certainly not pinning the weight onto my mother or my father.

This is my mess. My mind. My consequence. Plus, how bad can a state-run hospital really be?

Turns out. Pretty bad.

The last several days in this tiny, over-air-conditioned room, freezing compared to the Dallas sauna outside, have felt suspended from real life.

My one oversized window overlooks the rooftops of the entire medical plaza, but you wouldn't know it. The glass is almost completely hidden behind floral arrangements, balloons, and half-opened cards propped upright. Bouquets from Dallas friends. From faraway friends. From family. Bright colors pressed against sterile walls.

I've had a steady stream of visitors. Some expected. Some surprising. Greer and Addy have been here every morning, without fail. My mom rarely leaves. We've cried together. We've laughed until the crying turned into laughing again. As far as silver linings go, this time with them and the Twins' mom, Carol, has been a gift. They are human medicine.

My friend Tatum has come more than once. She grew up a few

doors down from me, though we were never in high school at the same time. She was heading off to college just as I entered ninth grade. We reconnected years later in London when Richard was finishing law school, and her husband was on assignment. She was working at the National Gallery then, the only American working with the Queen's Collection. She's brilliant, warm, and effortlessly funny.

I could talk to Tatum for hours, about everything and nothing at all. I'm not ready to tell anyone my future plans yet, but when the time comes, she'll be one of the first.

Some newer friends came in pairs. I don't blame them for wanting a buffer. Suicide is spooky. It makes people nervous, like all grief does or even cancer does, like something contagious might leak into the air.

Hayley arrived with a bouquet of zinnias from her garden, arranged in a pedestal vase that I've already asked my mom to take to my apartment. About 30 minutes into her visit, Hayley leaned in and told me she struggles, too, with her mental health. I would have never guessed.

Hayley is the epitome of composure, complete with shiny hair and bright teeth. She's the kind of woman who seems permanently centered. Hearing her speak so openly makes me feel less alone and oddly honored. My mess created space for her truth. It makes me wonder how many of us are secretly white-knuckling life.

My bombshell, dance-'til-dawn partner Maggie came, too, with her flowing red hair, chocolate in hand, then later an ice-cold Diet Coke. She has never put me on the pedestal Richard made up and never needed me to be the good girl. In less than two years of friendship, she saw me clearly. Fun but flawed. Loving but broken. Optimistic but damaged.

Rhett visited on the second day. I know he was there the first night, too. He drove Greer, but he respectfully stayed away from my room then.

When he did come in, he was gentle. Kind but guarded. I'm sure a part of me is unrecognizable to him. And I can't blame him for being unnerved. Before Brett, I never crossed a line. All those late nights at Bungalow 8, Butter, and Cain, the palm trees and celebrities and hours of dancing, none of us ever did anything shady.

I fully understand that when my marriage ends, and it will, my friendship with his wife will also shift the narrative, from beloved sisterhood to questionable influence. Just as I need to leave this place to survive, Rhett needs to build guardrails around his world. It's fair. I get it.

Beau, Greer's brother-in-law and a dear friend to Richard and me both, has been the biggest surprise visitor. I naturally assumed he would default to Richard's side. Not because he's cruel but because that's the code, right? "Bro before ho."

Instead, Beau's shown up every single day. More than Richard. Each time he comes with one of my favorite candies in hand, the kind of candy only liked by children and carnival workers—circus peanuts, candy corn, Swedish fish. He sits beside my bed and talks to me like I'm still me. The girl who danced on stage when Richard wasn't looking. The girl who helped him silk-screen custom T-shirts for a paintball tournament. The girl who convinced him to swap Nine Inch Nails for Carole King during Sunday brunches. Beau sees me as a sister. For now, that's holding. But I know that when I finally take the step to start over, really start over, the friendship will fracture. Another casualty. Another loss I'll have to accept.

I don't want to leave these people. They have shown up for me in ways I didn't know possible. Flowers, laughter, teeth-rotting candy, whispered prayers, hands wrapped around mine while machines beeped in the background. But I can't stay for them.

I wish I could pack our friendships into a suitcase and carry them wherever I land next. I wish loyalty didn't bend under the weight of divorce and scandal and mental illness. But I know otherwise. Sides get chosen.

In my parents' split, my mom was the chosen side. She stayed. My dad left. The narrative was simple enough for most people. Mine won't be complicated either. Certified crazy cheaters are rarely the side sane people choose.

Maybe time will soften it down the road. It did for my dad. Years later, many of the same family friends who froze him out now invite him to dinner again. He's oddly difficult to stay mad at.

I used to think that my dad didn't love me enough to stay, to want to work it out. For the first time, I'm considering something I've resisted my whole life: maybe he didn't leave to hurt us. Maybe, he left because he felt like he had to for his own survival. It's hard to hold that thought without flinching. Some of my wounds still feel fresh, even decades later. Fathers live on pedestals in little girls' minds. When fathers fall, the drop is far.

I never thought Dallas was my forever home. But my restlessness was never about the people. In such a short span of time, so many of them have opened their hearts and their homes to me.

That part is real. Leaving them will be real, too.

It's almost dusk by the time the "bed" they promised at East Pines actually materializes. All day, nurses have rotated in and out of my room, each one carefully explaining the next step. With every shift change, the story resets, as if I might somehow wake up confused again and need reminding.

Because it's an involuntary admission, I will be transported by ambulance. They say transfer like it's a polite relocation. A hotel upgrade. But the repetition of the word makes the ambulance feel less like medical transport and more like something reserved for inmates. Turns out there is no option to hail a cab to a mental institution.

By the time they wheel me out, my room has been returned to factory settings. The flowers are gone. The balloons deflated and removed. The cards boxed up. My makeup bag, toiletries, and stacks of soft pajamas are all sealed into plastic bags for my mom to take home. None of it can come with me to East Pines.

As they roll me toward the door, I glance back one last time. The machines are silent now. No beeping monitors. No IV drip. No tubes taped to my arms. The bed looks smaller without me in it.

I'm alive.

I take a slow breath.

Let's try to keep it that way.

Rhett offers to drive my mom and follow behind the ambulance. It's such a Rhett thing to do. He's practical, steady, and always steps in where needed.

Richard rides with me.

Whether it's out of obligation or for appearances or a suggestion from someone else, Richard is with me. And for this particular stretch of road, I'm grateful not to be alone. I'm usually fine alone. As an only child, I learned that skill at an early age. But not tonight.

I remember nothing about the ride to the hospital five days ago. This feels like my first conscious ambulance experience. Every image I've ever had of one comes from television, mostly from *Grey's Anatomy*. Bright white interiors, dramatic lighting, perfectly angled cameras.

This is nothing like that. It's dim. Metallic. Tight. There are no real windows in the back, just opaque panels and equipment bolted into every inch of space. Black-and-yellow hazard tape lines the edges and corners. It feels industrial. Contained.

I wait in a mandatory wheelchair. My chauffeurs for the evening are two very jacked paramedics, each taking an arm and guiding me onto the gurney. We may not debut as debutantes in Murray, Kentucky, but they would surely pass as suitable escorts at a coming-out ball. Broad-shouldered, polite, and efficient.

I smile and thank them as they strap me in, being careful and hyperaware to not sound even remotely flirty. Richard's tolerance for my friendliness has always been thin. A cheerful hello has earned me lectures before. Tonight, I aim for neutral. Monotone. Invisible.

The doors slam shut. And then, the sirens. The lights. The ambulance lurches forward. The wail slices through me. My entire body jolts at the sound. No one mentioned this part in the 10 separate briefings about my "transfer." Apparently, urgency is required. I suppose, my arrival at the "Cuckoo's Nest" cannot be delayed a second more. The flashing red and white lights strobe faintly against the interior walls.

Time is of the essence. Mustn't be late for my full body cavity search. The absurdity almost makes me laugh. Almost.

The drive feels endless.

Maybe it's the darkness, no windows I can see, and no sense of direction, that stretch the minutes thin. I have no idea which highways we've taken, whether we're heading north or south, or whether I'm still anywhere near the life I recognize.

For a split second, I flashback to my days in college. Blindfolded. Packed into a van. On the way to some random field as part of a hazing ritual for a secret society. I should have known better than to say yes to it. Every lesson my mother ever taught me about safety and common sense ignored in the name of belonging.

I know this isn't that. I know I'm not being abandoned in a field, or asked to eat a live goldfish to prove my loyalty. But something about surrendering control of where I'm being taken, unable to see, makes fear bloom in my chest for the first time. The spa-like "Canyon Ranch of Crazytown" is sounding pretty appealing right about now.

The ambulance slows and then makes a sharp turn. The ride

grows bumpier. Gravel under tires, maybe. A driveway. The sirens cut off. This must be the place.

The sun has fully set. Darkness presses against the windshield. I hadn't realized how much energy a day of waiting could drain from a person's body. Or maybe, it's the adrenaline finally leaking out and the anxiety of crossing this threshold seeping in.

What waits behind those doors?

When they open the back of the ambulance, the air is warm.

The building looks . . . ordinary. Like a strip mall you'd pass without noticing. Brown aggregate sidewalks. Beige, fake-stucco exterior. Fluorescent lights stuck under a long blue awning that reads "Admissions" beside the East Pines logo, a clip-art tree that feels almost comically generic.

No serene courtyards. No mountain views. No spa robes. Just a door.

One of the paramedics helps me down. As I step onto the pavement, my hair falls forward into my face. It smells faintly of Frédéric Fekkai, a rare shampoo splurge that my mom scored at TJ Maxx during a much-needed break from my hospital room.

One of the nurses told me this morning there are no hair dryers at East Pines. Not allowed. So, I washed and curled my hair one last time. A small act of control.

I'm wearing a new pink knit set my mom bought me from the same "Teej" trip, soft yoga pants and a matching long-sleeve top. Comfortable. Nothing fancy. Something I will likely burn later as a relic of this chapter.

I know what I look like won't matter to others here at East Pines. But it matters to me. If things are about to go low, and I suspect they are, I want to meet them feeling as intact as possible.

The double doors slide open. And I take a breath before stepping through.

The reception area lacks aesthetic appeal. I wasn't expecting marble floors and chandeliers, but it's the kind of bleak that feels preventable. The carpet is matted and vaguely stained. The chairs look like they've survived decades of restless hands and nervous pacing. Clean-ish would feel like a luxury upgrade. I understand the omission of photos in the brochure now.

Mom and Rhett trail in behind the paramedics and find two seats near a vending machine that roars like a freight train. The spiral racks inside are nearly empty, and the remaining snack packages look sun-faded, like they've been aging in there since the dawn of time. A fluorescent bulb flickers in the corner.

The cliché of it all is actually kind of funny. A nurse hands me a clipboard stacked thick with paperwork. It feels like I'm doing more signing than reading. Medical jargon makes legal language look breezy. I thank her with an oversized smile. It feels strategic. Allies could come in handy here.

I sit beside my mom on a rough blue tweed chair framed in brown laminate. A real beaut, Clark.

Humor is sandwiching each thought; it's my go-to coping mechanism. I can feel it. This is my life now. This is what happens when mania loosens your guard: You fall into a torrid affair with a devastatingly attractive New York man, and then you try to exit your own body in the most permanent way possible.

Consequences and I haven't been on speaking terms since April. We're reacquainting quickly.

While I lean into dark comedy, my mom is spiraling in the opposite direction. Her eyes are bloodshot. I'm fairly certain she cried the entire drive from Legacy Hospital. Rhett looks exhausted, the kind of tired that comes from absorbing someone else's panic for hours. He's been working overtime all week.

I'm not surprised he's here. Rhett is crisis ready. His whole family is wired that way. They show up for people they care about, even people they don't. They will show up for Richard when I'm gone, too. I know that.

The paperwork drags on.

Finally, Rhett stands and gives me a brief hug. "I'll wait in the car," he says, offering my mom an out. He'll drive Richard back to the apartment and take her home to their house. She flies back to Kentucky tomorrow. There's nothing more she can physically do for me here.

"Morgie, you don't have to stay here!" Mom whisper-shouts, her voice cracking. "This place . . . well . . . " Tears spill over. "We can find you somewhere better. You don't have to do this to yourself."

I understand what she's seeing. It probably looks like punishment. Self-hatred. But honestly? What is a fancy facility going to give me that this one can't? Over the last four years with Jet Set Lingerie, I've slept in five-star suites and roadside disasters alike. I know how to slum it.

Granted, I've never had a stranger for a roommate with no lock on my door and limited phone privileges, but I would still rather be here than at my apartment with Richard. That fact alone says everything.

"This is exactly where she needs to be, Mona," Richard says, firmly. "She needs to hit rock bottom."

His words catch me off guard. Not because of what he says, but because I forgot he was here. Clad in his three-quarter-zip, Richard is sulking in a chair out of my line of sight. Quiet. Possibly exhausted by the PR gymnastics bouncing around in his head. I know it firsthand. Spin takes brain power. Calculation. Performance.

Explaining his wife's mental institution stay is going to kick his undergrad degree in communications into overtime this week.

"He's not wrong, Mom," I say. "I can do this. I need to do this."

And I mean it.

I want more help. I want to understand my triggers. I want to recognize the warning signs before mania hijacks me. I want more than pills tossed at my symptoms. Would I prefer to do that in a place with Scalamandré wallpaper and Perrin & Rowe fixtures? Absolutely.

Instead, I'm likely headed toward ribbed vinyl wall coverings and a plastic Delta faucet shaped like a crystal snow globe with mildew at its core. Left for hot with a red arrow. Right for cold with a blue one. Assuming there is hot water.

My mom searches my face. "Are you sure you don't want me to stay?" she asks. "I can delay my flight."

"I'm sure," I say. "I'll be okay. Plus, look at this gorgeous luggage you and Greer picked out."

I lift the thin plastic Target bag. No real luggage allowed.

Approved items include:

- *Two cotton pajama sets, no buttons*
- *Two lounge outfits, no drawstrings*
- *A clear bag of non-contraband toiletries: ChapStick, lotion, bronzer, blush, travel toothpaste*
- *Shower flip-flops*
- *Sneakers (laces removed)*
- *Underwear*
- *Socks*
- *A journal, no sharp writing implements*

"Well," Mom says, reaching into her purse, "you're going to need these, too."

She hands me two packs of Virginia Slims 120s. Her brand. Two a day, every day of my life. A disciplined addiction. I stare at them.

"I'm told that these can be currency in here," she says evenly. "Use them to make friends."

I don't know where Mom got that intel, but I slide them into my plastic bag.

My next steps are through a series of secured doors. It's time for goodbye. I start with my mom. Face to face. Hand in hand. I slip off my Cartier watch and my engagement ring and place them into her palm. I don't know if they're allowed inside, but they certainly aren't needed here. She takes them without comment and tucks them into her purse.

Then she pulls me in, her grip tight enough to press the air from my lungs. She's smaller than me, but in her arms, I feel entirely enveloped. Safe. She holds on longer than necessary.

When she finally pulls back, she whispers quickly, "There are phone cards hidden inside the cigarette packs. Use them to call Brett whenever you want. And your dad drafted a medical power of attorney. You need to sign it tomorrow, so Richard doesn't control your treatment anymore. Greer is bringing me back in the morning before my flight. I'll bring it then. Good plan?"

I look at her. This woman. Always five steps ahead.

"Good plan, Mom," I say. "I love you so much. Thank you for being here."

My goodbye to Richard is brief. Awkward. A stiff hug. No kiss. He's trying. I can see that. I am, too. Maybe part of him feels validated leaving me here. Human nature doesn't disappear just because circumstances are tragic.

The doors buzz. Time for phase two of intake.

I walk through alone.

Chapter 19

THE CUCKOO'S NEST, PART II

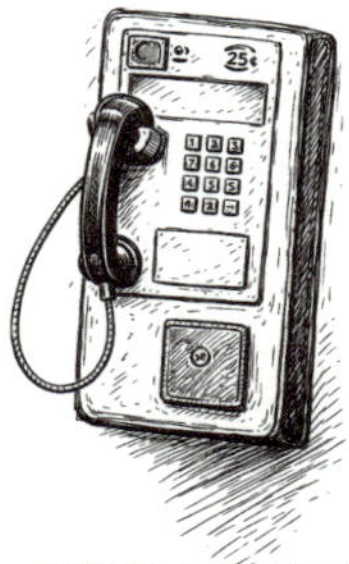

JULY 20, 2009
Evening—East Pines Hospital
Dallas, Texas

What awaits me behind door number two is worse than I imagined. The phrase "full body cavity search" gets tossed around casually on TV crime shows, like *Law & Order* and *CSI: Crime Scene Investigation*, as if it's just another step in the process. But no one ever really explains what it means. Somewhere in my brain, I'd translated "search" into "scan." I assumed I'd strip down and walk through something like an airport security machine. Nope.

The nasty carpet and busted lighting should have tipped me off. East Pines and Bush Intercontinental clearly operate on very different budgets. There will be no scanning. This is a manual search. Raw. Invasive.

As I enter, I'm greeted by my next intake provider, Angie, a brunette in street clothes. Black pants. Untucked polka-dot blouse, some ruching on the sides. Open blue cardigan with the sleeves pushed to the elbow. An enameled rainbow brooch ties the look together. She will finish my check-in and eventually escort me to my room. Angie looks like she's been shaped, in equal parts, by sun and routine. She's in her mid-50s, though she carries it with a kind of practiced brightness, the sort that comes from deciding, a long time ago, how she wants to be seen. She's sticking to it. Her hair is set just so, lifted and held in place with a devotion to hairspray that borders on architectural. Her hairdo doesn't move, even when she does. Angie takes my overstuffed plastic Target bag and hands it to the security agent, standing beside a conveyor belt like part of the fixture. The entire scene feels like a secondhand TSA checkpoint.

The security agent moves on autopilot. His thinning gray hair sits close to his scalp. Thick-rimmed glasses attempt to hide tired, red eyes. Blue shirt, dark pants, a scattering of unidentifiable badges clipped across his chest. A small metal detector works hard beside him, but apparently, it's not strong enough to detect through clothing layers, so he unpacks everything. One. Item. At. A. Time.

My mom's careful folding job dissolves instantly as pajamas, socks, toiletries, and flip-flops get tossed onto the conveyor belt, collecting cooties along the way. While he inspects every object I own, Angie guides me toward a corner of the room.

A flimsy privacy wall stands there, held upright by metal T-stands. The setup resembles a sitcom version of airport security, a low budget one at best. She points to a small nook and pulls a thin curtain around it.

"Go ahead and undress completely. No socks. No bra. No panties," she says. Then, attempting humor, she adds, "Just your birthday suit."

She gives me a few moments alone to disrobe, which feels silly given what's about to go down here. Why offer privacy when a full body inspection is on the menu?

"Ready?" she calls from the other side of the curtain.

"As I'll ever be," I reply, strangely upbeat, still clinging to the instinct to make a good first impression. Note to self: Morgan, no one here is fooled.

Angie pulls the curtain back. I keep my eyes down as she steps into the nook. Avoiding eye contact feels instinctive. I've seen my bruises already, in quick glances during showers or while swapping one pair of pajamas for another, but under the harsh lights they look worse.

Dark blooms along my ribs. Down my legs. Around my arms. I bruise easily. Always have. It's not the paramedics' fault. They saved me. Whatever they had to do to keep me alive, I'm grateful. But I won't be sad when these ugly reminders fade.

Richard hasn't seen me naked since I arrived at Legacy Hospital. For several reasons. The first being that he hasn't been around much. His coping mechanism, I assume. He's come just enough to play the role of concerned husband. Just enough to remind me that life after the hospital will look very different, that my freedom will depend on his permissions and proving my loyalty.

I made sure never to undress or shower while he was visiting. The bruises would have been further ammunition for his favorite narrative: how reckless I am with his reputation.

The morning after my mom secretly returned with her phone, Richard stormed into the hospital room like he'd sensed something had happened. Or maybe, he was just angry that the people around me were offering kindness instead of judgment. My mom was already there when he arrived, dropping off a stack of glossy fashion magazines. Her presence seemed to irritate him immediately. No hello. No good morning. For the second time, less than 24 hours from the first mention, he brought up an odd thought.

"You know, Morgan, if you had died, people would've thought I did this. Did you even think about that?" he asked. "What would that have done to me?"

"Richard," I said as calmly as I could manage, "you already scolded me about that yesterday. I assure you I didn't forget."

I swallowed every sharper response sitting on the tip of my tongue. Seriously, why does he keep bringing this up?

Instead, I said the only thing I could offer: "It's clear I did this on my own. You're off the hook." A pause. "But I am truly sorry," I added. "I'm sorry for all of it."

"We will start from the front," Angie explains. "Spread your legs wide and hold your arms above your head. This is my assistant, Mary, she will observe the procedure to ensure your safety."

Glad to see there's a solid checks-and-balances system on the "inside." I do as Angie says, thinking that maybe I should have read all the fine print of my admissions documents more closely. I clearly signed off on this. Not that I have anything to hide.

Wearing blue rubber gloves, she lightly pats down my entire body from the front while scanning every inch of me with her eyes.

"You may put your arms by your sides now," she says. "Please open your mouth as wide as you can."

I open so wide that the sides of my mouth crack open. Grateful to know I have the luxury of drugstore ChapStick waiting for me when I make it through this. Mary shines a massive flashlight down the back of my throat, while Angie prods around with a tongue depressor.

"No tonsils, I see," she notes. "Makes my job easier."

I appreciate Angie's commitment to small talk, but in this case, silence is golden. Am I supposed to respond to her? "Yes, Angie, this is such a wonderful and surprising silver lining to having a tonsillectomy during my senior year of high school, which led to my very poor decision to get a perm while still on the painkillers. Had I known this would work out better for you, Angie, then I wouldn't have lived with regret all these years."

This is just like when I'm at the dentist, and the hygienist asks me about my day, and I awkwardly try to answer her in spite of the tools and hands deep inside my mouth.

"Glad I could help," I tell Angie. Of course, it comes out garbled and muffled.

"Okay, it's time to do the back side," she declares. "This is more invasive. Let's have you come over to this table. Turn around, place your hands on the first set of marked arrows in front of you and bend over. Try to relax. That will make it easier on you."

Up until this moment, my sense of humor has been working overtime. Sarcasm has been my flotation device through most of this experience. The ambulance, the strip-mall psych ward, the vending machine relics. But there is no clever line waiting for me here.

My face burns. Tears start to gather before I can stop them, warm and salty as they slide down my cheeks. My hands press against the arrows taped to the wall in front of me. And then the most invasive part of the search begins. Angie starts with my bottom. There are bright lights, gloved fingers, metal instruments. Unlike a doctor's office, there's no lubricant, no gentle explanation, no attempt to soften the moment. Just procedure with a side of humiliation.

"Clear," she calls out to Mary across the room. For a brief second, I think it's over.

"Now, move your hands forward to the second set of arrows and bend a little further," she instructs.

I do as she says. But, my brain is somewhere else entirely. Growing up in the South, an intact hymen carried strange gravity, like an invisible badge of honor. A measure of worth that hovered over every conversation about girlhood. Thinking about it now makes my stomach twist. Who exactly was monitoring it? Why did it matter so much? Why did 13-year-old me worry that using a tampon might "break" something sacred?

Why did any of that determine whether a girl was still considered pure? The idea was everywhere. A girl could become "damaged goods" long before she understood her own body. And yet, boys never carried that same ledger.

Do I believe sex should happen in love and respect? Of course.

Do I believe people should wait until they're mature enough to understand the weight of intimacy? Absolutely. But the notion that a woman's worth is tied to the fragile status of a membrane, while men move freely through the world untouched by that metric? Nope on a rope.

And yet, as I stand here now, bent forward, exposed to a stranger's inspection, indignity rushes back anyway.

The physical pain from the probing behind me is sharp, embarrassing, and degrading. Opening myself to this stranger is worse. Allowing her to inspect the deepest, most private part of me for contraband like I'm hiding something dangerous inside my body is traumatic. It pulls me into a dark place.

A quiet voice in my head whispers:

This is it.

Rock bottom.

Richard would be so proud.

After that intense, deeply invasive process, I'm at a loss for why it took so long for them to find me a bed here. If this is the standard welcome at East Pines, I'm shocked anyone comes here at all.

Once I pull myself together, wipe the tears from my face, and get dressed again, the "tour" portion of intake begins. Angie recovers from our intimate encounter far faster than I do.

On my way out of what I privately label "Cavity Corner," I quickly thank Mary for her role in the matter, carefully avoiding eye contact. I cannot imagine performing that task day in and day out.

I slip my feet back into my childlike Velcro sneakers, shoelaces removed, of course, and Angie and I head off to the next "station." More fun people around every corner.

We exit the main building and step outside into an enclosed courtyard. In the darkness, it actually looks . . . pleasant. Four covered sidewalks form a square around a small open center, maybe a decent walking loop during downtime. In the distance, I see the perimeter clearly. Tall fencing surrounds the entire courtyard. Coiled wire on top, keeping people out. And in.

To enter the next building, we stop at a buzzer system beside a window of reinforced safety glass. A nurse sits behind it, controlling the doors. Employees scan in and out with security badges, but Angie opts for the buzzer to show me how the system works for patients. We wait.

"Morgan, this is Nancy," Angie says. "She runs the night shift desk. We're already past courtyard curfew tonight, but she's your go-to for outside access if you want to take walks or breaks. She records everyone's comings and goings. You always have to sign in and out."

"Nice to meet you, Nancy," I say. "You'll probably be seeing a lot of me. I plan on doing a good bit of walking. It's my saving grace."

Nancy gives me a polite smile. "Nice to meet you too. Morgan, right?" she checks. "You'll probably see more of my counterpart, Crystal. She runs the desk during the day. Good luck to ya."

Nancy seems kind enough and also completely numb to the environment around her. She distracts herself with what appears to be an impressive collection of desk flair. Coffee mugs with cheeky quotes and pens decorated with fake flowers taped to the tops so no one will steal them. Her nails are clearly a major priority—long acrylics, each one painted in a slightly different design. The patience required to sit still for that kind of manicure makes me anxious.

I offer Nancy one last polite smile and hurry to catch up with Angie, who is already halfway down a long white hallway. At the end is another door. Clear glass. Wide enough for a wheelchair. Frosted for privacy, and almost certainly shatterproof.

I'm not sure what waits behind it. But I feel confident it will not resemble a Southern sorority door song welcoming me with fanfare. Angie stops beside the door.

"So, this is the main event, Morgan," she says. "Through here are the nurses' and doctors' station where all your appointments and treatments will be scheduled. The common area is just beyond that. Group therapy and private rooms wrap around the back side of reception."

She gestures as she speaks, pointing like a flight attendant giving the pre-flight safety demo. Her hand signals are a little off. After years working Jet Set Lingerie events, I could teach her a thing or two.

My eyes drift past her toward the common room. A giant coffee table sits in the middle of the space, surrounded by four oversized sofas, only two of which actually match. The table itself is covered in construction paper and crayons. It looks like a preschool craft station. All it needs is a pile of macaroni noodles and a bottle of Elmer's glue.

A sudden thought hits me. Oh my God. Are there children here, too?

The lights are low. The room is empty. Music, surprisingly loud, spills from behind the nurses' counter, where one nurse sits on watch. She's reading a paperback with a glossy cover: the kind of cheesy murder mystery often left behind at all-inclusive resorts. It looks worn, possibly abandoned here by a former inmate. I mean, patient.

The entire day feels suspended in time, but the clock above the doctor's station reads 10 p.m. Angie mentioned earlier that curfew is at 9 p.m. That explains why the room is so quiet, the dark doorways lining the back wall like hollow mouths.

But something catches my attention.

"Angie, excuse me for interrupting," I say, "but where do all these doorways lead? The ones without doors?"

"I was just gettin' to that, hon," she says, her drawl thickening as the night drags on. The same thing happens to me. The more tired I get, the more Kentucky slips out of my mouth.

"These are the rooms," she continues, gesturing down the row. "Yours is right there." She points toward one of the dark openings.

"Number 11. I'm sure your roommate's already asleep. We're an early-to-bed, early-to-rise community here."

Roommate. That part hasn't fully sunk in yet. As we start toward my new accommodations, chaos erupts. A large man bursts from one of the rooms, shouting something unintelligible and charging toward the nurses' station. His voice echoes off the walls, frantic and jagged.

His pajamas are ratty and mismatched, one sleeve torn, the pants hanging unevenly. Suddenly, my carefully prepared outfits feel absurdly out of place and over the top.

My mom and Greer clearly packed me for the five-star version of this place, not the state-run situation I'm standing in now. Hopefully, it doesn't make me a target. Then again, maybe that's what the Virginia Slims are for.

"Friendship currency." Just like my mom said.

Before I can process what's happening, a security guard appears seemingly out of nowhere. The nurse must have a panic button under the desk because there's no way the tiny woman reading her murder novel can manage this situation on her own. The guard is dressed in a strange hybrid uniform: half scrubs, half police officer. He approaches the man calmly, like this scene is routine.

The man, who is obviously a patient, is now dancing erratically, shouting fragments of off-color remarks. It's hard to understand him, but he's noticeably upset. Confused. Completely unmoored. And he's enormous. At least 6-foot-4, broad in every direction.

For a moment, my mind goes back to a boy I grew up with who had Tourette's. Is that what I'm seeing? Is this a tic? A breakdown? Or something else entirely? Before I can even begin to understand it, the guard diffuses the situation with surprising ease. He speaks calmly to the man, like they're old acquaintances, gently guiding him away. The two disappear through a door that Angie never mentioned during the tour.

Angie doesn't even pause. She keeps walking as if nothing happened at all. "Shall we get you settled in?" she asks cheerily.

Oh sure, Angie. I'll be able to drift off after that, no problem.

"I guess I didn't realize there would be men sleeping, or not sleeping apparently, in the same wing as the women," I say, noticeably troubled by this revelation, "Especially, since we have no doors."

"Don't you worry about a thing, Ms. Morgan," Angie assures. "You saw how quickly Dwayne handled Rufus. The big guy, that's Rufus. Dwayne is always waiting in the wings should anyone get out of line. Plus, your roommate is a girl. Now, time for you to catch some zzz's."

WTF? Was there a chance Rufus could have been my roommate? I keep that scary thought to myself, though, as I step across the threshold into my room. The bed on the far wall has a body in it. Even in the darkness, I can see that the entire wall above her bed is plastered in tear outs from *Teen Beat* magazine. It seems Zac Efron will be watching over the two of us for the next week or so.

My empty, single bed is positioned closest to the door and less desirable, for sure, with views of the comings and goings, and, of course, more light peering in than my roomie's bed. Angie points out my desk space and closet, more like a kindergarten cubby. If shoelaces, mechanical pencils, and tweezers are banned items, then hangers are a clear no-no.

An instant unpacker, I start putting away my things. I stack my new loungewear duds smack in the middle, neat and straight. I place my clear bag of toiletries on the top shelf, my stash of ciggies just below, and my shower sandals on the floor next to the cubby. Lastly, my journal and two books: *The Help* and *The Widow Clicquot* on top of my desk.

"Okay then . . . your bathroom is that way," Angie says. "I suggest you keep everything of yours in your own space. You never know what might happen to it around here. There is a pocket door for privacy in the restroom, but please note it doesn't have a lock. No locks."

Comforting, Angie. You're really selling me on this place.

"Now, I'm going to need that plastic bag," she says, holding out her hand.

"My luggage, you mean?" I laugh. She doesn't. Tough crowd.

"Alrighty then, breakfast starts at 7 a.m. sharp," Angie informs me. "And you will meet with your doctor right after, around 8 a.m. He'll set your schedule and treatment plan and address any additional needs or questions you may have. I'll be gone by then, of course, but everyone is here to help, so just ask." And as she heads toward the door, she adds, "Oh, I almost forgot. The pay phone banks in the common area are yours to use during free time. Phone cards or collect. There are no official time limits, but please be respectful of those waiting to use them. Sleep tight, hon."

And then, she's gone.

I slowly undo my sneakers, trying to not wake up my mystery roommate with the obnoxious sound of Velcro. I slide them under the bed, pull back the covers, and fall in. I'm too tired to give much thought to the scratchy sheets and the bodies that have laid in them before me and the weird foam blanket that provides no warmth or security at all. My eyes flash to the ceiling, a popcorn finish. Of course.

July 21, 2009, Morning—East Pines Hospital, Dallas

Sunlight wakes me, and I'm genuinely surprised I slept at all. Except that yesterday drained me so thoroughly. My body must have simply shut down. I have no idea what time it is, but my stomach insists it's breakfast. Angie said the buffet starts at 7 a.m., though there's nothing in this room that could confirm it. No clock. No cords. No glass. No batteries. Anything remotely breakable or hangable has clearly been removed. Honestly, I'm amazed we even get a flat sheet.

I slip out from under the covers and tiptoe toward the doorway in my socks, careful not to wake my roommate. She's still completely out. I lean just far enough into the hallway to see the clock mounted near the nurses' station.

5:30 a.m. Which means it's 6:30 a.m. in New York. Brett's time.

He might already be out for his morning run. I picture him moving through the unruffled Manhattan streets, earphones in, sweat forming. I wonder if he's thinking about me. Wondering where I am. Waiting for me to call.

What am I even going to tell him?

This is the longest we've gone without speaking since he flew back to the States last week. If I move quickly, maybe I can get ready and call him before heading to the dining hall.

I rush to switch into my shower flip-flops and grab my tiny collection of supplies: today's clothes, my toothbrush, and the handful of makeup items they allowed me to keep. I twist my hair into a giant top knot with the single scrunchie I was permitted to bring. One lonely hair clip survived intake as well.

Inside the bathroom, two towels sit folded beside the sink. A tiny bar of soap. A sad-looking bottle of 2-in-1 shampoo, quite the fall from Frédéric Fekkai. A travel-size hairbrush completes the spa experience.

Since my plastic shower cap was confiscated at intake, I twist one towel into a turban around my hair. The other, barely larger than a glorified hand towel, I wrap around my body before sliding the pocket door closed.

The shower itself has only a half door: a fixed panel of wavy glass framed in rusty stainless steel. The drain is sealed halfway with orange foam caulk. No rods. No curtains. Nothing remotely capable of supporting a rope or cord. Safety first.

Naturally, there's no way to turn on the water without spraying yourself directly in the face. Lucky for me, it's freezing.

After standing there shivering for three minutes while the water warms, wrapped in a towel roughly the size of an Hervé Léger bandage dress, I give up and step in. The water has graduated from arctic to lukewarm.

Faster than the military-style showers my grandfather forced on us cousins aboard their houseboat every summer, I hit the essential areas, spending a little extra time reclaiming my dignity after last night's invasion. Cold water or not, it feels good to wash yesterday off my body.

My shower shoes squish against the tile as I return to the sink area to get dressed. I move quickly through the tiny ritual of putting myself together: moisturizer, a bit of bronzer, blush, lip gloss.

It's quite a different primping process than my fashion week shenanigans with the Twins. Back then, we'd sprawl across hotel rooms with makeup stations, accessory buffets, and racks of clothing popped up on every wall.

Here: one blush, one gloss, one outfit. No accessories.

Then again, pay phones don't have video, so who am I really trying to impress? The lip gloss is purely for my own sanity. I slide the pocket door open and nearly collide with my roommate.

Meggie.

Angie mentioned her name last night, though this is my first real look at her. She's not at all what I expected. We seem roughly the same age. She might even be a little older than me. Which makes the *Teen Beat* magazine obsession even more confusing. I'd assumed they bunked me with a teenager.

She speaks immediately, her voice bright and childlike.

"Hi! I'm Meggie," she says. "What's your name and how old are you? Do you have a favorite color? I love turquoise."

"Oh, hi, Meggie," I say, matching her enthusiasm as best I can. She seems so sweet, so innocent. I can't imagine what brought her here.

"My name's Morgan," I answer. "I'm 28. And yes, I do have a favorite color . . . well, two actually. Pink and chartreuse."

She beams.

"How long have you been here, Meggie?" I ask.

She pauses, thinking hard.

"I can't really 'member. A month maybe?" she answers, tilting her head. "I've had a lot of ECT though." She smiles cheerfully.

ECT? I make a mental note to figure out what that stands for.

"Okay if I use the potty?" she asks sweetly.

A month. Holy hell. I'm very new to the whole institutional experience, but a month feels like an eternity.

"Of course," I say.

As she heads into the bathroom, I quietly slip out of the room. Something tells me conversations with Meggie are going to be difficult to exit gracefully.

The hallway clock reads 6:30 a.m. It's 30 minutes before breakfast. Just enough time to try calling Brett.

The phone card in my hand reeks of tobacco. The Virginia Slims pack was the only place mom could hide the cards, but the smell is so strong. I haven't used phone cards in years. Maybe since the late '90s, wasting my time calling a high school boyfriend from a Parisian phone booth, when I should have been living my best life, frolicking up and down Rue Saint-Honoré with Greer, Addy, and our moms.

A few people are up and about. Reading, staring off into space, or playing a board game without an opponent. It's solid people-watching, for sure, but I'm on a timed mission. I pick up the phone to dial the 800 number on the back of the card. The cord gives me a quick case of arm whiplash. It's 10 inches long at most. This will take some getting used to.

I kneel down and punch in a never-ending stream of numbers, followed by Brett's. After the third ring, I start to give up. But then . . .

"Hello?" Brett answers. He's out of breath. Definitely on a run. I forgot that I'm calling from an unrecognizable number.

"Hey," I say softly, trying to not call any attention to myself in this room. "It's me."

"Hiiii!" he says. "I was hoping it would be you. Sorry, it took me a minute to answer. I'm out for a run, but I didn't want to risk missing your call. I was crossing the West Side Highway when it started ringing, and my phone was in this dumb zipper pocket of my running shorts, and I couldn't get it out."

If the situation requires five words to describe a scenario, Brett will use 75. It's endearing, but long-winded at times.

"Sorry, sorry, not important," he pants. "How are you? Where are you? Are you okay?"

"I'm okay," I answer. "I wouldn't say great, but I'm here in my new home for a bit. In terms of a star rating, I give East Pines a one, but I haven't had a meal yet. It could easily plummet below a single star." I laugh, returning to humor for survival purposes.

"I hate the thought of you in a non-perfect place," Brett says. "I hate the thought of you anywhere but with me actually." He's less out of breath now.

"I hate it, too," I agree. "Hopefully soon. I'm about to be assigned to a doctor, and then my therapy will fully begin. Until then, I don't know how long I have to be here."

"Well, as soon as we know that, I'm on a plane," he says. "Straight to you."

I think he means it. Still, a small part of me struggles to believe it's true. There is a lot I don't know about him. As much as I want every piece of him to be real, who he is, how he feels about me, I know I will survive without him if I have to.

Though certainly, life will be better with him in it.

We spend the next 20 minutes trading flirty banter. He walks me through his checklist for the day, most of it revolving around finding a tenant to sublet his apartment. Apparently, that involves meetings with the co-op board and an exhausting amount of New York red tape.

I fill him in on a few of the more bizarre details of my current situation, knowing the list will only grow longer as the day unfolds. The story that really sends him over the edge is my mom and the Virginia

Slims. He laughs so hard I can barely get the rest of the sentence out.

Something tells me those two are going to get along famously someday. That thought alone feels like a small gift, waiting for me somewhere in the future.

When it's time to hang up, he hesitates. He trips over his words for a second, gathers himself, and then says steady and sure, "Morgan, I'm falling for you." It's not quite the three little words, but the impact lands just the same.

Standing at a pay phone with a cord barely 10 inches long, too short to hang a Barbie doll, this gorgeous, hilarious, successful man, who could clearly have his pick of women, has chosen me.

The bipolar blonde calling from a mental institution.

With a little extra bounce in my Velcro-clad step, I head toward the dining hall in search of food. My expectations are modest: watery scrambled eggs, greasy link sausages, or maybe a stale cereal bar. Honestly, anything will do. I'm starving.

I'm startled by the explosion of color in the cafeteria. It's not exactly tasteful, but it's miles less depressing than the common room or patient quarters. Neon accents, laminated tables, mismatched chairs. The whole place feels oddly like The Max from *Saved by the Bell.* If only Kelly and Lisa were here to join me for breakfast.

More patients are up and moving now, and there's already a line forming along the buffet. No two people look alike. I find myself discreetly studying everyone, wondering what brought them here. Not in a judgmental way. Just sheer curiosity.

Is anyone else here like me?

I grab a tray from the rack and collect a place setting and silverware before sliding into the line. To my surprise, the options are actually . . . decent. Hard-boiled eggs, safe and predictable. Granola, yogurt, and fruit for parfaits. Turkey sausage, not greasy at all.

East Pines just earned itself half a star. Things are looking up.

Unsure of the social protocol, I choose a table by myself. Normally eating alone doesn't bother me, but here, I suddenly feel self-conscious. I don't want anyone to think I'm being rude. Or worse . . . that I think I'm better than them.

I'm already overdressed and a little too put together. Imagine if I'd shown up in my real clothes, say my vintage Carolina Herrera tuxedo jacket from the Memorial Sloan Kettering thrift shop, paired with a bold red lip. I'd feel more like myself. But it might also paint a target on my back.

The whole situation reminds me of the first day of ninth grade at a new school. I was never the new girl, but I imagine it must be terrifying, even if it looked exciting from my point of view. I still remember when Kirsten Hammonds moved to Murray in seventh grade. She was gorgeous, and the entire school went completely ga-ga over her novelty. Eventually, the excitement faded, and she blended into normal school life like the rest of us. But those first few days? From the outside, looked like a blast.

I finish breakfast quickly and head back toward the nurses' station so I won't be late on my first official day. Still trying to make a good impression. Likely a pointless instinct, but there's no harm in trying to make the most of my time here.

My doctor's office is impressively small, like it was added as an afterthought or carved out of a larger room that had better plans. It's a far cry from the sprawling private practice spaces I've come to expect. No soft lighting, no candle, no curated calm, certainly no velvet fainting couch waiting to catch a dramatic unraveling. Just two firm chairs placed a little too close together and a self-assembled desk with a box of tissues wrapped in a crocheted cover resting on top.

In the corner, a fake plant in a terra-cotta pot topped with flat glass marbles gathers dust with quiet determination, doing nothing to convince anyone it's alive, but also not quite ready to give up the role it's held since the '90s.

And yet, there it is. Framed, centered, and impossible to ignore hangs a degree from Johns Hopkins University. Crisp and authoritative, it's a reminder that, despite the setting, someone in this room is very, very qualified.

It's a strange pairing: diminished square footage and elevated credentials. But I'm not here to admire the decor. I'm here to heal. There's no cure for what I have. Only treatment. So, let's find the best one. In the midst of underwhelming decor, I find hope.

My assigned doctor is Dr. Ahmad Khan.

He appears to be in his early 60s, has kind eyes, a round belly, and a clean-shaven face. He's wearing a French blue button-down, no tie, pleated trousers, a white doctor's coat that does the heavy lifting, thick-soled Newport-style shoes with dark socks, and a gold wedding band.

He settles into a very specific posture, my paperwork in hand, one leg crossed neatly over the other, ankle balanced on his knee like he's been doing it this way for decades. His glasses rest low on his nose, clearly promoted to "reading only," and he peers over them rather than through them with earned authority. Swap the white coat for a blazer with elbow patches, and he'd be halfway through a lecture on something obscure and deeply important.

My immediate impression is that he's serious but not cold. Someone who takes his work home with him but doesn't waste time with unnecessary niceties. He's not here to make friends. He's here to help me learn how to live with this diagnosis.

"This is not a death sentence, Morgan," he says in a soft Indian accent. Then, he pauses. "But, and this is very important, the quality of your life will depend entirely on you. What you learn here. How you take care of yourself. And what you surround yourself with." He lets the last part hang in the air. "People included."

Chapter 20

THE RELEASE

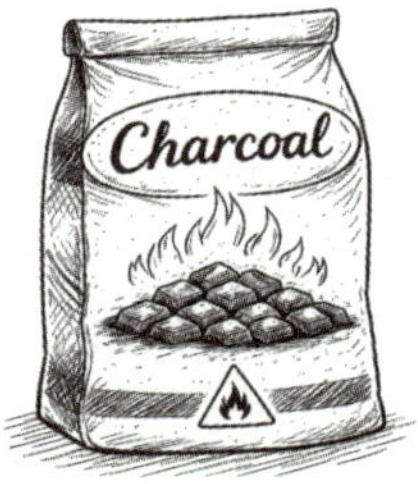

JULY 27, 2009
Midmorning—East Pines Hospital
Dallas, Texas

On the seventh day at East Pines, Dr. Khan tells me I'm stable enough to be released back into my regular life. Whatever that means right now. It's been quite a week. The cast of characters here has opened my eyes far wider than I ever thought possible from little old Murray, Kentucky.

The patients' outbursts don't announce themselves; they build and then break. A schizophrenic voice down the hall rises too fast, too loud, arguing with someone no one else can see. Doors slam not in anger but in panic. A woman, so desperate for a way out that she turned to nearly 200 extra-strength Tylenol—the only thing within her reach.

And then there's the drops. The kind that happen mid-sentence. Shoulders folding in, eyes going vacant, like the person just stepped out of themselves without warning. Tears that don't fall neatly but spill in hot, frustrated tracks, almost angry at their own existence. You can feel it in the room when it happens, the way everything tightens and then goes still.

Most surprising is the laughter. It comes out of nowhere, from almost every patient. It's impossible to explain but necessary for coping.

Nothing here feels exaggerated. If anything, it feels stripped down. Unfiltered. The versions of people we usually manage to keep hidden are suddenly right there on the surface. Each patient has a story to tell, to live, and to somehow survive. It's brutal but valuable in ways I can't fully understand yet.

For me, it's been an immersive crash course in bipolar disorder, not just the diagnosis in a clinical sense but the lived reality of it. The edges of it. The parts that don't make it into tidy explanations. And, uncomfortably, the parts I recognize as my own.

My official diagnosis: Rapid Cycling Bipolar I.

Over the course of the last week, so many things have finally clicked into place. Behaviors and warning signs stretching back to my late teens suddenly make sense. The list of little things I shoved under the rug or ignored is borderline embarrassing. Or maybe my behavior was simply what I thought was expected of me as a girl. Suck it up and smile. That's often the socially acceptable response to female struggle.

The significant progress I've made under Dr. Khan's supervision, with 24-hour observation and multiple private and group therapy sessions each day, is priceless. I'm not leaving this place on a manic high (the kind doctors frown upon and the kind I've admittedly enjoyed from time to time), but I am leaving with something better.

Hope. And a plan.

At the moment, only two people know the full outline of that plan: Dr. Khan and Brett. Soon, my mom will know as well. But first, I need to get out of here.

The fastest way to do that is to allow the hospital to release me to my husband, who they've determined is the most appropriate person to take responsibility for me. They ask me repeatedly if I fear for my safety with Richard and whether I believe he might physically harm me.

The honest answer is no. Never.

Richard is furious. And he has every right to be. He's hurt and embarrassed. Blindsided by how quickly our life unraveled. Yet, I would be lying if I said this week hasn't given me perspective. Comparing my situation to the trauma and severity of symptoms the other patients carry makes me feel more capable. Even slightly validated.

I don't think my life with this disorder has to be defined by survival alone. I think I might actually be able to thrive with it.

My sweet roommate, Meggie, has the emotional and cognitive capacity of a 12- or 13-year-old tween girl. Years of electroconvulsive therapy used to treat severe childhood trauma and sexual abuse have permanently altered the way her brain functions. She will likely spend her life in institutions like this one. Her body will keep aging. Her mind never will.

It turns out that Rufus, the gentle giant who caused the chaos on my first night, has severe Tourette's layered on top of multiple developmental disabilities. The likelihood of him living independently is almost nonexistent, and his support system outside these walls is minimal.

My favorite person I met this week, though, is Shelly. Shelly loves the ocean. Everything about it. Dolphins, sea turtles, coral reefs. She smiles constantly, like she lives in a quiet, joyful aquarium inside her own mind.

During our first group therapy session together, Shelly and I sat next to each other in a wide circle of patients. The therapist asked us to share a moment when our illness, addiction, or personal struggle overtook our core values and led us somewhere destructive.

For me, there are plenty of options. But I don't choose the affair.

Even though I'm ashamed of my infidelity, part of me knows I would make the same choice again and again if it meant meeting Brett, and that story feels . . . complicated for the group session. Almost like a happy ending disguised as a mistake. And compared to the stories being shared around this circle of addictions, assaults, and years of abuse, my moral crisis about sleeping with someone outside my marriage, only the second sexual partner of my entire life, feels strangely small.

Too innocent.

I can't find a way to tell it without sounding judgmental or naive about the way I'd been raised to think about sex. So instead, I talk about the overdose—the night my neurotransmitters completely misfired. The truth, the hard truth, is that I didn't want to die.

Still, it's the hardest part to explain, especially to my family. It sounds implausible, but it's real. I wasn't depressed in that moment. I needed a release. I needed relief from the electrical buzzing inside my body. I needed out of my own skin.

Of course, I tried to explain that when I was at Legacy Hospital, to my mom and the Twins. I didn't bother trying to explain it to Richard. I don't think he would have heard me anyway. I hadn't navigated my dad through it either.

Since everything happened, I've only spoken to my dad twice.

But my mom tells me he's called her every single day. Checking in. Asking questions about me. Offering to come immediately. Offering help in any way he can. Their relationship has been complicated since the divorce—careful, sometimes strained, but this much has always been steady: my dad loves me, as much as he loves anyone.

The first time Dad and I spoke was back at Legacy Hospital. At the time, I was still foggy and in recovery, the room too bright, machines humming softly around me. But I remember Dad's voice, grounded, and familiar. No edge to it. Just there. Holding.

I make the second call while at East Pines.

I have little competition for the pay phone banks. Apparently, no one else's mother is slipping phone cards into cigarette packs. After a few long calls with Brett, with my knees pressed into the hard concrete floor to accommodate the short telephone cord stretched to its absolute limit, I learn to pull up a chair when we talk. That 10-inch cord is relentlessly unforgiving.

The hallway whirs around me, full of distant voices, a television playing something indistinct, a rerun of a terrible show that basic cable runs into the ground, the occasional sharp echo of a door closing down the corridor.

When Dad answers, I can hear it immediately—the relief. It smoothes something in his voice.

"Morgie," he says, and I can picture him in the kitchen, leaning against the counter, standing, one hand pressed on the cold marble like he does when he's trying to stay steady. "Has it happened before?"

"Yes, a few times," I admit, "but it was different then."

"You've cheated before with different people?" Dad continues, not accusing, just trying to understand, trying to get it right.

"What!? No! I've never cheated. But," I say, pausing and feeling the weight of it settle as I say it out loud, "I have tried to commit suicide before." I take a breath and continue, "Just not with pills. That's what I meant by 'different.'"

There's a long silence.

Not empty, it's full. I hear Dad breathing unevenly. A small, involuntary sound he's trying to hold back. I've only heard him like this once before.

It was when he told me about Becky for the first time. I was 8 years old. We sat on the upstairs balcony off my parents' bedroom, just the three of us, the original unit, before anything was fractured. I remember the air being still and the way the world seemed to pause around us. I dropped to my knees, screaming in a voice I didn't recognize as my own.

And my dad, 6 feet tall, solid, composed, already donning a full head of silver hair, far before his time, folded with his head in his hands and his shoulders shaking. I thought he was laughing. It didn't make sense.

But it wasn't laughter. It was heartbreak. A grown man, undone by the pain of his little girl. And so—he stayed. He announced he would call things off with Becky. Somewhere deep inside him, I think he believed he could. I actually think he really tried.

Now, through the phone, I can hear it again. Fainter now. But still unmistakable.

"Oh, Morgan," he says finally, his voice breaking just slightly, "I've had it all wrong. I thought this was over Richard. But it's not."

"No, Dad," I say, my own voice steadier than I feel. "It's not."

We talk on the phone a while longer. He tells me about my Aunt Beth, his only sister, who was diagnosed with bipolar in her early 20s and spent nearly four decades managing it with lithium. He tells me the stories slowly, like he's turning them over in his hands before offering them up. How brilliant Beth was. How stubborn she was. How fiercely she protected her independence, even when the illness tried to steal it from her.

There's something about the way my dad listens, even over the phone, that makes it easy to keep going. He doesn't rush to fill the space. He lets things hang just long enough for me to step into them. I can see why he's so good at being a lawyer; why people sit across from him and tell him things they didn't plan to say. There's a steadiness to him, but also a surprising lightness. A lift in his tone, a small warmth that slips in just when you expect him to stay formal. It disarms you. Makes you feel safe enough to be honest.

Dad and I talk about my treatments at East Pines. The medications they've adjusted, the structure of the therapy sessions, the things Dr. Khan has helped me recognize in my own patterns. I can hear Dad moving on the other end of the line; he is probably pacing, one hand on his chin, the other potentially pressed to his belly.

And then, carefully, we talk about my plan. I can't tell him everything yet, not before I tell Mom. But he reads between the lines well enough to understand one key detail: Richard is not going to be a part of it. Dad lets out a soft, knowing chuckle, low and brief.

"That doesn't surprise me," he says.

There will be no love lost between the two of them.

For the first time in a long while, the conversation feels easy. Honest. Like we've stepped out of something formal and into something more natural, two adults, no longer navigating around old family landmines. Finally.

And then, without really planning to, something I've carried quietly for years slips out.

"I wish," I tell him, my voice more subdued now, "that on my wedding day . . . you had asked me if I wanted to run out the back of the church."

There's a pause on the other end. I can hear him breathe in, slow, measured. The kind of pause that makes space for something real. And oddly enough, saying it out loud doesn't feel like reopening a wound. It feels like opening a window. Letting air into something that's been sealed shut for years. For the first time in a long time, my dad and I are just talking. No defenses. No scripts. No pretending. Just honesty.

"I wish we did this more often, Dad," I tell him.

"Me too, honey. I'm here. Any time. Just call."

While I've been at East Pines this past week, my mom has spent most of her time back in Kentucky, but she did stop by once on her way to the airport. This time, Richard wasn't with her, which meant I could finally sign the medical power of attorney over to her, granting her the legal authority to speak for me if I couldn't speak for myself.

Richard's anger, justified or not, shouldn't give him the power to lock me away in an institution without my consent.

Visiting hours were closed when Mom came by, so I didn't get to actually see her, but I was able to sign the paperwork with the appropriate witnesses present. Even without a hug or a conversation, it gave both of us peace of mind.

Visitation at East Pines is strict: one hour per day, only during dinnertime and only on Mondays, Thursdays, and Sundays. Greer has come every single time allowed. Richard has come once.

I cannot imagine what the East Pines cafeteria has been like for Greer's pregnancy nose. Sweet Greer deserves an Academy Award for pretending the smell of fried salmon patties, steamed broccoli, and onions and potatoes didn't bother her.

Our time together this week has been brief, but I have cherished every visit. The days she came seemed to move faster.

Between calls with Brett, which have been two sometimes three a day, my treatment sessions, three scheduled meals, journaling, writing apology letters in crayons, and the endless miles I have logged pacing the courtyard, one small square at a time, I've kept myself busy. But nothing has healed me the way laughing with Greer has.

We have tried to keep things light during her visits, but there are certain topics we haven't been able to avoid. Like our business.

For almost four years now, Jet Set Lingerie has been our shared oxygen. Talking shop is second nature to us. And right now, we need a plan, one that is fair to everyone, one that accounts for my recovery and the Twins' pregnancies.

Another presentation for Maidenform has been looming over us. Our first meeting in June with them went incredibly well. But the follow-up presentation, the one where acquisition might actually be on the table, is approaching quickly. There is simply no way that I will be emotionally ready, or that anyone will believe I'm ready, to walk back into that level of pressure.

So, the Twins, and their growing baby bellies, will have to take the lead. I know they'll nail it.

With both of their maternity leaves approaching, we decide to treat my recovery in a similar way. I'll take six weeks completely off. No expectations. No in-person commitments. If a major decision comes up that requires all three of us, I'll step in remotely as best I can, just as they will during their leaves. It feels fair. Practical.

In the quieter moments of Greer's visits with me, we laugh about the surreal turn our lives have taken, particularly mine. From five-course tasting menus at Jean-Georges . . . to soggy dinners at East Pines, on the kind of trays filled with lukewarm, plastic plates with lids fogged over, everything tasting faintly the same.

We don't laugh in a way that diminishes what has happened, or what is still ahead, but in the only way we know how to survive hard things. It's the same medicine we've used since middle school.

By her third visit, Greer clearly notices I've been busy making friends. Patients drift over to our table, lingering, saying hello like we're all part of something shared. Fluorescent lights flicker overhead. It makes Greer giggle that I've bothered with makeup, that I still try to look like myself in a place where most people have stopped trying altogether.

"Pip," she laughs, "you know they don't crown a Homecoming Queen in here, right?"

I laugh back. I know exactly what she means.

Greer has always been able to draw out my truths faster than almost anyone. Which probably makes this whole situation especially confusing for her. How has she not seen me? How has she not noticed that my marriage wasn't a happy one? How has she missed the signs?

Simple. I didn't let her. That answer is still hard for me to admit.

But, it didn't happen all at once. A comment softened. A story redirected. A feeling turned into a joke before it could land any other way. At first, it felt protective, like I was sparing her something unnecessary. Then, it became about protecting me and, eventually, Richard. Then, it became habit. Finally, it became pure instinct. And ultimately, I didn't know how to unwind it.

Where do I even start? With the first lie, when I reported that Richard and I had a great honeymoon? The first omission, when I pretended Richard truly loved them and was thrilled when I wanted to start a business with them? Is it the first time something felt off, and I chose not to name it? Like the times Richard pulled me aside at a party to tell me I'm too loud and I dress too slutty and I'm just overall "too much."

It was easier to keep going once I started hiding myself. Like a hamster wheel I didn't mean to step onto, but I keep running because stopping requires an explanation I don't have the energy, or the courage, to give.

During what turns out to be our final visit, though neither of us knew it at the time, I think about telling her everything. That I'm leaving Dallas for good.

The words rise, sitting just behind my teeth. But I stop myself. Again. For her.

Her plate is already overflowing. Addy's, too. The two of them are leaving for New York in two days for the Maidenform meeting, the final push for an acquisition. They don't need one more piece of my chaos pulling their focus away.

A nurse wheels a cart past us, the metal rattling slightly over the tile. Someone down the hall calls out a name that isn't answered. The air feels unsettlingly still.

Once I'm out of here . . . once they're back from New York . . .

Then, I'll tell them everything. I'm ready for that now. Brett is ready, too. And we have a plan. It's layered and complicated and built around protecting my health first. But it's there, fully formed.

Just waiting for me to step into it.

In my circle therapy sessions at East Pines, the patients are encouraged to ask each other questions if we feel we might learn something from the person sharing. No one is required to answer, and no one is pressured to speak beyond what they're comfortable with.

In a room filled with people of different ethnicities, socioeconomic backgrounds, genders, and upbringings, we somehow come together in the same place with one shared purpose: understanding our mental health journeys.

It's been a beautiful thing. No stigmas. No judgment. I didn't walk into East Pines with a "woe is me" mindset about my diagnosis. But spending time here, hearing stories, witnessing struggles so different from my own, has left me feeling deeply grateful.

Grateful for the life I have. Grateful for the treatment options available to me. Grateful that my illness, while serious, is something I can manage. Something I can choose to live with.

My last appointment with Dr. Khan is short and sweet. He writes my updated prescriptions, with a few tweaks and a new med to try. He goes over the doses and the rules. At one point, I swear I almost catch him laughing when I ask him where my Klonopin script is.

"Surely, after this many hours with me, you know that dark humor is one of my favorite long-term coping mechanisms, Doc," I say, attempting a wink but nailing the smile. "In all seriousness, Dr. Khan, thank you. Thank you for everything. You made me feel safe and heard. I won't forget what I've learned here."

A nurse waits for me outside. She walks me to my room, holding a large, drawstring plastic bag. My homeward bound luggage.

"Okay, I hope it was a great last visit with your doctor," the nurse says. "Now, let's get you packed up for your pickup. Your husband is outside in the car waiting to take you home."

Nice of Richard to come inside, I think sarcastically.

I walk into my room. No more *Teen Beat* posters on the walls. Meggie was moved to another hospital yesterday, closer in proximity to her family. We had a long hug goodbye, and she shared a few more fun facts about Zac (Efron) before she left. It's bizarre to know without question that you'll never see a person again, after experiencing something truly life-changing together. I doubt I would even recognize Meggie in the "real world" on the off chance our paths would ever cross.

The nurse hands me the bag to fill with my things. I stuff it with all the clothes, the drugstore toiletries, less the ChapStick that I put in my pocket, and my shower shoes. Inside my copy of *The Widow Clicquot*, I slide my stack of letters, handwritten in crayon as personal thank-you notes to everyone who visited me at Legacy Hospital.

"This is trash," I say, handing the full plastic bag to the nurse.

She doesn't question me. I walk out, feeling lighter, with only my book in hand. Lighter indeed.

As I step across the threshold of East Pines, I pause. The involuntary part of my life ends right there. For a moment, I stand still, letting the weight of it all settle in. Then, I turn and look back over my shoulder at East Pines one last time.

Don't forget this. Don't be ashamed of it. This is part of your story now, Morgan. A story to share. To tell without shame.

I've heard it said, "What doesn't kill you makes you more interesting at cocktail parties."

I smile to myself.

Damn. I'm about to be a big hit.

Richard is leaning against my car, parked right at the front entrance. The scene might feel like something out of a romantic comedy, albeit a slightly dark one if he was the person I actually wanted to see, but he isn't that person.

We exchange simple hellos, both of us clearly unsure of what to say next. Then, we hug. A real hug. The wall between us is tall and thick now, but for a moment, maybe out of exhaustion, maybe out of simple familiarity, we hold each other the way we once did. Not as the people we've become, but as the 19- and 20-year-olds we once were before everything complicated us.

"I brought you something," he says, a small smile forming. Before he can explain, I hear a rustling sound from the back seat. A scruffy black puffball stands on hind legs, wet nose mashed against the window.

"Normie!"

I rush to the door and fling it open. Norm launches himself into my arms, showering me in frantic puppy kisses.

"Oh my God—hi, buddy!" I laugh, burying my face in his fur. "Thank you, Richard. Thank you."

It's a genuine act of kindness. And the reason he didn't come in.

Of course, Richard is capable of kindness. He has many wonderful qualities. Unfortunately, I seem to bring out the worst in him more often than the best.

"My parents brought him back while you were in here," Richard explains. "And the Duvalls offered us their ranch, so we can all stay there. I arranged for us to go there this afternoon. My parents, too. Just for one night."

I blink. A forced family weekend with my in-laws? At someone else's ranch? It's not exactly the gentle re-entry I imagined after leaving a mental institution. This feels more like re-entry by fire.

I haven't seen Richard's parents, Susie and Dusty, yet, but I feel avoiding them completely will only make things worse. And I don't want to disrupt the fragile peace forming between Richard and me. For now, steady is the goal.

"Oh . . . not exactly what I expected," I say carefully. "But we didn't really talk about plans, so . . . that's fine. It'll be nice to get outside." Then, I quickly add, "We'll come back tomorrow though, right? I'm pretty tired."

"I'm sure you are," he says. "Yes, just one night."

A pause.

"I invited Aaron, too." Richard adds.

What the actual hell?

Aaron is Richard's childhood best friend, the kind who predates context and, apparently, boundaries. He's also someone I've always cared about, in a familiar, long-standing way, since my sophomore year of college. But tonight, the last thing I have in me is small talk.

Especially with Aaron.

He's 6-foot-4 in that unmistakable, all-American way with broad shoulders, easy posture, and blonde hair that somehow still reads varsity, even years later. He's the kind of man who has never had to wonder if a room would receive him well. Women who are drawn to athletic charm tend to orbit him without much effort on his part, a long and well-documented history he carries lightly, like it's just another thing that happens to him.

And then, there's the other part.

Aaron has made it very clear, openly, confidently, that he doesn't believe mental illness is real. Not misunderstood. Not complicated. Just . . . not real. Which feels like a particularly bold stance to take while standing in front of someone actively living with a diagnosed mental illness.

I'm not asking for understanding, or any type of forgiveness for that matter. That would be generous. But a basic willingness to believe my diagnosis exists doesn't feel like too high a bar.

Still, here he is.

And I can't shake the feeling that Richard's inclusion of Aaron tonight isn't accidental. It feels purposely placed. Strategic. A small, deliberate way to make my release back into the real world just a little harder.

And the truth is, I don't have anything left to fight it. I've spent the last twoish weeks talking my brains out—therapy sessions that pull and stretch and turn everything inside out. I am, quite literally, out of words. And I'm emotionally wrung dry. If Aaron is expecting charm or lightness or even polite engagement, then he's going to be disappointed.

If Greer and Addy were going to be with us tonight, maybe it would feel easier. But they're already in New York preparing for the Maidenform meeting. So, what exactly are the five of us supposed to do? Sit around a campfire making s'mores while they debate whether bipolar disorder is real or not? This has disaster written all over it.

"Where are your bags?" Richard asks as we get into the car.

"Nothing was worth keeping," I say, buckling my seatbelt. "I tossed it all. Time for a purge."

I glance over at him. I wonder if he knows he'll soon be part of that, too.

The drive back to our apartment is nearly silent. Richard fiddles with the radio, flipping through stations that never quite stick. I sit quietly, letting Norm curl into my lap, calm and cozy against me.

"You know, I've been thinking," Richard says. "I really think you should take up hiking. I think it would help you. A lot."

I can't decide if he's being cruel, clueless, or if he is kidding. Does he really think extreme hiking will somehow cure me?

Hiking? Me? Has this man ever actually met me?

Seriously, Richard. No. Just no. Hiking and camping are not going to cure me. In fact, they might encourage me to wander off a cliff. I am not a hiker. I am not a camper. I have no desire to become one. Not for you, not for anyone, not even for Brett. For goodness' sake, I have a poster of Phyllis Nefler in my office. That should tell you everything you need to know. Brett has known me for two months and figured that out within two minutes.

"Hmmm . . . sure, maybe," I say lightly. "But, you know, I've never really been that kind of outdoorsy girl."

I don't want to lie, but I also don't want to argue. I have 24 hours of small talk with my in-laws and Aaron ahead of me. No need to burn through my quota already.

We arrive at our apartment building and pull into the garage. I carry Norm upstairs. I'm not ready to let him out of my sight or arms.

Walking back into the apartment feels strange. Heavy. Questions drift through my mind that I don't want to ask. Did they carry me out? Did they wheel a stretcher through here? Were the paramedics men or women? Did the neighbors watch? Did Richard cry? Was everyone frantic or calm? I'll probably never know. And maybe that's okay.

Although, in a world where I was taught to write a thoughtful, handwritten note for every gift I've ever been given, down to a Vera Bradley curling iron holder, it's utterly ridiculous that I will never be able to properly thank the men and/or women who saved my life that night. (But also, thank you again, Ms. Keller, for the gorgeous curling iron case. I never left campus for a weekend getaway without it.)

As soon as we're inside, Richard says, "My parents just left for the grocery store. You can pack a little overnight bag. Plus . . . I thought you might want a minute in the apartment."

I head toward the closet to pack for the ranch. I know my carry-on is still sitting there, half-packed for the New York trip that never happened. I'm not ready to open that bag. I'll just grab a tote bag instead. Fill it with denim, Frye boots, a cute eyelet top, pajamas, and workout clothes for a walk. A sundress for the drive home tomorrow.

"Wait," Richard says suddenly. "Don't go in there yet. I have a gift for you."

"What? You do?" I ask, surprised.

I have a moment of doubt. Maybe, I've misread everything. Maybe, he's trying to repair things between us. Maybe, starting over feels overwhelming for him, and this is his way of throwing one last Hail Mary.

"Yes," Richard says. "I wasn't sure what the right welcome-home gift is for this situation. New territory. But I think this is it. It's in the closet."

The way he says the word gift doesn't quite sound right, but I follow him anyway.

Our bedroom closet feels smaller than I remember. The air is still, faintly stale, holding onto the scent of cedar shoe forms and expired lavender sachets. The door stays open behind me, but it doesn't feel like an exit. It feels like a frame.

My mind jumps to possibilities. A soft robe. New pajamas. Given his hiking obsession, maybe some misguided outdoor gear.

I step inside, scanning the shelves. Nothing.

"I'm sorry," I say, turning slightly. "Is it hidden? I don't see anything."

"Just look up," Richard says, a sense of pride in his voice.

I do. And there it is.

Wedged between two pristine shoeboxes—one wrapped in navy, stamped with Prada and one in pinstriped kraft paper with Louboutin printed in white—sits a giant bag. Blue bottom. White top. A red oval logo pressed almost flush to the ceiling, the popcorn texture brushing against it.

It takes me a second. Then, I recognize it.

I pull over a step stool, its metal legs scraping and catching the yarn of the carpet, and drag the bag down. It's heavier than I expect, dense and unyielding in my hands. At least 15 pounds.

Charcoal.

The same charcoal the ER doctors pushed through tubes up my nose at the hospital. Thick, gritty, impossible to swallow. Coating everything. My throat. My mouth. My memory. Designed to absorb, to neutralize, to pull the poison of the overdose out of me whether I wanted it or not.

"A bag of charcoal?" I ask, my voice much flatter than I feel. "That's my welcome-home gift?"

"Yep," Richard says, a small, satisfied edge to it. "To remind you what you put us through. Now, put it back up there and face it forward. I want you to have a daily reminder of what you did."

The space tightens.

Not physically, but in that way where your body becomes suddenly aware of its own edges. My shoulders feel too close to the walls. The air seems thinner. Richard's presence behind me, just outside my line of sight, feels heavier than the bag of charcoal in my hands.

It's been less than 20 minutes inside these walls with him, and I can already feel it. The suffocating weight of what a life with Richard actually is.

But not for much longer.

I lift the bag back onto the white, ventilated metal shelf, my arms straining slightly, and nudge it into place. The coated paper crinkles under my hands as I shove it forward, aligning it carefully between the boxes. Presentable. On display.

"Is that forward-facing enough for you?" I ask. I don't wait for an answer.

I grab fresh clothes and move past him, out of the closet, the air shifting again as I leave it behind. Norm follows close at my heels into the bathroom, his nails clicking softly against the tile. I close the door behind us.

The shower comes on too hot at first, steam rising quickly, filling the small space. I step in anyway, letting the water hit the top of my head, running down, washing over everything. My first proper shower since Legacy Hospital. I wash my hair slowly. Deliberately. Letting the heat sit on my skin, trying to feel where my body begins again.

No tears come.

Instead, I picture the bag of charcoal, heavy, ridiculous, and deliberate, set loose on a river. The current taking it away slowly at first, then farther, then smaller, until it's just another object drifting out of sight.

I'm still not completely convinced cognitive therapy works. But I'm committed to my health. I'm committed to using every tool in my box.

And besides . . . in 36 hours, everything will be different.

I must endure 36 hours. I can do this.

But also . . .

Fuck Richard.

And his fucking charcoal.

Chapter 21

THE RESCUE

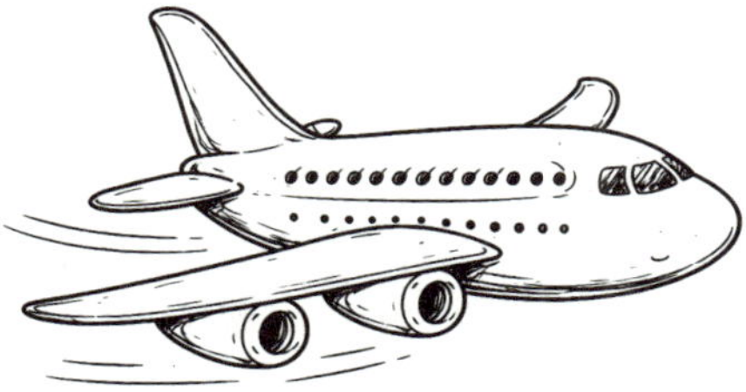

JULY 28, 2009
7 p.m.—Our Apartment
Dallas, Texas

The night we get back from the ranch, Richard hands my BlackBerry back to me. In his mind, I suppose, I'd earned back the device somehow, by spending time with his parents and never once asking for it. I suspect he also realizes that having a wife with absolutely no way to communicate with the outside world is more inconvenient than he originally thought. My mom helped push that realization along by calling his phone to check on me . . . frequently. More frequently than necessary.

Brett and I have been communicating mostly through email on my laptop, but we have kept it light. During our last phone call, when I was still at East Pines, we finalized the details of his trip to Dallas.

Originally, we both had hoped he could come the day after I was released, but without knowing my exact discharge date, it was impossible to plan precisely. Two days after my release was the closest we could get.

I've never been naïve about Brett. I know he's lived a full life before me. There's history there, as there should be. I've never needed all the dating details. They're not the point. He's human. Imperfect. And he's not some knight arriving to rescue me. That part, the saving, belongs to me.

As awkward as the ranch visit was, I appreciated the chance to see Richard's parents again. They have always been incredibly kind to me.

When Susie and Dusty returned from the grocery store before our drive to the ranch, they set their bags down on the kitchen island and immediately wrapped me in a hug. They forgave me before I even asked for forgiveness, which, of course, I did. They live their faith in a way that truly means loving your neighbor as yourself. It's remarkable. A small part of me hopes their kindness toward me might last after I leave for good, but I know that's impossible. It's a good thing really. It will make room in their hearts to welcome the next person who comes into Richard's life with open arms. Which I'm sure will happen quickly.

Dusty couldn't take any more time off work, so on our way back from the ranch, we dropped Richard's parents at the airport. Once they were gone, I settled Norm into my lap and closed my eyes, pretending to sleep. It made the ride serene. Shorter.

Before long, Richard and I were back in our apartment. Very few words were exchanged. We put on pajamas. We popped microwave popcorn. We watched a few episodes of *Mad Men*.

Our usual weeknight routine. For a moment, it almost felt normal. I tried to appreciate it as the last time we might do this together. But on my way to the bathroom, I passed my closet. The giant bag of charcoal stared down at me from its perch.

Richard was right about one thing. It's definitely a reminder. Just not the one he intended. Instead, it's a 15-pound reminder that I don't have to stay here anymore.

Life makes no promises. I hope Brett is part of my future, but if he isn't, nothing really changes. I'm not leaving Richard for Brett.

I'm leaving Richard for me.

Meeting Brett has been a bright spot in an otherwise dark chapter. A silver lining. A catalyst, perhaps. But he's not the reason for my divorce. He's not the reason for my illness. And he's certainly not the reason for my suicide attempt. Brett is simply someone who appeared in the middle of the storm. But he's also still an unknown.

I return to the couch and watch the final minutes of the episode with Richard. When it ends, I scoop up Norm, grab my phone, and head to bed. I set my alarm for 6 a.m. Sleep comes almost immediately. Maybe, it's the new medication. Or maybe, it's finally having a little bit of peace.

July 29, 2009, 6 a.m.—Our Apartment, Dallas

I wake up before the alarm goes off. Too excited to stay asleep. I reach over and switch it off before it can buzz, leaving my phone on the bedside table.

In the bathroom, I wash my face, moisturize, and add a touch of makeup: a little undereye concealer, bronzer, blush, and a swipe of mascara. Brett or no Brett, I do this before any walk or run. It's silly, but it also takes less than two minutes to not feel like a complete hot mess.

With my current title, "Crazy Hot Mess," in the biggest small town in the world, anything to help me feel less like one is worth the effort.

I pull my hair into a messy high ponytail, the curls from yesterday still bouncing. Then, I change into tailored white running shorts and a pink halter yoga top, no-show socks, and sneakers. Into the bottom of my crossbody bag, I roll a slinky coral sundress and a pair of sandals, along with a perfume sample and a pretty pink lipstick.

I grab my car keys, wallet, and phone as quietly as possible and head toward the front door.

Richard is still fast asleep, on his back, snoring. On the back side of a bill sitting on the counter, I scribble a quick note:

Went for a run on the loop. In case I miss you before you head to work, have a nice day. –Morgan

Out of habit, I add a small heart. The second I draw it, I feel like a fraud. Of course, the heart isn't the fraudulent part. The run is. I'm not going for a run. I'm going to the airport. Brett lands in less than 45 minutes, which is almost exactly how long it will take me to get there.

I'm equal parts nervous and excited. It's been almost four weeks since we've seen each other in real life, since I dropped him off at the Newark airport. A lot of life has happened since then. So much, in fact, that it almost sounds made up.

His friends are confused. My friends are in the dark. Between China, mental institutions, my marriage, and a failed meet-the-parents mission, Brett and I have a lot to untangle. It all sounds insane. Because it is. But it's real. There is no reason for a man to fake falling in love with a girl who just spent time in a looney bin. What possible benefit could that have?

Just as my nerves start to overwhelm me, I pull my car into the arrivals pickup line at the airport. It isn't overly crowded. It takes only seconds to spot Brett. Fitted, distressed jeans. A signature white button-down. A worn tan leather duffel slung across his body.

He spots me at the same moment. His smile spreads wide across his face. Mine mirrors it instantly. Now, I have to decide whether to stop the car and let him jump in . . . or get out. Letting him hop in feels anticlimactic. I'm getting out. That's what he would do.

I pull up beside him and shift the car into park. He reaches for the passenger door handle and then notices I'm climbing out. He drops his bag beside the car and walks around toward me.

We meet at the back of the car. He doesn't say anything. He simply lifts me into his arms, nose to nose, eyes locked, and kisses me. Just like our first kiss all over again. For a moment, I can almost feel rain on my skin.

"Hi," Brett says, setting me back on the ground. "I like when you're little." He means when I'm not wearing heels.

"Hi," I laugh. "I know you do. Let's go, handsome."

"Okay, perfect girl," he says, grabbing his bag. "What's on the agenda today?" So casually. Like nothing about this is odd at all.

"Well," I say, glancing at the time, "seeing as it's only 7:30 in the morning . . . breakfast?"

I slide back into the driver's seat. "Room service, perhaps?" he suggests.

I type the name of his hotel into the GPS and pull away from the curb. As we drive, he takes my hand and lifts it to his lips, pressing a quick kiss against it.

We talk the entire 20-minute drive to Hotel ZaZa, far from my apartment, far from Richard's office. It's not lost on me that what I'm doing is wrong, but I'm not trying to rub it in anyone's face. And besides, the day after tomorrow, I'll be gone.

Brett has arranged for the hotel room to be ready early by paying for the previous night as well. The check-in process is lightning fast at this early hour, and before I know it, we are stepping into the elevator. Just the two of us.

He can't help but touch me, gentle and sweet at first. His hands cup my face as he kisses me, then slide down my back, settling at my waist as he pulls me closer. By the time the elevator doors open on our floor, I'm pressed against the mirrored wall, Brett's lips trailing down my neck.

He takes my hand and leads me down the hallway toward the room. Outside the door, he kisses me again while waving the key card over the sensor. The lock clicks open.

Before I can even step inside, he scoops me up in his arms and carries me across the threshold into our beautiful suite.

A tray of champagne in ice chills on the cocktail table beside a carafe of orange juice and a bowl of fresh strawberries. Sunlight pours through open curtains, illuminating the room. Mint-colored lacquer trim frames the doors and windows. A tall chocolate-brown headboard stretches halfway up the wall beneath soaring 12-foot ceilings. He tosses me playfully onto the bed and jumps beside me, bouncing the mattress so I lift into the air. Lying there, meeting my eyes, he says softly, "I just can't stop smiling when I'm with you."

For a moment, life feels right, like the way it's meant to be. And then my phone rings. I ignore it and lean over to kiss him. "I can't stop smiling with you either," I agree.

My phone rings again. And again. I glance at the screen.

"It's Richard," I say. "I think I have to get it."

"Get it," Brett says calmly. "You've got this."

It's embarrassing to admit, but I need Brett here. I need his steady encouragement, his constant reminder to be strong, to be honest, to choose myself. He has never once asked me to choose him. Only to choose myself. Now is my chance.

"Hello?" I answer, standing at the foot of the bed. The soft, cool duvet brushes my leg. My bare feet press into the plush silk rug. My left hand nervously finds my lips, I pull at the skin until it breaks, allowing me to peel off thin layer after layer. The longer Richard speaks, the likelier I'll draw blood.

"Morgan, where are you?" Richard snaps. "Don't say the loop. I know you're not there. I've driven around it three times already."

"No," I reply evenly. "I'm not on the loop. I'm at Hotel Zaza with Brett."

I say it calmly. Matter-of-factly. Richard is anything but calm. I feel Brett move closer before I see him. My head stays down, fixed on my freshly painted red toenails, focused on Richard's words. Brett's presence settles in behind me. His breath is warm at the back of my neck, close enough to register. His hand finds my upper arm, a quiet, grounding squeeze. Not hurried. Familiar. Then a soft kiss on top of my head. Calming.

"What the hell, Morgan?" Richard asks. "What are you doing? I'm calling your mom. I'm calling the Twins. I'm going to tell everyone."

I don't have anything to say to Richard. There is nothing left. My left hand falls to my side, away from my mouth, as the stress of his voice fades.

"Okay," I say.

He hangs up. The room is cold, Texas air-con style, but the initial shock waves moving through me, subtle but constant, warm me from the inside out. The air smells like cologne, strawberries, and coffee, an odd, disorienting mix that somehow works.

I feel myself expanding, like Alice in Wonderland after the growing potion, suddenly too large for the room, for the moment, for the version of me I'm supposed to be. I should probably feel scared. Or sad. Or worried. But none of those emotions show up. Only two words come to mind.

The End.

It's going to be over now, but I need Richard to officially say so. Maybe that's the coward's way out. But this won't work any other way. Everyone in our lives will try to push Richard and I toward counseling, toward trying again and again for the sake of our marriage vows. They'll blame it on me having bipolar. And I'm afraid I might kill myself trying to please everyone. The people I love. The people who believe so fiercely in marriage that they can't imagine letting one go.

I believe in marriage, too. Deeply. But I won't survive if I stay with Richard. This isn't a healthy place for me. And that's not his fault. We bring out the worst in each other. He's not the support system I need. And that's okay. I've been done for a long time. And now, it's clear Richard is done, too.

"Wow. That was fast." Brett responds. He's standing right in front of me. Surprise flickers across his cute face, still somehow boyish.

"Yep. It sure was." I say, falling into his arms.

I think I might cry, but instead, I start laughing hysterically.

"Are you okay?" he asks. At first, he assumes I'm sobbing. When he realizes it's laughter, he freezes for a moment, unsure what to do.

"Sorry," I manage to apologize between breaths. "I'm fine. I actually don't think any of this is funny or insignificant, but I have a toxic trait of reacting the opposite way sometimes. I get the giggles at funerals, too, which is why I hate going to them." I cover my face with my hands and stare at the floor.

"Ha ha! Me, too!" Brett says, laughing with me.

"You do?" I ask, looking up at him in shock, and that only makes us laugh harder.

Eventually, his laughter softens. He gently lifts my chin so I'm looking straight at him. My own laughter fades.

"I know I haven't officially said it yet," he says quietly, "but I came here to get you."

"Well," I smile up at him, "I kind of assumed. And as much as I love hearing that, and as much as I prayed it might be true, this rescue mission is really for myself. Me choosing me. You and I . . . as an us . . . that's icing on the cake."

I can see relief pass across his face. He never wanted to be the villain in someone else's marriage. The guilt of it has haunted him. Apparently, a good Catholic upbringing leaves a lasting imprint. He doesn't want to be the reason a marriage failed.

Greer and Addy have assumed he's been in it for the chase. As girls, we're practically trained to believe that's how men work. Play hard to get. It's supposedly the surest way to win men over.

Being a married woman is about as hard to get as it gets. But Brett has hated every second of the secrecy and the lies. He hasn't been interested in a game. The fact that I've been "hard to get" has been his least favorite part about me.

"God, that makes me so happy to hear, Morgan," he says.

The way he says my name completely undoes me. He leans down and kisses me.

The buzz of my BlackBerry interrupts us. This time it's my mom. Richard must have gotten her first. Lucky her.

"Hi, Mom," I answer, my voice slightly perkier than it should be. I'm not naïve. I know difficult days are ahead. But I'm ready to face them now.

"Well, Morgie," she says matter-of-factly, "I think it's time you let me in on the full plan. So, let's hear it."

Years of chaos have turned my mom into a master of crisis management. My mom is basically a female version of Job from the Bible. Life tests her endlessly, and she keeps moving forward. She's also a doer. If she wants a new brick patio, she builds one herself. If she doesn't like a wall in the house, she knocks it down herself. Sometimes, that causes . . . complications.

Like the time she demolished a wall only to discover the main water pipe ran right through it. We ended up with a freestanding sink in the middle of her newly expanded bathroom for months until she could afford to hire a contractor. She dressed the sink in a Laura Ashley pleated skirt, and we all joked about the "skirted centerpiece" for years.

I've just taken a sledgehammer to my life.

Now, we have to skirt the sink.

"Mom, I'm sorry you had to hear it from Richard," I say. "Though I'm sure he relished the moment. It's the least I could do for him." The sarcasm oozes out of me.

"Oh yes," she says dryly. "He thoroughly enjoyed asking me, 'Do you know where your daughter is?'"

When my mom impersonates Richard, his voice somehow turns into the wicked old lady from *Snow White*. Now, I'm picturing him in a black hooded cloak holding a basket of poisoned apples.

"He got to you fast," I say.

"Yes," she says. "I was his first call. Lucky me. But, Morgie, he plans to work his way down your entire list of friends unless you'd like to get to them first."

"Nope," I say. "I have zero desire to do that. If I learned anything at the Cuckoo's Nest, it's that everyone is carrying their own load. People don't have that much energy left over for someone else's drama. And once you've been in one of those places, the jig is pretty much up anyway. People can think what they want. I'll survive it."

"Okay, Boo," she says. "So, what's the plan now? How long can Brett stay in Dallas?"

I explain as best I can. My immediate plan is to come back to Murray. Get my footing. Start the divorce process properly. Brett has to return to China in three or four days. Today, we'll try to pack a few suitcases of my personal belongings. I'm not taking anything that belongs to Richard. Just my things. Mostly the fashion. Everything else he can keep.

"Mom," I add, "could you come get me? No rush. Brett will stay with me until you arrive. And . . . I'd really like you two to meet."

"Of course," she says. "I can be there tomorrow morning. Does that work?"

"That's perfect," I say, relieved. "Thank you."

"You don't have to thank me," she replies. "I'm your mother. What you should have done was stash away the cash I've given you over the years. But I suspect that money was converted into shoes." She pauses. "Morgie . . . do you have any money at all?"

The honest answer is no. Managing money has never been my strong suit. Champagne taste on a beer budget. And this summer's mania obliterated whatever savings I had left. I'll pay for that recklessness by moving back in with my mom and selling whatever I can. But I will not pay for it by asking Richard for money. I don't want anything that might complicate or delay our divorce.

Texas has a 60-day waiting period for uncontested divorces. The goal is get out quick.

"Not much," I admit, thinking of the $40 in my wallet.

"Morgan," she says firmly, "go to the ATM today and withdraw a little. Nothing major. No more than half of what's in the account. Just enough to get you out of Dallas."

We hang up so she can start packing for the drive. Brett has been waiting patiently, but I can tell he's anxious for an update.

"She'll be here tomorrow afternoon," I say.

"Good," he replies.

I smile. "What are we going to do until then?" I say playfully.

He laughs, scoops me up into his arms, my legs wrap around him, and he carries me toward the bed.

My phone has been blowing up for the last hour, but I'm not interested in explaining myself to the list of friends to whom Richard is tattling. When Greer and Addy call, I will answer, but not until then.

I know they're in the Maidenform meeting now. I don't want to do anything to unnerve them, although I'm sure Richard couldn't give a shit about that. He's already made the call to Greer and Addy. I'm sure of it.

Brett hovers over the bottle of champagne like he's trying to decide if it's appropriate to crack it open as my marriage officially dies.

"I can see you're struggling with a decision right now," I say. "To pop or not to pop? The answer is no. It's absolutely not appropriate. But we can't let a good bottle like that go to waste, right?"

He kisses me softly just after our glasses clink.

"Let's make this our thing," I suggest.

"A kiss after every toast?" he asks. "I love it."

A tradition born.

The day becomes a strange kind of roller coaster, with long stretches of bliss with Brett, interrupted by stressful drops of shame-filled phone calls.

I try to stay steady in my decision. I will never be proud of my failures or my many flaws, but I have to find a way to move forward without sliding back into the gutter again.

The inevitable call from Greer and Addy is the hardest. Letting them down is the last thing I ever want to do. And of course, this is a huge disappointment to them.

They're hurt. Confused about why I wasn't fully honest with them sooner. I try to explain, but it's the kind of conversation that really needs to happen face-to-face. Words over the phone feel clumsy and incomplete. At one point, I attempt to ask how the meeting went, but the question sounds ridiculous in the middle of everything else going on.

Richard called them repeatedly during the meeting until they finally stepped out of the conference room and answered. It's painfully obvious that my situation is spilling into everyone else's lives. When we hang up, I don't feel great about where things stand between us. This will take time to repair. Years, probably. But I'm willing to do the work.

My relationship with Greer and Addy may never return to exactly what it once was, but it was already destined to change with their babies on the way. This just adds another layer, of complexity, of hurt. And I get it.

Brett and I are starving. I'm not sure if it's the bubbly on an empty stomach or the surrealness of the day, everything carrying that light, untethered feeling of a champagne buzz, but we both need to eat. We step out into the streets of Dallas in search of food and an ATM.

The Texas summer greets us immediately. Not just warm. Dense. The kind of heat that feels like it's rising from every direction at once, pressing in from above while the sidewalk radiates it back up through the soles of our shoes. The skyline hovers above us, glass and steel shimmering slightly in the distance. My skin catches it quickly, a light sheen forming, glistening at my collarbones, along my arms, my upper lip. Everything feels amplified. Slowed and intensified at the same time.

We pass a bank just outside of the hotel. The air conditioning inside the phone-booth-sized ATM machine is aggressive. We fold into the small space together, our bodies close, warming the air inside quickly. I enter my pin number and wait for the balance of the checking account. $2,000. I take out $1,000. Exactly half. Per my mom's suggestion.

Brett steps up to the ATM after me, pulling out his card. I assume it's to get cash for lunch, something quick, practical. We're both too hungry to overthink it.

"I don't want you to worry about money. We'll figure this out as we go," he says, handing me $3,000.

I blink at it, disoriented. "What?" I ask. "Wait—no. You don't need to do this. I can figure all of this out."

"Yes, you can. And you will," he says, slower than his usual pace. "But I can help. So maybe let me, just a little."

The way he looks at me when he says it—steady, open, something unmistakably kind about it—settles far deeper than the money itself. There's no hesitation in him. No performance. Just a certainty that he wants to be here, in this, with me.

Outside again, the heat wraps around us like it's been waiting. We lace our fingers together and start walking, no real direction, just movement. The city pulses around us, cars, voices, something distant and metallic, but it all feels slightly blurred at the edges.

Brett's pace slows, and I step ahead without noticing. Then, gently, he pulls my arm, spinning me back into him like we're about to dance. Our chests collide abruptly. His arms come around me easily, instinctively, wrapping around my waist tightly. I feel safely cocooned. Our sun-soaked scents meet and settle together. Sweat. Skin. Salt.

"Morgan, I'm in love with you. I'm all in," Brett declares. He basically shouts it from the rooftops, Ron Burgundy style.

"I'm in love with you, too, Brett. I'm in," I say, without having to think about. It just rolls right off my tongue.

Like clockwork, almost as if he can sense my happiness from miles away, Richard calls to ruin it.

"Morgan, you took all the money out of the account?" he asks. "Seriously, what is wrong with you?"

"Hi, Richard," I reply calmly. "No, I didn't. I took half. The other half is yours. And I don't want anything else except my clothes."

"I've drawn up a temporary division of assets!" he shouts. "Come get your shit so I can get our divorce officially started." He hangs up.

I stare down at my phone. I have no idea how Richard found the time to draft legal paperwork in between his marathon rounds of tattling to everyone about my life choices, but I'm not even going to try to understand him anymore.

Short of my clothes and a few sentimental items that belong to my family, I have zero interest in any of the things in our apartment. I know my lack of interest will infuriate him. I'm not trying to provoke him, but right now, it feels like a small bonus.

I look over at Brett.

"How would you feel about some fast food to hold us over?" I ask. "I might be on borrowed time before Richard burns all my Chanel. Those treasures might be my meal ticket someday, so I really can't mess around." I laugh nervously.

"Are you kidding?" Brett says dramatically. "I'll eat anything to save the Chanel!"

He's teasing me a little, but it's adorable. We hurry back to the hotel and head down to the parking garage. I toss him the car keys.

"Brett," I admit, "I'm actually a terrible driver. And my sense of direction is garbage. I was a complete ball of nerves getting us from the airport to the hotel. Honestly, the main reason I prefer Uptown New York is 80% because it's a grid and 20% because of the shopping, and well . . . Bemelmans, of course." I drop my head in my hands. "I get lost everywhere I go," I continue. "I know you just said you love me . . . but knowing this . . . are you still sure?"

He grins. "Never been more sure of anything," he says.

Then, he starts the car.

"Let's do this," he says. "First stop: Whataburger. Next stop: Chanel rescue."

With greasy fries in hand, Diet Cokes in the cup holders, and Phoenix blasting on the radio, Brett and I cruise into the parking lot of my apartment building.

"You're good to hang here, right?" I ask.

"Of course," Brett says. "But call me if you need anything, and I'll be right there to whip some ass."

He's laughing so hard he can barely get the sentence out.

"You're on speed dial," I tell him.

I step out of the car and walk toward the front doors of the building. Instead of waiting for the elevator, I take the stairs up to our floor. My heart is beating faster than it should be. Before heading to the apartment, I stop by my storage unit down the hall and grab two giant suitcases.

When I reach the door, I pause. Maybe I should knock. It doesn't feel like my home anymore. But instead, I just turn the handle and walk in.

Norm greets me immediately, jumping up with a flurry of puppy kisses. The feeling hits me like a gut punch. I already know the first thing on Richard's list will be Norm. And I'm certain Norm won't be placed in my column of assets.

I stand there for a second, unsure of what to say to Richard. Or whether I should say anything to him at all. Then, I realize I don't have to. Richard isn't here. The apartment is empty.

For a moment, I consider calling Brett and asking him to come upstairs, but I decide against it. What if Richard just stepped out for a minute and comes back?

On the kitchen counter, I spot two handwritten copies of a "division of assets" document Richard has drafted. A pen sits beside the papers, along with two carefully placed sticky notes shaped like arrows that read "sign here."

I imagine he probably had the stickers in his work bag already, though the thought of him racing to Office Depot to make it feel more official than necessary makes me laugh. Attached with a paperclip to one copy is a brief handwritten note.

Morgan,

Assuming this list is acceptable to you, please sign both copies. For the items we still need to specify, we can do that tomorrow, assuming the window from 4-6 PM works for you. We will also need to discuss liabilities at that time.

Richard

I look over the list. My instincts were right. At the very top, in the right-side column, Richard's column, is *NORM*.

His side of the list continues with:

- *All his earnings from The Providence Group and retirement funds*
- *Morgan's car*
- *All personal effects, clothes, etc., including Cartier watch*
- *All apartment furniture, except an antique buffet*
- *All art, except the painting of Petros the Pelican*
- *The Christmas china and all Waterford crystal*
- *Christmas ornaments of his choosing*
- *All cookware and small kitchen appliances to be distributed evenly*

Holy shit. Did he literally just open all the cabinets and make a full list of the contents of our apartment. I seriously couldn't care less about any of these items. I move over to my side of the list. Not as robust:

- *Morgan's stake in Jet Set Lingerie*
- *Engagement and wedding rings*
- *All her personal effects including her Cartier watch*
- *Monogrammed Wedgwood china*
- *All family sterling silver*
- *See Richard's list for additional division of items.*

I pick up the pen and notice. ironically, that it's from The Carlyle. If this isn't intentional, then it's an uncanny coincidence.

Norm is at my feet, staring up at me with his signature underbite. A single tear hits the paper and smears the line about Christmas ornaments. Signing away Norm is almost too much to bear, but I'm not fit to be his mom right now. And fighting Richard over him is not something I can emotionally handle. Norm has never been Richard's dog. Norm has always been mine. I'm his main caretaker, but there are so many big unknowns about my life. Where will I live? What will I do?

So, I sign both copies.

I pick Norm up and carry him with me into the closet while I pack as much as I possibly can into the two large suitcases.

In the first bag, I place my designer handbags, blazers, shoes, and my bangle bar. Brett has been dying to see my bangle collection since the first time I visited his apartment. In the second suitcase, I pack my favorite outfits, stuffing it so full I need all my weight to get it to zip.

Then, I clear out the bathroom drawers and cabinets, tossing everything into one giant tote bag: makeup, toiletries, meds, my underthings, a few pairs of pajamas, and a stack of swimsuits.

Norm hates the sight of suitcases. He's a nervous wreck now, glued to my side as if he knows exactly what's happening. My heart breaks. The guilt is real. Somehow, leaving this little dog is harder than leaving the human I've spent nearly a decade with. It's a brutal truth.

I roll the suitcases toward the door. They each weigh well over the 70-pound airline limit, but luckily Mom doesn't charge for overweight baggage in her car, and she definitely doesn't judge it.

I kneel down to Norm's level and give him one of his favorite treats.

"I'll see you tomorrow, buddy," I whisper, kissing his nose, knowing it will probably be the last time I ever see him.

When I open the door, Richard is standing right outside it. My face is covered in tears. They're all because of Norm, but maybe, it's better if Richard assumes they're about him. It softens the blow.

"So sorry," I say quickly. "I was rushing to get out. I assumed, since you weren't here, you didn't want to see me."

He doesn't respond right away. He just looks me up and down as he steps by me to enter the apartment, making sure Norm can't slip past him into the hallway.

"Have you had that on all day?" he says it with a level of disgust.

I'm still wearing the same basic workout clothes I put on this morning when I left to pick Brett up from the airport.

"Yes," I say, confused.

"You never changed when you went to see him?" he presses, his voice getting sharper.

"No. Why?" I ask. I genuinely don't understand why this matters.

"It's just not like you," Richard snaps. "You're always overdressed, always trying to impress people. I can't believe you went to see him looking like that."

At first, I think he's insulting how I look. I wouldn't blame him. Unkind words feel inevitable right now. But then, I realize what he's actually saying. His comment isn't about my clothes. It's about the fact that I'm not trying to impress Brett.

It's the same reason he was furious when I described Brett as an unemployed accountant from Ohio. Richard has imagined I'm chasing some glamorous fantasy or some ridiculous fairy tale.

Instead, I showed up in running shorts.

"I guess I just didn't think it was real," he says quietly. "That you'd actually be this comfortable with him."

I don't know what to say. And I don't want to be cruel.

"I'm sorry, Richard," I say gently. "I wish I had told you I wanted to leave before any of this happened."

"But you would still leave?" he asks, almost rhetorically.

"Yes," I answer. "I mean . . . I pretty much did when I got the New York apartment for the summer. But then, the Twins' birthday came up, and I couldn't extend the lease, and I didn't know what to do. I know I didn't handle it the right way. Obviously, I know that."

I gesture toward the paperwork on the counter.

"But Richard . . . you clearly want out, too," I continue. "No one draws up a division of assets that fast."

For a moment, it feels like we might hug goodbye. But it passes.

"I'll come back tomorrow, during the 4 to 6 window you suggested, to get the rest of my things," I say.

I roll the two suitcases into the hallway and toward the elevator. I manage to hold the tears back until I reach the car. Brett takes one look at my face and immediately jumps out, grabbing the bags from me and pulling me into a hug. I bury my face in his chest and cry.

"That bad?" he asks softly.

"It was saying goodbye to Norm," I explain. "And Brett," I choke through the tears, "it was a decade of my life." I take a breath. "But I'm relieved, too," I continue, "and grateful for whatever comes next."

"I know this is hard," Brett says. "What can I do?"

I think for a moment.

"How about you take me on a proper date," I suggest.

"Funny you should say that," he says. "I made us a reservation at a downtown steakhouse." He opens the car door. "Tonight calls for Manhattans and surf-and-turf. Don't you think?" he asks.

"It most certainly does," I agree.

He loads the bags into the car, rolls down the windows, and opens the sunroof. Soon, we're cruising, with Christopher Cross's "Sailing" filling the air, soaking in the feeling of my brand-new freedom.

Chapter 22

A MOTHER & A MARRIAGE MYTH

JULY 30, 2009
10 a.m.—Hotel ZaZa
Dallas, Texas

My mom and Brett have never spoken. Never even seen each other before. But they already share something powerful, a love for me. And in their own ways, both of them survived the past few weeks and the emotional roller coaster that I, with some help from my disease, dragged all of us through.

"Well, it's not every day you meet your married daughter's boyfriend," my mom says, laughing as she walks into the hotel room.

Brett doesn't miss a beat. He steps forward and hugs her immediately. Two pieces of my life clicking together perfectly.

I'm slowly getting better at acknowledging the suicide attempt as part of my bipolar disorder. It doesn't sit entirely on my shoulders. The affair, though, that one does. I can't let myself off the hook there. I need to own it, if I'm ever going to heal and move forward. Naturally, my mother thinks the entire thing is Richard's fault. But that's what mothers do. Once a mama bear, always a mama bear.

Brett, on the other hand, tends to be more levelheaded about it. Though knowing my mom, she could probably rile him up and recruit him to her side, if she really wanted to.

"Great to meet you, Mona," Brett says warmly. "And 'boyfriend,'

I like the sound of that." He glances back at me and pulls me into a sideways hug.

I'm still in my nightgown, wrapped in the hotel's robe with slippers on my feet, and I fit perfectly into the crook of his arm. I slip out from his embrace and fall straight into hers. I haven't seen her since I've been out of East Pines. What a swing of events. To her, I must look like an entirely different person.

And Brett, he truly feels like my boyfriend now. It seems like we've been together for much longer than we actually have. It's funny how 24 hours can completely change the direction of someone's life.

July 29, 2009, 5 p.m.—Hotel ZaZa

When we get back to the hotel after picking up the first round of my things from the apartment, the mood is light and easy. The ease feels like a gift. Nothing about the past few weeks could be described that way.

Brett puts on "Then Came You" by The Spinners through a Bose travel speaker, a gadget I'd never seen before, and suddenly, the whole room feels like a dance floor. We twirl around the suite, sometimes holding each other so close it feels like we are one person, other times spinning apart and being silly. He pours champagne while keeping time with the music, and I run a bubble bath and lay out a special outfit for our dinner date.

We finish the bottle of champagne we'd opened earlier that morning and then abandoned mid-chaos. The hotel kindly keeping it chilled for us in a giant ice bucket. It feels like it belongs to the moment.

We soak in the tub afterward, each on our own respective end, skipping the *Pretty Woman* pose entirely. The bathroom fills with steam while we talk about everything and nothing. Eventually he looks at me more seriously.

"Okay," he says. "There's something big we need to talk about."

"Geez, you're scaring me," I laugh nervously. "What is it?"

"We have to book your ticket to Beijing," he says. "I can't leave here without knowing exactly when I get to see you again."

He pulls me gently toward him by my knees and kisses me quickly before sliding me back to my side of the tub.

"No funny business until we get the date locked down," he adds with a grin.

"Well," I laugh, "my schedule is suddenly pretty wide open." Then, I grow more thoughtful.

"But I really need to talk with Greer and Addy first," I explain. "We still have a lot to figure out with the business. They want me to take six weeks to get my feet back under me. After that, I'll probably need to step in more since travel will be harder for them with the babies coming."

I did the math out loud. "It hasn't even been a week yet . . . so that probably leaves a five-week window where I could come visit you," I say. "What do you think?"

"I want you on the plane with me in two days," he admits. "But I know that's not what's best for you. You need time to breathe. Time that's just yours."

He pauses and suggests, "How about two or three weeks from now?"

Part of me doesn't know what to think. Being away from him already feels hard. When I am with Brett, I feel free to be exactly who I am. But the idea of flying to China for a man I've only known for six weeks, two of which I just spent in a hospital, is a lot to absorb.

He senses my hesitation.

"Morgan," he says gently, filling the silence, "there's no rush. I'll wait as long as it takes."

I believe him. He has never once pressured me or made me feel like I have to prove anything, about myself, or about my feelings for him.

I slide back across the tub toward him. "Let's do it," I say finally. "The third week of August sounds perfect."

He places his hands on my lower back and pulls me into him.

"Perfect, I'll book your ticket tomorrow," he says softly, as he leans into my ear. Wrapped in warm water, his mouth brushes my neck and moves to my collarbone. I love that he knows exactly where to touch me, how to touch me.

July 30, 2009, 10 a.m.—Hotel ZaZa

"Mona, can I get you a coffee? How do you take it?" Brett asks.

"Yes, perfect," she says. "Just black, please."

"Like your men, I assume," Brett says, quoting *Airplane!*.

It's a slightly risky joke to make the first time you meet someone's mother, but it hits perfectly with Mona. She loves that movie. Brett is constantly quoting something: a song lyric or a line from a show or a famous sports moment, and somehow, he slips them into conversation so naturally it never feels forced.

He pours my mom a cup of coffee from the pot he ordered earlier with room service. I'm not a coffee drinker. I've always preferred my caffeine in the form of Diet Coke and Toblerone. Brett's morning routine, though, feels incredibly grown-up: black coffee, eggs and bacon, and a copy of *The Wall Street Journal*. I settle for tea and a yogurt parfait while he reads bits of the morning headlines out loud to me.

I can already imagine this becoming our ritual. In my mind, we're in his New York apartment, but I could get used to the idea of us in Asia, too. For now, though, my focus is on me. On getting healthy.

"Alright, you two," my mom says, settling into her chair with the coffee. "What's the plan? How do we get Morgie out of here?"

My mom has never liked Dallas. I don't think it's really about the city though. She always knew I never wanted to leave New York. More accurately, she knew I didn't want to move here with Richard. If I have a daughter someday, I hope my maternal instincts are as sharp as hers.

"Brett leaves on a five o'clock flight back to New York tonight," I explain. "Then, he is back to Beijing early tomorrow morning."

"I was thinking," Brett adds, "we should go find some good old Texas barbecue before I have to head to the airport. Are you two game?"

"Sounds good to me," Mom says. Then she grins. "But, if possible, could we sit outside? Maybe in the smoking section?" She laughs. "I might need a cigarette today. My nerves are shot."

"I hear you," Brett says, laughing. "Maybe, I'll even join you."

He glances over at me, already anticipating my reaction.

"Way to be a great influence, Mom," I tease.

I can tell Brett is a little nervous at lunch. Between bites of brisket, he talks quickly, almost too fast, and I'm not sure my mom can fully keep up. She isn't interrogating him exactly, but she's naturally curious about everything. Why is he in China? What're his parents like? Is he sad to leave New York? And then, she gets to the real question.

"Brett," she says calmly, "based on your actions, it really seems like you're in this for the long haul. Is that true?"

"Mom!" I interrupt. "Brett, you don't have to answer that."

I pat his knee under the table. He takes my hand, lifts it gently, and kisses the top of it.

"Happy to answer," he says. "Of course, I'm in. I wouldn't be here if I wasn't." He smiles and glances at me.

"She's not wrong to ask, Morgan," he continues. "I'm sure I seem too good to be true." He laughs, clearly trying to lighten the moment. Then, he turns back to my mom and places his other hand gently over hers on the table.

"Mona," he says sincerely, "I've fallen in love with your daughter. It's been a bit of a crazy start, to say the least. But it's real. And I'm here to help her get back on her feet however I can."

He pauses and adds, "Then, hopefully we can think about the

future. But not until she's ready."

At East Pines, Dr. Khan, and practically every nurse in the building, talked constantly about the importance of a support system. They said it mattered just as much as medication and therapy.

Richard was never going to be that kind of support for me. He didn't want to hear how bad things could get with my illness. He didn't want to carry any of the weight. And now, he doesn't have to.

For a reason I may never understand fully, Brett doesn't see my illness as something burdensome. He doesn't treat it like a flaw that needs fixing. He just sees me. In a strange way, maybe him meeting me while I was in a manic episode made my honesty unavoidable. There was no polished version of myself to present to him. No careful mask. Take me or leave me. And he took me.

"I'm very happy to hear that," my mom says to him. "But I want her to have some downtime first. Time to really take care of herself, somewhere I can be nearby and keep an eye on her."

"Of course," Brett says.

Then, he says to me directly, "I'd like to help out financially, so you don't have to stress about that part. I know you're willing to sell your Chanel collection to start over, but I don't want you to have to."

He smiles slightly. "Although," he continues, "if you want to sell those wedding rings and that Cartier watch Richard gave you, I won't object."

After our long lunch, we head back to the hotel so Brett can pack. The closer we get to the hotel, the sadder I feel knowing he's about to leave. When we're together, everything feels right, even when the circumstances around us are a complete mess.

Mom and I decide to drive him to the airport to squeeze out a little more time. On the way out of the hotel, he quickly stops by the front desk.

"Alright, ladies," he says casually, turning back toward us after speaking with the clerk, "I took care of the room for tonight, so you don't have to move or anything. My card is on file if you want to order room service or need anything at all."

It might be cliché, but it feels really nice to be taken care of. Acts of service, that's definitely Brett's love language, just like my mom.

Brett drives my car to the airport. The ride is filled with stories, our stories. The ridiculous, chaotic ones from those first few weeks together. He tells my mom about some of my more manic moments, the times when he first started realizing just how wound up I really was.

Like the night I asked him to meet me at the same karaoke bar when I was out with Richard so we could sit in separate rooms and sneak off to see each other.

"Our girl was a little reckless, to say the least," he says, laughing at the memory. "And it was exciting for a while, but eventually, I realized something more was going on."

He squeezes my hand and continues, "I'm just grateful the end result is this, and mostly that she's safe. That message she left me from the hospital, that was one of the darkest moments of my life. The thought of never seeing her again . . . " He trails off. "Brutal."

By the time we take the airport exit ramp, my eyes well with tears. I'm not ready to say goodbye to Brett. It feels like we've just begun.

He pulls his leather duffel from the trunk, and I step out onto the curb beside him while my mom moves into the driver's seat. Of all people, she's most familiar with my less than proficient driving skills.

Brett takes my face in his hands.

"We're going to figure all this out," he says softly. "Don't worry. Just rest. Enjoy time with your mom. Sit in the sun. Float in her pool."

He smiles and assures me, "Two and a half weeks will fly by. We'll talk, text, email, whatever you want. No limits now."

Then, he lifts me by the waist and kisses me. Slowly. Deeply. He looks straight into my eyes.

"I love you."

"I love you, too."

Then, he turns and walks toward the entrance, his duffel slung over his shoulder. Just before the automatic doors close behind him, he turns back one more time, waves, and blows me a kiss.

"See you in Beijing, my perfect girl!" he calls out.

To meet Richard's time window, Mom and I drive straight to the apartment. Exhaustion starts to settle in. We're already dreaming of hotel robes and room service cheeseburgers. But first, I get to do the thrilling task of dividing up stainless-steel cookware.

Mom follows me in her car to the apartment. On the way, we stop at a car wash so I can vacuum mine out. I'm leaving it with Richard today, and I don't want to hear any complaints about saltine crumbs in the cupholders. Of which there are many. Four quarters and an industrial vacuum fix the problem nicely.

This time, when I arrive at the apartment, I knock. With Mom standing beside me, it feels like the right thing to do. It isn't really my apartment anymore. Richard opens the door and steps back to let us in. Every surface is covered with things. Objects are in mid transition, like the room itself hasn't decided what it is anymore.

The dining table is buried under Christmas ornaments, their glass orbs catching the light in small, fractured flashes. The kitchen island is crowded with All-Clad cookware, serving trays stacked unevenly, a scattering of gadgets that feels suddenly excessive. Nothing is where it belongs. It's all laid out like a rummage sale.

I roll in two more suitcases, their wheels catching slightly on the threshold, while Mom carries two plastic bins from my storage unit down the hall; her breath is just a touch heavier than usual.

We know for certain that these bins, plus the two giant suitcases I packed yesterday, will fit in her car. We'll try to wedge whatever else we can into empty corners, but beyond that, I'll have to come back another time.

There is no greeting. It's straight to business.

"Let's get the ornaments out of the way," Richard says.

Norm appears at my side immediately. I pick him up instantly and let him lick my cheek. Something I never used to allow but can't resist today. I make my way to the table, riddled with Radko.

Knowing my mother won't handle this part well, especially since she bought most of the ornaments scattered across the table, I gently ask her to go into my closet and start packing whatever is left of my clothes into the suitcases. She clearly doesn't love the assignment, but she reads my body language and disappears down the hallway.

"Happy for you to go first," I tell Richard. "And hello," I add, trying to make nice.

He picks the Zeus ornament. Mom gave it to me after Richard and I spent a summer studying abroad in Greece. It's beautiful hand-blown glass, painted in careful detail, glitter catching at the edges. A Bergdorf's find. One of my favorites. But it's an ornament. It can break. It won't break me. I place it in my cognitive river and let it drift.

My turn. I reach for a Christopher Radko piece, a New York City Rockette, circa 2000, all sparkly and red, tiny top hat still perfectly intact. It feels lighter than I remember.

But the moment has already passed for Richard. When I didn't react to Zeus, something in him shut off. "Look, there are about 100 ornaments," he says sharply. "Just take 50, and I'll pack up the rest after you leave. Same with the stuff on the kitchen counter."

"Richard, please, take whatever you want," I say gently. "It really doesn't matter to me."

I meant it kindly. But I realize immediately I should have said it differently.

"I think that's clear, Morgan," he says, his voice tight.

The room feels smaller for a second.

The only thing on the kitchen counter I actually want is the black enamel KitchenAid mixer. Not because I bake, but because it carries something else entirely—Mama Jean's hands guiding mine through making pavlova, biscuits, mashed potatoes. The kind of learning that lingers.

"Would you mind if I take the mixer?" I ask carefully. "The one Mama Jean gave me?" I hope for a yes, but I know I'll survive a no.

"Sure," he says. "I'd like these pieces of All-Clad." He gathers a small stack of practical pots and pans.

"Works for me," I say, packing his leftovers into one of the plastic bins. The granite countertop, the finish my mother lovingly refers to as "wet dog," begins to reveal itself again.

"Maggie wants to buy the antique buffet," I tell him. "Mom and I will move everything else we can't take today into my storage unit, so you don't have to deal with it. When I know where I'm landing permanently, I'll work around your schedule to come back and clear the rest out. Does that work?"

"Sure. Whatever." He sounds bored and walks toward the TV, a yellow legal pad and pen in hand, as if he is personally recording each item we pack away.

Then, almost as an afterthought, he asks, "Morgan, do you even know where you're going? Are you seriously moving back to Murray?"

The smug edge in his voice finally ruffles my feathers.

"Yes," I say calmly. "I'll be in Murray for a bit. I'm actually looking forward to a slower pace."

I could have stopped there. That would have been the high road. But I don't. I fluff my feathers right in his face.

"Then, I leave for China in two weeks for a three-week trip," I add. "After that, I'm moving back to New York full-time."

Most of that is true.

The New York part isn't quite as finalized as I made it sound. It's my plan. Brett and I have talked through it in detail. At first, we thought I might move into his apartment, but the sublet paperwork has already been signed by his new tenant. Now, the idea is to find a lease starting in September.

My tone suggests it's all signed, sealed, and delivered. It isn't. And it's a low blow that I should have kept to myself.

"Well," Richard says flatly, "I guess you're his problem now."

"Nice, Richard."

At this point, my mother deserves an Oscar for Best Performance in a Silent Film. She finished the closet in record time and now stands quietly wrapping my share of glittery ornaments while pretending not to hear every word between us.

I pack the remaining kitchen clutter into a bin and move over to the buffet to gather my sterling julep cups, trays, and place settings. Then, I help Mom wrap the last few ornaments.

As quickly as we can, Mom and I haul bins and suitcases out to the car. I run a few extra boxes down to the storage unit. We cannot get out of this depression-soaked apartment fast enough.

The only thing slowing me down is the small black fur ball glued to my side. Norm. I know this will be the last time I ever see him.

Finding Norm was quite literally "how much is that doggie in the window?" The tiniest Brussels Griffon. Solid black. Scruffy little beard like a tenured philosophy professor. Slightly judgmental eyes. Completely irresistible. He was the only kind of dog I ever wanted.

I can still see him in the front window of that fancy Upper East Side pet store on Lexington, between 62nd and 63rd, just around the corner from our New York apartment. Hiding in a sea of white crinkled paper, surrounded by squeaky toys, blinking out at the world like he owned it. And then he looked at me. Really looked at me. It felt mutual. Immediate. Love at first sight.

Richard and I bought him on the spot. No planning. No research. No thought given to what raising a puppy in a fifth-floor walk-up would entail. Just a leash, a tiny collar, and us carrying him home like a prize.

Very quickly, one thing became clear. Norm was my dog. My responsibility. Mine to take to work. Mine to arrange daycare for. Mine to coordinate boarding whenever Richard and I traveled. Mine to wake up with at 6 a.m. for freezing New York winter walks.

Richard made that boundary clear. And honestly, it was totally fair. I pushed to buy Norm. Richard was grinding through 12- to 14-hour days at the law firm, trying to prove his value and climb the corporate ladder. Getting a dog didn't fit into his version of forward motion.

There were moments when I missed Richard during that time. When I felt proud of his ambition. When I believed we were building something together. It's hard to access those feelings now.

But at that time, they were real. It wasn't always this fractured. It's just with every new rule Richard invented, spoken or implied, deserved or not, I retreated a little further. Not in a way anyone outside could clock.

But internally, in the quiet corners of my heart and mind, I moved away. Not all at once. Just inches at a time.

And yet, 10 years with someone, trying to grow up beside them, attempting adulthood together, sharing apartments and cities and losses and tiny black dogs, that means something. Even if it no longer means forever.

I know Richard will send Norm to live with his parents the moment I'm gone. Norm will probably have a wonderful life there, and I'm grateful for that, but it means I'll never see him again. I'll never see his little snaggle tooth. I'll never smell his puppy breath. I'll never wake up to him curled against my feet or catch him watching *Meerkat Manor* when I walk in the door. Norm will never understand why I left and didn't come back. My tears come fast and hard. I'm sobbing like I've lost a family member. In a way, I have.

Mom is crying, too, not because of Norm, but because her heart is breaking for me, her only daughter.

Eventually, I force myself to pull away. I reach into my pocket and give Norm one of his favorite treats. As expected, he trots happily to his "spot" beside the sofa to enjoy it.

I walk over to Richard. A hug feels like the right thing to do. I honestly have no idea when, or if, we'll ever see each other again. An uncontested divorce in Texas is simple. We don't even have to be in the same room to sign the papers.

The hug is stiff and cold. Like two cardboard cutouts trying to embrace. Neither of us cries. I leave my car keys on the counter. It's his car now.

"Bye-bye, Normie," I whisper, my voice cracking.

Then, I look to Richard and say, "Please send the final divorce papers to my mom's address."

And with that, I closed the door on seven years of marriage.

I check my phone as soon as we get back to the car. Brett has been texting nonstop, asking how it went, making sure I'm okay. I fill him in quickly. We have one more stop in Dallas before I can leave for Kentucky.

This one is going to be rough.

Getting a drink is out of the question, so Mom and I meet Greer for ice cream. I wish Addy were here so we could do this all together, but she flew back to Knoxville after the Maidenform meeting. Greer is already sitting outside at a small café table when we pull up. The second our eyes meet, as I step out of the passenger side, we both start crying.

I run to hug her, though her growing bump keeps a little space between us. It's a strange feeling. Greer has always had the flattest stomach of any human I've ever known.

"Pippy," she cries, "you're really leaving me for good. What am I going to do without my Pip here day in and day out?"

"What am I going to do without you?" I ask.

The truth is, I haven't known adult life without Greer for almost seven years now, pretty much my entire marriage. Leaving her is harder than leaving Richard.

The workdays side by side. The lunches. The travel. The laughs. Sharing every thought and every idea.

"Everything is going to change, Pip," she says through tears. "It'll never be the same. No couples' trips. No double dates. It's all ending, and I'm just not ready to say goodbye to all that."

"Boo," I say gently, "I'm still going to be me. We still have the business to figure out. I'm still here." I tap my chest. "I just won't physically be here."

Then, I rest my hand on her belly. "But it was always going to change," I say softly. "It's going to change so much when this sweet baby gets here. We don't even know how much yet, but it's going to change."

I know the explosion of my life will probably always be seen as the catalyst for whatever happens next with our friendship and with the business. But there are so many variables. So many unknowns. I'm willing to carry whatever part lands on my shoulders.

After half an hour of sad goodbyes, tears, and the kind of ridiculous jokes that only best friends can make in the middle of heartbreak, Mom and I know we have to get back to the hotel. A good night's sleep is a must.

One last bear hug.

"I love you, Greer," I tell her. "We'll find our way."

Chapter 23

THE RESPITE

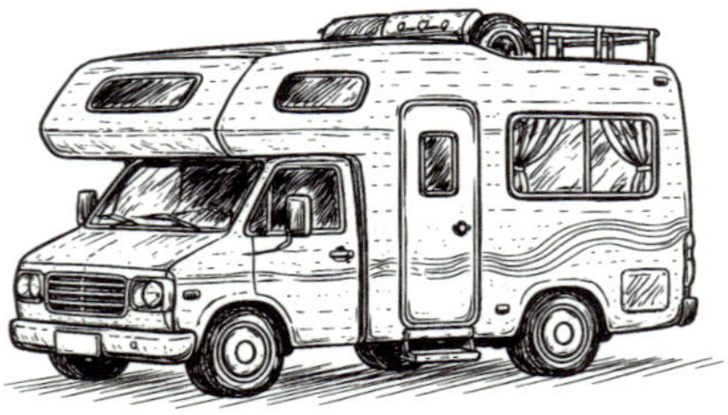

AUGUST 1, 2009
Early Morning—My Childhood Home
Murray, Kentucky

They say you can't go home again, but so far, my sweet little hometown has offered a remarkably soft landing. The first night back in my childhood bed brought the best sleep I've had in years, more than eight uninterrupted hours without waking a single time.

It's a dramatic contrast to my usual rhythm of three to four hours, broken up by restless waking every 90 minutes or so. Maybe my brain has finally settled after the chaos of the past eight weeks. Maybe it's a mini remission. Or maybe it's the quiet of country life. The sounds of nature, or sometimes the absence of sound altogether, is exactly what my brain has been craving.

Brett and I check in every morning and again each night. Living in opposite time zones is strangely fascinating. When I wake up, his day is winding down. When I sit down for dinner, his workday is just beginning.

Every call seems to involve planning something. First on the list: my trip to China. I leave in just two weeks. He's taken care of nearly everything, including my plane ticket, my visa, and a growing list of things he wants to show me once I arrive. My excitement and my nerves are running neck and neck.

The total time Brett and I have actually spent together is still far less than the three consecutive weeks we're about to share in China. This trip will be a moment of truth for us.

Between Brett's calls, my days quickly fill with visitors from nearly every chapter of my life. Apparently news of a suicide attempt followed by a stint on a funny farm generates quite the meal train of casseroles. My mom's house has become a revolving door since the first week.

My dad shows up bright and early, doughnuts from Sammon's Bakery in hand, the morning after we arrive. He hugs me longer and tighter than he ever has before. Something between us has shifted, understated but unmistakable, and it feels like one of the greatest silver linings of this entire ordeal.

My own perspective has softened, too. When Dad married Becky, I was only 17, less than a year after he left our family. A part of me will always wish the three of us had stayed intact, our sacred unit. But my capacity to understand and forgive has grown enormously.

You only get one dad.

I don't want to miss out on my relationship with him. Life is far too short. Besides, I don't want to miss out on his amazing storytelling. He has a gift for turning the simplest stories into bestsellers. Even my mom admits it. I think part of her is secretly happy that this whole experience has revived the friendship they once shared.

After Dad's visit comes a parade of my mom's friends, the women who helped raise me. Murray is a little like Mayberry from *The Andy Griffith Show*. Everyone knows everyone's business. There can be a dark side to that, but my mom manages to avoid the shady crowd entirely. Her group of friends shows up with nothing but open arms and zero judgment.

My recent life explosion seems to have tipped some invisible scale. In their eyes, I'm no longer just "Mona's daughter." I've crossed over into their ranks, an adult woman with my own storm to weather, now welcome into what they jokingly call their "pity parties."

On my second day home, six of them arrive together with wine bottles and trays of food: homemade pimento cheese with crackers, spinach dip with Fritos Scoops!, and tiny chicken salad sandwiches.

We gather around my mom's pool overlooking the watershed. A bluebird day above us while we talk for hours. And not just about me. They begin telling their own stories. The failures, heartbreaks, mistakes. Things I never knew about these women I grew up seeing as second mothers. Their honesty surprises me. Encourages me.

They offer kindness in generous handfuls, trailed with laughter. And they ask a lot of thoughtful questions. A lot. I answer them all. At this point, nothing feels off-limits. Once you publicly admit to a stay in a mental institution, there's no point tiptoeing around the things that got you there.

More than once, my mother gently reminds me that I only have to share what I'm comfortable sharing. I sometimes wonder if she means what she is comfortable with me sharing. In the South, airing your dirty laundry is generally frowned upon. But I'm not uncomfortable. I'm healing.

My next visitor is not nearly as accepting of my new direction. In fact, she makes it quite clear that she disapproves within five minutes of her arrival. Naturally, she frames that disapproval in the language of faith. At one point, she asks me, quite seriously, if my plan was to sleep with Brett, wake up the next morning, ask God for forgiveness, and then repeat the cycle all over again.

The question stuns me. And tickles me. To think we might only have sex at night, and furthermore, that I only pray in the morning. A very missionary outlook.

Ashleigh is a childhood friend. From middle school through high school, the four of us, Greer, Addy, "Ash", and I, were inseparable. We shared the messy milestones of adolescence together: first crushes, first sips of alcohol, first awkward make-out sessions. We all tested boundaries in one way or another.

And through all those years, when Ashleigh was figuring out the edges of her own life, I never once interrogated her morals the way she's doing to me now. Truthfully, I don't feel that I need to ask God for forgiveness every single day for loving Brett. We are adults. We are committed to each other. Yes, there isn't a legal document binding us together yet, but our relationship isn't built on casual sex.

Of course I have asked God's forgiveness for the adultery itself, for the lies I told to hide the affair, for the secrets I kept, and for the pain I caused both Richard and my family. I struggle to believe fully in the grace that God promises. I always have, and especially lately. I don't feel worthy of God's forgiveness. But every morning, I wake up and try to be the best version of myself that I can be. But what strikes me most about Ashleigh's probing is the cruel timing.

Barely a week after my release from East Pines, she chooses to drive two hours to come here to visit me, with a clear plan to lecture me about my morality. It's obvious that I've dropped my basket. I'm not denying that. I'm owning my mistakes openly. But hearing this judgment from someone who has dropped her own basket once or twice in life felt . . . heavy.

Her message lands like a lead balloon between us. I keep my composure during her visit, but after she leaves, I know our relationship will never be the same. Right now, my self-preservation has to matter more than preserving my friendship with Ashleigh.

During group therapy at East Pines, we talked often about the ending of relationships. About how healing sometimes requires accepting that not everyone in your life can move forward with you. Some people simply can't walk the next stretch of the road beside you.

I will always hold a very special place for Ashleigh and the memories we shared together in my heart. This isn't easy. It's painful. But for now, it's necessary.

The next visit from an out-of-town friend is more than welcome.

Brandace is one of those rare, unicorn friends. The kind whose presence is instantly good for your soul. We became fast friends from the very beginning of college, both of us small-town girls who believed life might be bigger and broader than the places we came from.

She's the kind of friend with whom time apart doesn't matter. Months, or even years, can pass without seeing each other, and when we reconnect, it's as if no time has moved at all. The conversation simply picks up where we left off.

She arrives with a beautiful bouquet of flowers in one hand and a good bottle of wine in the other. We spend hours sitting on the edge of the pool, our feet dangling in the cool water while the sun warms our shoulders.

We take a long walk along the country roads, stopping to visit cows and horses, wandering down dirt paths toward old barns and through fields of tobacco, with endless conversations about every topic under the setting sun. About her life. About my future. About the past, and how I got so much of it wrong with Richard. About the next chapters waiting for both of us.

She never judges me, but she has questions, of course. And just like Greer and Addy, she is most surprised by the polished marital façade I'd maintained for years. She doesn't make me feel bad about it though. She accepts it for what it is. During Brandace's 48-hour visit, we cover everything.

When the time comes for her to leave, I find myself wishing she could stay longer. Life feels calmer when she's around. Lighter. More fun.

Between visits, calls with Brett, and trying to sort through my future, I spend hours with my dad's mom, Mama Jean. Living only 10 minutes away, she's been a constant in my life.

As her only granddaughter, we share a special bond. As I was growing up, she was there with us on every Christmas morning for the frenzy of gift opening. Wednesday night spaghetti dinners were our standing ritual. We connected over hats, furs, and vintage brooches, vintage to me, anyway.

My grandmother has always been a proper woman. She never leaves the house without lipstick. She is always well-dressed and always composed. Three times a week, you can find her in church, her blonde coif perfectly set as she sits in the pew.

For as long as I can remember, she has been enormously proud of me, happily bragging about my modest accomplishments to her friends. But now, here I am, a hard fall from that pedestal she placed me on. Fresh out of the psych ward and headed toward divorce. I wondered if she will ever see me the same way again.

It's a frivolous thought. The truth is, she never knocked me from the pedestal. Just like my mom, Mama Jean loves me completely, warts and all. She made that clear the very first afternoon I visited her after coming back home.

"Morgan, my only granddaughter," she said, "there is nothing, and I mean nothing, you could ever do that would make me stop loving you."

Then she added, with complete certainty and a smirk, "And the truth is, we all know this is Richard's fault."

The first part is true. The second is simply the perspective of a fiercely loyal grandmother.

She made us tea and biscuits, and we sat at her kitchen table for hours. That afternoon, I learned more about Mama Jean than I had in my entire life. Somehow, my own story gave her permission to open up, to tell me things about her past that she had never shared aloud.

At first, she was hesitant, careful not to reveal too much. But slowly she softened. She told me about a physical affair she carried on for years, 10 years exactly, she said, before it ended suddenly one day. Then, she spoke about another relationship, more emotional than physical, that also lasted a decade. To me, it sounded more like a deep friendship, but she confessed that it never quite sat right in her heart.

Part of me wondered if she was suggesting that love comes and goes in waves of 10 years, but that marriage stays. After all, she was married to my grandfather for 55 years before he passed away.

"Mama Jean," I asked carefully, "are you suggesting I should have stayed with Richard? Or that romantic love only lasts 10 years? I just want to make sure I understand."

She smiled gently.

"Sweetheart, I'm not suggesting anything," she said. "But none of us knows how long we have on this earth. I want my only granddaughter to know the real me. And I want you to know it's okay to make mistakes. We all have . . . and we all will."

I will never forget those talks with her. I'm forever grateful for her vulnerability and her love. Growing up in the Church of Christ as she did, where women are judged for sport, our conversation could have gone in a very different direction. But my grandmother understood something deeper than the mechanics of religion. She understood the two simple messages that sit at the heart of the Bible:

Love the Lord with all your heart. Love your neighbor as yourself.

Simple. Direct. And yet, most humans somehow manage to complicate those two instructions every single day. She never did. She lived them.

The first two weeks back in Murray have passed much faster than I expected. For the most part, the time has been restful, encouraging, even invigorating. For the first time in a long while, it feels like my whole life is still in front of me. A chance to start over. To manage my illness head-on. To take care of myself in a way that might keep me from hurting myself or the people I love ever again.

Brett and I have already been deep into planning what comes next, though always with me in the lead. He is careful about that. His role, as he puts it, is simply to support me.

The plan is for me to return to New York in September, after my visit to China. Together, we find a tiny jewel box of an apartment on the Gold Coast, Fifth Avenue and Ninth Street, a dreamy location. A little under 500 square feet of furnished space, colorful and cheerful, with a tiny kitchen and a renovated bathroom. Perfect for my new life as a party of one.

Meanwhile, I start selling off anything I no longer need. The Cartier watch. My engagement ring. Designer clothes. I even cash in some childhood savings bonds that have just matured, lucky timing. Every dollar counts.

Brett quietly handles some of the bigger things without being asked. The lease. The plane tickets to get Mom and me to New York so I can move in, since he won't be able to make it back. A credit card for emergencies, and, as he calls it, a little "NYC Mad Money." (We laugh at the unintentional pun.) But not every moment in Murray is as peaceful as the visits with friends and family.

My divorce is moving forward in earnest, quickly. Dividing the assets was one thing. But there are debts, too, mostly mine. The result of manic spending sprees, reckless shopping, and financial commitments to Jet Set Lingerie that I simply hadn't been able to afford. Commitments, nonetheless. Credit cards with interest rates that could make your eyes water.

About 10 days into my stay, the hospital bills start to arrive at my mom's house. Richard has them forwarded. Even at the cheapest, most rundown psychiatric hospital the doctors could find for me, the total cost is staggering, more than $150,000 and climbing.

Then comes the letter from my insurance company.

Denied.

They're covering zero dollars. The reason: self-inflicted injury.

Covering nothing from Legacy. Covering nothing from East Pines. For me, it's a gut punch. For Richard, it must feel like an emotional victory.

Naturally, he is furious when the hidden debts surface, about $20,000 spread across a few credit cards, accumulating interest at the speed of light. One more layer of secrets I have kept.

Richard's proposal during the settlement negotiations is simple: I take the hospital bills, and he assumes the credit card debt.

After talking it through with my dad and his legal brain, and with my mom, we decide to take the gamble. My dad is convinced the insurance company is out of line. Years of experience has taught him that "no" is often just the opening move for insurance claims this large. He begins fighting the denial immediately.

I agree to Richard's proposal. A lawyer in Dallas, mutually agreed upon by both sides, drafts the final paperwork. On the 31st day after our initial filing for separation, the documents will be sent to the District Clerk's office. Our marriage will officially be over.

Not long now.

As the final agreement takes shape, Richard and I set a date for me to return to Dallas to pick up the rest of my things. Conveniently, he will be leaving for a hiking trip that same week, so we won't have to see each other.

For a moment, I consider just leaving everything behind. Letting it all go. But then, I picture my vintage collection, years of garnering each beautiful piece, each with her own story. I can't bear the thought of these treasures ending up at Goodwill. Or worse, in a landfill.

One afternoon by the pool at my mom's house, I tell my parents about the trip and ask how we should get everything back to Kentucky. I suggest renting a small U-Haul.

"How about a family trip in my RV?" my dad says.

I completely forgot he owned an RV. He and Becky bought it when my little brother was born. At first, I think he is joking. He isn't.

"I've been thinking about it since you mentioned needing to go back last week," he explained. "If we leave at six in the evening and each take a four-hour driving shift, the three of us can get there by six in the morning. No stops. Bathroom on board. Becky can pack meals for us."

He continues mapping it out.

"We load your stuff. There's plenty of room in the back, and we get back on the road by 10 a.m. Another round of shifts, some sleep in between, and we'll be home in Murray by 10 that night."

My mom bursts out laughing.

"Wow, Mark," she says. "In 33 years, I've never seen you plan anything like this. Remember when you didn't even reserve a hotel room the night before you took the bar exam!?"

He smiles and shrugs.

"It's my daughter," he says simply. "And it's my turn."

It is touching. And also, completely hysterical. The original three, back together again, for 36 hours only, to retrieve my stuff.

August 15, 2009, 5 p.m.—My Mother's Driveway

Four days after we agreed to the RV plan, and just five days before my flight to Beijing, my dad's beige RV, stripes wrapping around it in various shades of taupe, rolls into my mom's circular driveway at five in the evening with about four hours of daylight left. Half of me expected Snot and Ruby Sue to tumble out of the back.

The first couple of hours are quiet. Dad drives. Mom sits in the cushy passenger seat. I stretch out on the back sofa, wedged between the removable table and its four cupholders, giving the whole space a distinct pontoon-boat vibe. From my spot in the back, I can feel their silence.

But when it comes time for the first round of snacks, the tension breaks. As mom hands out sandwich bags, filled with Doritos distributed evenly, the nerves settle, and conversation slowly creeps in. They reminisce, stories about friends from long ago, good memories, little anecdotes about me as a kid. The mood changes.

As an only child, hearing my parents laugh together for the first time in more than a decade feels rare and precious. Maybe the cliché is true; time does heal certain wounds.

I take the second driving shift. Neither of them seem thrilled about seeing me behind the wheel of this enormous vehicle, but I manage. I remain laser-focused on staying between the lines. Besides, I have the youngest eyes for the darkest part of the night.

A couple hours in, I spot flashing lights.

"Guys," I say cautiously, "I think we're being pulled over. There are lights and sirens in my side mirrors."

Mom has been snoozing in the back, under a blanket with cats printed on it. She immediately sits straight up, a pillow crease on her face.

"Stay calm," Dad says in his slow, steady lawyer voice. "Turn on your blinker so he knows you see him, and slow down. We need to be under 20 miles an hour before you move to the shoulder."

Calm is not what I am feeling. I definitely hadn't been speeding. This thing couldn't break 70 mph even if I tried. Somehow, I manage the maneuver without incident, easing the RV safely onto the shoulder. The officer approaches the passenger side.

"License and registration."

Dad reaches for the glove box, pulling out the registration along with his driver's license as the owner. I dig frantically through my tote bag, overflowing with toiletries and snacks, trying to find my wallet.

"Officer," Dad says politely, "may I ask why you pulled us over?"

"Sir, I'll tell you when I tell you," the officer replies curtly.

Feisty.

He walks back to his patrol car with our paperwork.

"What on earth could this be about?" Mom asks.

"Everything's current," Dad says calmly. "Just renewed the plates. Had the taillights checked yesterday."

A few minutes later, the officer returns and knocks on the side door. Mom slides it open.

"I need all three of you to step out of the vehicle," he says.

We climb out and stand together on the pitch-dark shoulder of the highway. Giant grasshoppers leaping around our ankles.

"It's like we're in Egypt," Dad says dryly. "Eighth plague."

Dad's biblical knowledge is impressive, leftover from that Church of Christ upbringing. He made the move over to the much more relaxed Methodist variety back in college upon realizing he liked the taste of bourbon.

We watch as the officer searches every corner of the RV. Dad knew this was within the officer's rights, one of the exceptions to search warrant rules for vehicles, so we simply wait in the humid summer air. Then come the questions.

Where are we coming from? Where are we going? Why are we traveling together?

"Mom, Dad, let me take this," I say.

The officer allows us back inside the RV where the lights are on and the bugs are not.

"Sir," I begin, "these are my parents. They've been divorced for 10 years. My dad married his secretary; I only mention that to clarify that it was not an amicable divorce. I'm 28, currently going through my own miserable divorce, and I just got out of a mental institution two weeks ago."

I take a breath.

"These two have generously agreed to spend 24 hours straight together in this small RV, driving from Kentucky to Dallas and back, just to help me retrieve the rest of my belongings from my soon-to-be ex-husband."

I pause.

"Any chance you can tell us what this is about and then let us get back on the road?" I ask.

The officer's eyes widen until they look like dinner plates.

"Is this true?" he asks my parents.

"Yep," they say in unison, barely containing their laughter.

"Well damn," the officer says. "That's the craziest story I've heard in a while."

He shifts his hat and explains, "We've got an Amber Alert tonight. Protocol says we have to stop any large vans or recreational vehicles until the girls are located."

He hands the paperwork back and says, "I'm going to let you folks get back on the road. Sounds like you've got quite the adventure going already."

I climb back into the driver's seat to finish my shift. Dad resumes his role as co-pilot, and Mom slides the side door closed behind us.

Then, once the officer is safely out of earshot, the RV explodes with laughter.

An adventure indeed.

We pull into Dallas just before six in the morning.

The packing itself turns out to be surprisingly easy. Most of my clothes are already hanging on rolling racks, and the rest of my things are neatly stacked in plastic bins. The slowest part is the shoeboxes, dozens of them, stacked floor to ceiling in the storage unit. My mom surveys the towering wall of footwear.

"I can see where all that rathole money I gave you went," she says.

"Don't shoe-shame me," I laugh.

As we load the final stack onto the dolly Becky smartly insisted we bring, Brett calls to check in. I fill him in on the overnight adventure, the police stop, the plague-sized grasshoppers, the RV logistics, and tell him we are about to get back on the road.

It took us less than three hours to pack up the remnants of my seven-year marriage. Remarkable, really. Or sad. Depends on how you look at it.

I put Brett on speaker so he can say hello to my parents and thank them for making the trip, something he joked he should have done himself.

Then he casually adds, "Mark, you should top-shelf Richard."

"What on earth does that mean?" I ask.

He laughs.

"Honestly, I'm not sure this is a second-conversation-with-your-parents kind of topic," Brett says.

There's a pause.

"Let's just say," he explains, "it's of German descent and involves a . . . bodily deposit . . . in the top part of the toilet tank. Creating a smell people usually can't locate for weeks. Urban-legend fraternity prank."

Running on almost no sleep and about 16 hours of continuous travel, the RV erupts in laughter yet again.

"Well," Brett says through the phone, "glad I can bring some levity to the situation. The least I can do. Call when you're back in Kentucky," he adds. "Love you."

"Love you, too," I say, still giggling. "Sleep tight."

It's well after bedtime in Beijing.

The three of us each do one final loop through the apartment and the storage unit to make sure we've left nothing behind. Dad checks last. I drop the apartment keys at the front desk, which just opened, and climb back into the RV.

Five minutes of navigating, and we are back on the highway. For a while, no one says anything. Then, as we cross the city limits and Dallas slips into the rearview mirrors, my dad breaks the silence.

"I went ahead and top-shelfed him," he says.

Chapter 24

THE BIG APPLE BACK & FORTH

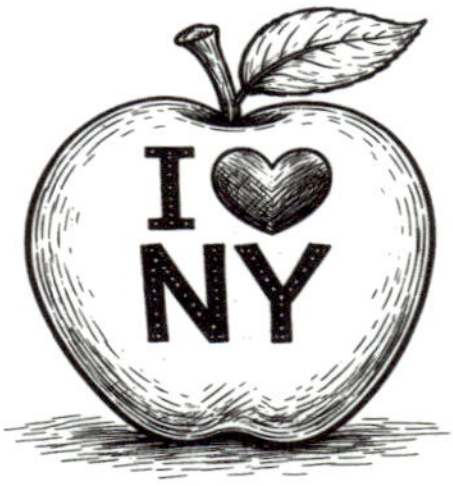

AUGUST 19, 2009
EWR to PEK

With an hour and a half left in my 14-hour flight, I kick my glam routine into high gear. Luckily, the rest of first class is still fully reclined and asleep. I have free rein of the larger of the two restrooms.

I grab my thoughtfully packed beauty bag, complete with a change of clothes, and slip inside the tiny space. Then, the process begins. I brush my teeth, wash my face, wipe down my body with a baby wipe. I change into fresh Jet Set Lingerie and pull on a chocolate silk mini dress embroidered with blue and white flowers. I apply a new face of makeup and dry shampoo the heck out of my hair.

Less than 20 minutes later, a polite knock on the door signals that my time is up. I wipe down the counter like a good houseguest and scoot back to my seat.

Aside from the nervous excitement of seeing Brett again, the flight passes in a blur. I've had my fair share of domestic upgrades to first class, but this is my first time flying internationally in the front of the plane. The Häagen-Dazs sundae cart alone is enough to make this country girl never want to sit in coach again. I soak up every second.

Now, it's time to pop two Tylenol, in the off chance my excitement raises my body temperature. The last thing I want is to get pulled out of the arrival line as a suspected bird flu patient.

When the wheels finally touch down, my whole body buzzes. But, this time, it's not because I'm manic.

This is something better, excitement in its purest form. The kind that feels clean and bright, like the real me. Moments of remission are rare for me still. Land mines exist around every corner, and I know that's part of my life. But today, I'm soaking in the joy of this moment. A moment where I feel . . . normal. Of course, my meds play a huge role in this. But, who cares? No one judges a diabetic for taking insulin.

I race through the temperature check and head toward immigration as fast as my legs will carry me. I know Brett is waiting for me on the other side, and I can't bear one more minute apart.

As my turn approaches. I shuffle up to the counter and slide my passport across with a smile. The agent scans my photo and studies my face. Then, he ruffles through the pages until he finds my visa. I stand there, trying not to look anxious, silently praying for the heavy-handed stamp.

Thump. I'm in.

A man with my name on a sign greets me at baggage claim. Asian airports always nail this part. It was the same in Thailand for Jet Set Lingerie factory visits. I'm grateful for the help and relieved that I won't look like a sweaty pack mule when Brett lays eyes on me for the first time in weeks. So far, the only Mandarin words I'm comfortable uttering out loud are *xie xie* (thank you), but it's exhilarating to use the language for the first time.

I closely follow the kind gentleman, dressed in the same grey uniform as the sea of workers, assisting arrival guests at every turn. Carrying only my small purse, I round the corner to proceed up a long ramp, crowded with locals waiting for their loved ones.

Brett is there, at the very top of the ramp. He's holding an embarrassingly large bouquet of flowers that covers most of his body, impatiently waiting behind the marked line. I start to skip towards him. The bouquet drops to the floor, and he scoops me up in the air, wrapping me in his arms. We slowly spin as he kisses me. Time suspends. Secrecy is over. I am no longer committed to anyone but him. Peace washes over me.

"It's so good to hold you," he says, smiling ear to ear.

We head straight to the hotel from the airport to drop my bags and freshen up for dinner. We hardly come up for air on the drive.

After one final sweep of hospitality—with all my suitcases perched on luggage racks—the bellman exits. The hotel door clicks shut behind us. Alone at last. For a moment, neither of us moves.

The room is softly lit by gilded lamps. Views of Beijing fill the floor-to-ceiling windows. It has the subdued hum of a five-star kind of luxury. Our time apart went by fast, but in this moment, it feels like a lifetime. How do we get back to the ease of it all? Brett makes the first move, breathing me in like something essential. Familiar. Necessary.

"You're here," he says, his voice low against my hair.

"I'm here," I playfully whisper.

His first moves are almost careful. Three weeks of missed touch pressed into a single breath. The kiss deepens. Not urgent, but sure. His hands drop to my waist. I slide mine up his chest.

"Three weeks . . ." I say.

"I counted down every day," he says.

He kisses me again, slower this time, deliberate. His hand moves to my cheek, then into my hair, anchoring me. The world outside the windows keeps going, taxis moving, crowds of people shuffle about, but inside our room, time folds inward. I gasp when he lifts me, surprised and delighted. He carries me a few steps to the sofa, as if the bedroom is too far away. Taking the hemline of my dress in his hands, he lifts it over my head, taking in each bit of my body.

"How very Chinese of you," he laughs, noting my matching red bra and panties as he slips them off. His fingertips trace my skin like rediscovery. A pause here. A breath there. Every kiss intentionally placed on me.

I slowly undress him, my mouth grazing him. Our bodies collide, skin against skin. His hand laces with mine. The chaos of the city just beyond the glass acting as a witness.

"I missed you," I say against his mouth.

He answers by pulling me closer, deeper. And then, my body gives itself over completely. Like he was made just for me.

In this luxurious room, high above the rickshaws, street markets, and traffic jams, it's not the hotel that feels five-star, it's the connection between us. It's going to be brutal to leave this man in 16 days.

My first trip to Beijing solidifies one thing. Brett is all in. Not that I doubted him, but I'm grateful for the reassurance. I'm confident in his commitment, yet I don't feel rushed or pressured to be anywhere other than where I want to be. Obviously, that includes wanting to be with him, but I need to be with myself. Beijing may very well be my future, but New York, on my own, is where I'm meant to be now. I still have a lot to figure out. Jet Set Lingerie and the Twins are two of the big ones. Plus, Beijing seems to be a different animal. I need time to adjust.

I typically consider myself well-traveled, especially for an American. At 28, I've covered a good amount of ground. I've got the majors under my belt. A solid chunk of Europe: Italy, France, England, Spain, and Greece. Plus, a few outliers: Netherlands, Czech Republic, and Ireland, among others. In the States, I've made the appropriate rounds, from East Coast to West Coast, with cool mountain towns in between. North to south, from Michigan to Miami. But nothing prepares you for Beijing. It's a place all its own.

For starters, I didn't fully anticipate the vastness of the language barrier. For example, Starbucks. I didn't realize I would need three entirely new words just to get to a coffee shop. And I never dreamed only 10% of the staff of a five-star hotel would speak English. Americans are spoiled. Myself included. We're coddled with our language, spoken fluently almost everywhere. Not here. This level of foreign is something I've never encountered.

Brett takes both Fridays off during my stay and keeps his work hours far lighter than usual. Even so, I have plenty of free time to entertain myself—and I make the most of it.

At first, I explore on foot, sticking close to the hotel and the familiar streets nearby. The smells overwhelm me—fresh herbs, damp vegetables, lychee skins, and cardboard boxes. Alleyways in the hutongs carry wafts of laundry detergent, bicycle grease, and sometimes the sharp smell of pickled cabbage fermenting in giant crocks. Passing by luxury hotels or temple courtyards, brings notes of sandalwood incense, expensive perfume, and fresh flowers.

After a few days, I feel ready to hail a taxi and venture out to the street markets scattered across the city. It isn't easy. The only way to manage, short of speaking fluent Mandarin, is by asking the hotel's concierge to make me stacks of flash cards with addresses written in Chinese characters to show the drivers.

The markets in Beijing are a full sensory event, equal parts treasure hunt, comedy show, and competitive sport. Rows and rows of tiny stalls spill into each other, stacked from floor to ceiling with handbags, silk scarves, pashminas, sunglasses, belts, and watches. The energy is electric.

Vendors call out to you the second you make eye contact, as they pull bags and shoes from hidden cabinets, unzipping secret compartments full of even more merchandise. Bargaining is not optional; it's the main event. A simple question like "How much?" begins a dramatic dance of calculators, head shaking, laughter, fake offense, and theatrical walkaways. Prices start high enough to make you gasp, and if you're doing it right, they eventually fall somewhere closer to reality. Colorful RMB exchanges hands and everyone smiles at the successful transaction.

During my mornings with Brett, getting ready as if we're an old married couple, my souvenir buying phrases in Mandarin improve greatly:

Duōshao qián? (How much?)

Tài guì le! (Too expensive!)

Wǒ bú yào. (I don't want it.)

Hěn piàoliang! (So pretty!)

My solo adventures fill me with a sense of pride, especially my negotiation skills, and I love recounting the stories to him each night over dinner. I love every second of our time together. Some days are carefully planned, spent at extravagant restaurants and glamorous bars. Others are more simple, curled up on the sofa watching terrible movies with subtitles. But each day starts and ends the same. Wrapped up in each other.

During the second weekend of my visit, Brett books a getaway to the Commune in Mutianyu, the place he mentioned on our call in Miami, a one of a kind resort built adjacent to the Great Wall. The plan is for him to pick me up after work on Thursday, but I secretly arrange for the driver to pick me up first. I surprise Brett at the office, dressed in a long red gown, makeup and hair perfectly in place, holding a beautiful picnic basket with cold champagne and two coupes for the drive.

I'll never forget the look on his face when I strolled into his office, completely unannounced, dressed for a masquerade gala, mask and all.

"God, you're fun," he says, his eyes studying every part of me.

The best word. Beauty goes. Youth is fleeting. But fun, that's magic. Fun lasts.

Our weekend at the Great Wall, wrapped in mountains on all sides, exceeds every expectation of what a holiday getaway could be.

Hidden in a ribbon of stone, rising and falling with the spine of the hills, stretching endlessly, we share moments of lightness, peppered with deeper conversations about our pasts, our hurts, and our hopes.

We rush nothing. If we miss a dinner reservation. No sweat. Something else awaits us. We walk for hours on the wall, to parts completely abandoned and only accessible through the resort, grown over with bushes and weeds, crumbling and cracked in certain parts. Some moments feel surreal. But the weight of his body, the squeeze from his hand to mine, the taste of him, his fingertips against my face prove otherwise.

The rooms at the Commune surprise me. Modern. Fresh. Each villa is designed by a different Asian architect, so that no two buildings are alike. One house is all glass and sharp angles; another looks like it was folded out of concrete, and another disappears into the hillside like it grew there.

Inside, everything is minimalist in that intentional, expensive way. Clean lines. Pale wood. Cool stone floors. Furniture that looks sculptural but somehow still comfortable. There is very little clutter, which makes us and our connection feel like the real decoration.

After a few days away from the crowds and the horns and the buzz of Beijing, we make our way back. The flurry of plans makes the week go by in a flash. Soon, it's my last night.

We won't see each other again before my birthday, so Brett wants to celebrate early. He books dinner at Maison Boulud, Daniel Boulud's restaurant inside the original U.S. Embassy, a masterpiece of a building near Tiananmen Square.

The interiors alone are mind-blowing. Soaring ceilings. Grand staircases. Tile and molding details to die for. Delicious food. Even better company.

We sit side by side in the booth, his shoulder pressed against mine. He tells me how excited he is for me to have my own space for the first time. He makes it clear that nothing would make him happier than having me in Beijing, living everyday life together as a team, but he understands it has to happen on my terms. My timeline.

"Morgan," he says, "I know you've been hustling to sell your things, stockpiling money for your fresh start. It's amazing, really. You have such grit. I knew it the moment I met you."

He pauses, taking both of my hands in his. "You have no fear," he says. "I'm sorry you've been living with clipped wings. But you're free now." He smiles, mostly with his eyes. "There will never be another box. The world deserves to get everything you've got to give it."

With his right hand, he pulls my left arm closer to him. Holding it gently, his other hand appears from behind his back, slipping a black, diamond bezel J12 watch onto my wrist.

"It's set to Beijing time. I'll be here. Whenever you're ready," he says. "Happy birthday."

When the perfect words don't form in my head, I give way to the physical world, pressing my lips against his. He pulls me into him, our feet tangled beneath the table, tucked away in the darkest corner of the restaurant as if we are the only two people in the vast dining room, dripping in candlelight. Full of French wine and *fromage*.

Even while I wrestle with the sins that have brought me here—my adultery, the wreckage behind me—I find myself quietly thanking God for Brett and for this fresh start with every breath. Noting in my prayers that I would have been equally happy with a colorful Swatch watch.

The next morning at the airport, we stand together laughing, talking, kissing until the very last second before I have to go through security. His hands roam from my waist to my lower back and back up to my face.

Before I step through the security gates, we finalize plans for my next visit in October. He wants me to come back to help him find a permanent apartment. Apparently, hotel living, and the cost of laundering socks, has finally gotten to him.

But first, it's time to make a space just for me.

September 17, 2009—My Jewel Box Apartment, NYC

I slide the key into the doorknob, my heart beating fast. I'm about to cross the threshold of my very first solo apartment.

As of today, I'm 29 years old, and yet, I have never actually lived alone. Straight from my mom's house to the freshman dorm at college, then to my sophomore-year apartment with my roommate, Jaimie, then to the sorority house, with goodness knows how many girls under one roof. And then after graduation, directly into married life.

Behind this door lies something that belongs entirely to me. My own small nook in the best city in the world. With my mom behind me, each of us dragging three oversized roller bags stuffed with clothes, shoes, handbags, and the necessary knickknacks of a life in transition, we step inside. The apartment is tiny, but every inch of it has been carefully considered. A small entryway opens into a galley kitchen on one side and a wall of doors on the other, each leading to generous closet space, New York gold. Beyond that is the studio itself.

A cheerful chartreuse sofa sits in the living area, paired with a large storage ottoman in front. The television is framed inside a sleek wall unit with shelves and compartments that will soon house my small army of bags and shoes. Just a few steps away stands a queen bed, surrounded by tall windows overlooking Fifth Avenue. We'll dress it with fresh monogrammed linens.

Coming from sprawling Murray, Kentucky, my mom must feel like I am moving into a mouse hole. But she is perceptive enough to see the joy written all over my face.

"Well," she says gently, looking around, "it's perfect."

"Yes," I say, smiling. "It really is. And it's just mine."

She tilts her head and asks, "Is that a knock at the door?"

In 10 steps, I'm in front of it, pulling it open.

A delivery man, dressed in a blue workman's blazer, stands in the hallway, holding a giant bouquet of pink English roses arranged in a beautiful green vase, wrapped with a wide grosgrain ribbon and sealed with a gold wax stamp. I didn't need to read the card to know who had sent them.

Twenty-nine roses for your twenty-ninth year. I am so lucky that you were born. I have dinner reservations for you and your mom at Il Mulino and two tickets to Wicked are waiting at the box office. Wish I could be there to celebrate! So happy you're "Back in the New York Groove." Happy Birthday! I love you, Brett

Damn, he's good.

After five days of observing me in New York, my mom felt confident enough to leave me alone. She isn't stoked about it, but she knows it's the right thing. I'm well beyond the age of being able to live alone. I've got this.

I spend my first week playing in my neighborhood. Finding the closest Duane Reade, the best Chinese takeout, splurging on fun treats from Citarella, just around the corner, and strolling the streets in search of local vintage. I know the neighborhood on a surface level from living in the city before, but now, I have the time to dig deep and find all the hidden treasures. I invite friends from every corner of the city to join me for lunch, dinner, and drinks, all in the name of defining my favorite spots.

Almost by design, an out-of-town guest asks to visit every other week. The staggered visits, most certainly calculated by a small group of the people who love me the most, are welcomed. I know they are checking on me. I don't mind. Every person, bipolar or not, should be so lucky to have this type of support system.

First up: Greer.

She texts from the taxi. *5 minutes away!*

I'm so excited to see her. We haven't had any time together, just the two of us, since the pill bottle hit the fan. It's the longest we've gone in years. I rush down the elevator to the curb to be there when she arrives. I want to properly welcome her to my new nook in NYC with a Diet Coke and a mini Toblerone in hand.

As her cab pulls up, I start to worry that the space between us, the weight of everything we have survived together may have altered the friendship. Will there be levity? Will there be jokes? Or worse, will there be judgment or doubt? Will I feel the need to prove my life choices to her for the next four days? Or hell, for the rest of my life?

I haven't thought of Richard much since we came to a final financial agreement for the divorce. But I should probably ask her about him. That's the right thing to do. I think. Assuming there is a proper protocol to addressing a soon to be ex-husband who still works for your best friend's husband.

Richard deserves to keep the Dallas crowd. It's his home now, not mine. It never was. Honestly, without the drag of keeping me in my box, he can finally start living his best life. Bless his heart.

All my worries subside the second her Chanel ballet flats step out of the taxi. We don't skip a beat. Rushing upstairs to drop her bag in my little gem of an apartment so we can hit one of our favorite downtown lunch spots. Over street corn at Café Habana, we play a game of 20 questions. Pretty heavy-handed on her end, but I get in my fair share as well.

She asks me all about my visit to Beijing, curious about my feelings for Brett. Wondering if anything has changed after so much uninterrupted time together, for better or for worse.

"Only for the better," I assure her, blushing. "But I'm in no rush. This is where I'll be for as long as I need to be."

Everyone who loves me is walking on eggshells, worried about overstepping with their advice, though they're not particularly good at hiding what they're thinking. Even if no one says it outright, I see the fear sitting just beneath the surface. They're all terrified I'm going to pack up and move to China. I thought signing a year-long lease in New York might calm their nerves.

Nope.

Greer is especially focused on Brett, on his commitment to me. I know the questions come from a place of concern, of protectiveness, and I understand that. But after years of hiding the truth about my marriage, I don't quite know how to make her believe me now. This part is my own doing.

Brett has done nothing but show up and prove himself. And yet, he's paying for my past, for the illusion I maintained of a happy marriage. The doubts people have about him aren't really about him at all. They're about me.

Many of my recent therapy sessions covered the topic of doubt in depth. After severe bipolar episodes, it can be incredibly hard for family and friends to trust again. Dr. Khan prepared me for moments exactly like this. But he was also very clear about one thing: I need to set healthy boundaries.

My mom. My dad. The Twins. Mama Jean. Their constant need for answers is rooted in love. But it isn't my responsibility to answer every question they carry. They lean on doubt because they're afraid of missing something—afraid they won't see the warning signs if things start to tilt again.

The people-pleaser in me wants to reassure them all with guarantees and proof. But the truth is, the best I can offer is this: that I'm taking my medication, that I'm doing my best to sleep six to eight hours each night, that I'm exercising, and that I'm staying in close contact with my doctors.

Beyond that, everything else is speculation. Only time will reveal what's real.

My six-week respite officially ended last week. Greer doesn't rush me, but she doesn't pretend, either.

"There are a few things coming up we should talk through," she says, easing into it. "Nothing we can really put off."

I nod, taking a sip of my Sancerre, and settle in.

We decided 30 minutes ago that this particular conversation would be a more positive experience with a change of scenery, so we popped down to Cru, the restaurant in my building, known for its wine, cheese, and cool Greenwich Village crowd.

"Maidenform is still interested, but dragging their feet to provide any concrete information," she continues, almost carefully. "Saks is waiting on the most recent shapewear samples. They haven't approved our current shade of nude. And QVC . . . QVC feels real now."

There's a softness in the way she says it—hopeful but measured.

"And Pornkiat?" I ask.

She pauses, just briefly. "He's . . . nervous," she says. "More than usual—about more than the economy."

Part of that makes sense. Part of it sounds like a clue only.

Pornkiat bought 25% of Jet Set Lingerie last year—our factory partner, our production lifeline. And right now, he's watching the U.S. economy unravel in real time.

Investment banks are collapsing. Others are only surviving because the government is stepping in. Homes are slipping into foreclosure. Brands are quietly folding. Real estate feels unstable in a way it hasn't before. At least not in my memory.

"It's a lot to watch from where he's sitting," she adds gently. "I think it's shaken him."

It's shaken everyone. It's the biggest financial crisis of my lifetime. The kind that makes even the most certain plans feel fragile. It's also why Brett took the leap to China. The U.S. feels like a dumpster fire, and he's not wrong.

"So, what does he want us to do?" I ask.

"We try to give him something solid," she says. "One of the three—something we can point to and say, this is real, this is moving forward. And we take it one step at a time," she adds, softer still.

There's a layer underneath it. Not pressure. Not quite. But something close. I can feel it all stacking: the babies, Brett half a world away, an economy in free fall, production already dragging. Too many moving parts. Too many things we can't control.

"I'm here," I say. "In New York. Or traveling wherever I'm needed."

She nods, like that's enough for now.

"And, Greer, it's where I want it to be," I add.

In between the stress and spreadsheets of work, Greer and I also squeeze in time to really catch up and have downtime with each other at a few of our favorite Uptown spots: The 21 Club and La Grenouille. Playing dress-up has and will always be a coping mechanism for me, a way to get out of my head. Some people like to paint, but clothes are my favorite medium.

There is nothing like hitting the streets of New York with your best friend, dressed in vintage finds and PR closet designer shoes while the crisp fall air surrounds you, protecting our curls without a drop of humidity.

At the end of Greer's visit, I think we are in a better place. We have a plan to navigate the next big steps for the business. I commit to staying put to see all the big ones come to fruition. It's clear we will never be able to go back to the way it was before. Change is life's only promise. And like every relationship in my life, this friendship is constantly evolving.

Fall in New York is my absolute favorite. The weather is peak, and the way the light hits the buildings, makes it seem forgiving somehow, more welcoming. The days get shorter and restaurants feel cozier. It's still warm enough to dine outside, but now, with a jacket resting over the shoulders.

Brett and I fall into a routine of Skyping twice a day, morning and night. Occasionally, if I have dinner plans, I'll set up my computer to face the TV so he can catch the Yankees in the playoffs. One thing made painfully clear during my time in Beijing is the lack of access to good Internet or American culture.

I can't believe how fast each day passes. I'm back to walking miles and miles a day. With my new meds, the steps are cathartic, not chaotic. I stroll through art museums to calm my mind. I protect my alone time, but I make enough plans for peace of mind check-ins, for me, and honestly, for my mom.

Before I know it, it's time to go back to Beijing. But this trip is not just to China. Brett is joining me in Thailand for a factory visit to see how production is coming along for the new shapewear and for QVC samples. My packing prep becomes more calculated with each trans-Pacific flight. Surprisingly, we are already comfortable with this extreme version of long-distance dating. He handles all my travel arrangements from the town car pickup at my apartment to my retrieval in Beijing. He's always standing at the top of the ramp at the airport when I arrive. A driver, waiting in the wings, is there to help with my bags and get us home. Every reunion is exhilarating. Mind-blowing really, with layers of built-up passion from the lack of everyday life we share. Each time we are together makes us long for more time, more normalcy. The thrill of long distance is fun, but we want the gritty real stuff, too.

Before we can pop down to Bangkok and Phuket, there is work to be done. He sends me on a mission to do something that goes against my life goal of living full-time in a hotel. Ideally, at The Carlyle. But for now, Brett needs normalcy; he needs an apartment to feel more settled, and he wants my approval. His time in Beijing is not temporary. Five to ten years is the timeline.

Admittedly, I gulped when he said it out loud for the first time.

To allow ourselves more playtime in Thailand, we decide that I should handle the home hunting while he gets his work done. With a driver who speaks no English and a realtor who speaks very little, I head out bright and early as he leaves for work. I dress in my new market finds, pairing them in ways that feel a little over the top—even for me. It's liberating to experiment with fashion in a place where no one knows me. I lean all the way in, with more Upper East Side Iris Apfel, than "off to Pilates" Dallas basics.

After the fifth or sixth place I tour with low popcorn ceilings, weird smells of unfamiliar spices, horrendously oversized furnishings in cheesy chinoiserie textiles, not properly reflecting the history of the print, and bathrooms the size of coat closets, I start to panic. I check in with Brett to share my lack of success.

"Love, you would never live in any of these," I say definitively. "I think something is off. Can we have your assistant explain that we want something more . . . elevated?" The "we" rolls off my tongue. The casual nod that I would also prefer not to live in a place like these is pretty obvious.

"Yes, let me get her on the line," he says. "Also, love that we."

In less than a minute, the problem is resolved. The USD to RMB conversion was done in reverse and the range of rent given was entirely wrong. The agent unnecessarily apologizes a million times, almost like she's from the South herself, and we make our way to the car to "start over." Starving at this point, I scarf down a bag of green-tea-flavored Lay's potato chips. Absolutely terrible, but I didn't want to be rude to this darling young girl who was already in a tailspin of embarrassment.

We see three more apartments before finding the ONE.

As soon as we drive up, a wave of excitement washes over me. A brand-new complex, built on the heels of the Olympic Games, of eight modern towers, each soaring 20 stories in the air, linked by glass skybridges. It is its very own village, plopped smack dab in the middle of the city, with on-site cafes and markets. At the base of the buildings, a giant, open-air park with large-scale sculptures, water features sprinkled with lotus flowers, and avant garde seating areas. It feels like Le Centre Pompidou, and I half-hope a mime shows up and escorts me through the rest of the tour.

The agent guides us into the building closest to the entry gate and we ride to the 11th floor. The doors open to a moody, dimly lit space, covered top to bottom in black slate. Quite the contrast from the white exteriors with primary color accents tucked inside window frames and under the sky tunnels. This floor only has two large apartments. Light floods the dark hallway as she opens the door to apartment 11B.

It spills across the wide-plank floors, bouncing off the white walls and climbing all the way up to the tall ceilings. Wrapped in glass, shimmering like it was daring us to fill it with a life.

The walls are blank and bright, a clean slate in the most literal way. No history. No marks. No stories yet. The floors are smooth and light, the kind that feel solid when you walk across them. The windows stretch from one end to the other, framing the city like a moving painting, traffic below, sky above, everything in motion.

I hadn't let myself envision a home with Brett yet. But this could be the first place to belong to both of us. The first place where our routines will intertwine. Where coffee mugs will live permanently on the counter. Where arguments will echo briefly off those white walls and then soften. Where laughter will bounce higher than the ceilings.

I can imagine it at night, when the lights go down inside and the city shines beyond the glass. It's stark now, but it won't be. I'll bring the color, the texture, the Morgan touch, even the bangle bar. It will become our own suspended haven, like a glowing lantern.

I dial his number and tell him, "I've found the one!"

He replies, "Perfect, I have, too."

Two days later, feeling happy about a signed lease, we hop on a flight to Bangkok. Brett booked the Peninsula. Positioned on the banks of the Chao Phraya River, the Wat Arun Temple stands just across, commanding the skyline.

It feels surreal to show Brett more of my world, more of the work the Twins and I have been building for almost four years. To walk him through the factory, to introduce him to the production team, to stand beside him while we reviewed edits for Saks and QVC.

We comb through the samples, flag adjustments that should have already been updated, but had not advanced since our last visit in February. They assured me it was "in the works," and on the surface, everything feels pretty productive. Familiar. Grounded. Later that night, we have dinner with Pornkiat.

It starts out pleasant enough, polite conversation, shared dishes, small smiles. But I feel it almost immediately: something tight beneath the surface. Though he never met Richard, Pornkiat understands very clearly that Brett is not the husband I've spoken of in the past. There's confusion in his eyes. Even concern. It's none of his business, but he's making it so.

The questions begin to pile up: about the Twins and about their pregnancies. How long will they take off? Will they return? What is our plan? How do we move the business forward? The tone is careful, but the implication isn't.

Suddenly, what happened earlier at the factory clicks into place. The samples for Saks and QVC, due in just a few weeks, are nowhere near where they should be. Progress has slowed, noticeably. And now, it's obvious. The slowdown isn't accidental. It's coming from Pornkiat.

I do my best to answer every question, steady and measured. I reassure him that the purchase order from QVC will be finalized in the coming weeks, assuming, of course, that the adjustments we requested weeks ago are made. I remind him that our timelines depend on his follow-through.

I make it clear our personal lives have no bearing on our commitment to the brand, and find myself wondering if anyone would be drawing that line at all if we were men. I emphasize that the Twins' pregnancies and my marital status don't dilute our dedication. If anything, they sharpen it.

He listens. Nods. Asks a few more questions, but less sharp this time. By the end of dinner, the edge seems to have dulled. I leave feeling lighter. Believing he intends to honor his promises and meet his production obligations.

Next stop, Phuket.

Pulling up to our private villa at The Banyan Tree feels like stepping into a film. The dark teak gates open slowly, revealing a secluded haven wrapped in lush green and endless sky. The level of service in Southeast Asia is unparalleled, almost invisible in its perfection.

For 48 hours, we barely leave our little sanctuary. Breakfast and lunch are served poolside beside our enormous private infinity pool, the water blending seamlessly into the horizon. The world beyond our villa fades away.

Brett makes sure every detail is taken care of. Not just the obvious luxuries—the chilled towels, the fresh fruit, the perfectly timed coffee, but also me. He checks in daily about my medication, about whether I am resting enough, moving enough. He pays attention in a way that feels grounding, not intrusive.

His playful ideas for "boosting endorphins," mostly involve our bodies tangled together in the heat of the afternoon. The air carries the scent of sunscreen and salt and skin warmed by the sun. His hands rarely leave me, a simple reassurance of his love.

We drift in and out of the pool all day, cooling off and returning to the warmth, suspended in a slow, tropical rhythm.

By evening, we dress properly. Brett is in a linen suit. Me in a silk, backless gown, colorful bangles stacked up my arm. We make our way to dinner under the stars at one of the seaside restaurants. The ocean waves crash nearby, candlelight flickers, and for a while, everything is suspended in twinkling light, indulgent and intimate. Like a dream.

It would be so easy to fall into this life, claiming it as real, but I know better. Life comes in waves. This is one hell of a good swell, but inevitably, it will crash. Hopefully, my mental toolbox is more equipped to handle whatever life throws at me now.

Come Monday, I'm back in New York. The chilly temps are rolling in now. A bed all my own in the teeny space I share with a few of Cinderella's mice friends awaits me. Turns out my thought of a "mouse hole" wasn't so off base. Apparently, living in a building with a restaurant comes with both convenience and a few uninvited roommates. But I love my tiny space and my newfound independence. It's the leaving Brett part, and the peace he brings me that is hard.

Luckily, this goodbye feels easier.

The Yankees just clinched the American League Pennant, securing their spot in the World Series. Suddenly, the timing shifts in our favor. Brett will head back to the U.S. a few days earlier than we originally thought, only 10 days after me.

And he has a plan.

His idea of winning over my dad isn't with a bottle of good Kentucky bourbon (although a bottle of Pappy van Winkle would do the trick) or forced conversation, it's baseball. He invites Dad to Game Two with us. My dad, an avid fan his entire life, has somehow never been to a World Series game. Some might call it bribery, but Brett doesn't see it that way. He sees it as setting the stage, giving them something shared to stand on before the harder conversations begin. A night under stadium lights. The roar of the crowd. A common language spoken in innings and statistics.

If he's going to earn a place in my dad's heart, he might as well start in the bleachers.

The plan is a success.

The cherry on top is that the Yankees win.

A few days later, Brett's parents arrive in NYC. After a failed attempt back in July, I'm thrilled and anxious for a second chance to meet them. Unfortunately, I don't have the equivalent of World Series tickets in my back pocket. Just little old me, properly medicated with fresh blonde highlights and a super cute (hopefully Ohio mom-approved) dress for a double date at Les Halles over lunch.

Another success. They could see Brett's love for me, his care, his constant attention. And I think their levelheaded, Midwestern attitude appreciated my candor. At this point, I have nothing left to hide.

I'm an open book. My pages are a little stained, corners well worn, but still, I'm a story worth reading.

The whirlwind of introductions continues when Greer and Addy fly in for a one-night-only meet-and-greet with Brett. For some reason, I'm more nervous about this than when I met his parents.

Brett has a certain way about him.

He's not a Southern guy. He doesn't dress like one. He doesn't sound like one. He has absolutely no idea what Croakies are, and he's never heard of Wallabees. I'm sure he owns a pair of Nantucket reds somewhere in a closet, but they're reserved strictly for the coast. You won't catch him wearing them around the city.

Brett shows up as himself. Tailored but effortless. Confident, and sometimes a little loud. The kind of man who will charm the entire table without trying and then forget to mention he just paid for it. I don't know what they'll think of him. I don't know if he'll pass whatever unspoken test we've all been trained to administer. And I wish I didn't care, but these girls, they're like family. I want them to love him. I want them to understand that it's real.

The bar on lower Park Avenue glows in low, amber light. Glasses clink, ice settles. The space is modern and newly renovated. We picked it for the bar area. Beautiful and big. No issues scoring a good spot.

Brett and I arrive first and claim a small corner of the bar, standing close, the white honed marble cool under my fingertips. I smooth my dress once, unnecessarily.

"You're nervous," Brett says, not looking up as he signals for drinks.

"I'm not nervous," I say, too quickly.

He glances at me with a quiet smile. "You are."

"I'm just . . . aware," I correct, tucking my hair behind my ear. "This is a lot of worlds colliding."

"Your worlds," he says easily.

Exactly.

Greer and Addy arrive together, already mid-laugh, their excitement cutting cleanly through the room. I spot them before they see me and lift a hand.

"There they are," I say, as if Brett couldn't spot the lookalikes or feel the energy shift in the room when they stepped through the door.

We run towards each other, as we always do. Loud. Mildly obnoxious. Completely unbothered by perception. Greer hugs me first. Warm, steady, a quick squeeze that says more than anything she could say out loud. Addy follows, a little tighter, a little quicker, already looking past me.

"And this must be Brett," she says.

He steps forward, easy, self-assured without trying. Slim jacket, open collar, no tie. He looks exactly like himself.

"Actually, it's Keith to you," he says, with a big grin on his face. Proud of his joke, he looks to Greer. "And clearly, we've spoken before." He winks. It's the perfect ice breaker. We all laugh. Awkwardly at first and then, at similar times, we all relax, leaning into what could have been uncomfortable, we choose otherwise. And the laughter becomes real, natural.

"It's really great to finally meet 'the Twins.' I've heard so much about you," he says. Nodding towards me, he adds, "This one is always saying how you're family to her."

Drinks arrive, champagne for Brett and me. Soda waters with lime, served in wine glasses for the double buns in the oven. We don't sit. We hover, shifting slightly to make room as the bar fills in around us.

"So," Addy says, leaning in just enough to be heard, "tell us about yourself, Brett."

There it is.

Brett doesn't hesitate and asks, "What do you want to know?"

Greer smiles. "Careful, that's a dangerous question with us," she warns.

"I can handle it," he says, with a hint of a grin.

And he does.

He answers without overselling and asks questions back that feel real. Within minutes, Addy is laughing—fully, not politely. Greer watches him in that pensive way she has, taking it in, measuring without making it obvious.

I let myself step back just slightly, watching the exchange.

At one point, Addy tilts her head and asks, "But you've never been to the Derby right?"

"No, but it's always been on my list. Should we all go?" he asks.

Greer and Addy exchange a look. It's one that says they would love to, with an undertone that it will likely never happen, certainly not in the near future. Too many wounds waiting back in Texas.

But even so, the bar feels warmer now, or maybe, it's just us. The space loosens. Brett catches the bartender's eye at some point, subtle, practiced, and when the check comes, it disappears just as quickly. No announcement. No pause.

Of course.

I catch Greer's eye across the small circle we've made. There's something at rest. Addy studies Brett a beat longer than necessary, then nods, almost to herself.

"Well," she says finally, "I get it."

He passed. I try not to smile too obviously. Because I did want this. I wanted them to see him the way I do. To understand it's real. But also, if you don't like Brett, that's not his problem. It's yours.

Over the next few weeks, things start to slip. Not all at once. Like slow-motion dominoes. Greer calls first.

"Saks is out," she says, her voice careful in that way that tells me she's already processed it but realizes that I have not. "They're not taking on any new shapewear right now or any new brands at all."

I close my eyes, pressing my fingers lightly to my temple. "Okay," I say. "That's okay. We still have . . . "

"Maidenform paused acquisitions this morning," she adds, smoothly cutting in.

I let out a breath that feels thinner than it should. "Of course they did," I say.

Another pause.

"And QVC?" I ask, even though I already feel the answer forming.

She hesitates.

"Morgan . . . Pornkiat missed the final sample deadline," she says.

The words land slower this time. Heavier.

"They pulled the PO," she confirms.

"Greer," I begin, "I hate to say it, but I had a feeling this might happen when we were with him in Thailand. He was so hesitant, resistant even, to prepare the exact samples in final production quality as they demand. He didn't understand the process, though I really did plead with him. I promise you."

A week ago, we were celebrating it—calling it our turning point. Something that proved we were moving forward. And now, it's gone.

"I know how hard you worked in Bangkok," she says." I know you thought it helped."

I swallow. "I did think that."

"I did, too," she says quickly.

But it didn't. Neither of us know what to say now. The uncertainty hangs in the air. We hang up a few minutes later. The room is suddenly too quiet, too still. I sit for a second, staring at nothing. It feels like the end of an era. And now, all the reasons I said I would stay have vanished almost overnight.

While the Yankees playing in the World Series was a bonus visit for Brett, we always knew that he would be in the States in early November for the wedding of his dear friends in Connecticut. He arranged a car service to drive us out. We packed one bottle of fancy Dom for the happy couple, and one bottle of yellow label Veuve on ice for us to drink during the ride.

About 20 minutes outside of the city, my phone rings. It's my landlord. At first, it alarms me. I fear something is wrong with the place. Cheryl is a dream and the kindest woman. She and her husband bought the property as a long-term investment, but in the interim, their daughter, Kelsey, was able to live there during school at FIT. She is on a small sabbatical for some reason, hence the sublet. The reason for Cheryl's call is simple. Kelsey wants to come back to school in the spring, starting January. Cheryl assures me that the lease is mine for as long as our contract reads, but if there is a chance that I want out early, they will be happy to move Kelsey back in, versus finding her another temporary spot.

"One second, Cheryl," I mute our side of the call. Brett already heard everything she said on speaker phone.

He looks me right in the eyes. "Move to Beijing," he says. "Be with me. Every day. Every meal. Every moment. Let's do this . . . for real."

Everything in my body wants to say yes. Is this mania? Is this me? I hate having to question the two. For a moment, I wonder if I'll ever be able to definitely tell the two things apart. Will I ever be confident in making grand life decisions? And then, I let my shoulders relax. They drop inches, and I take a deep breath. What if a part of my mania is my superpower? What if it allows me to take bigger risks than others ever will? What if it opens me to a world I may have never dreamed of?

I unmute the phone. "Cheryl, Kelsey can have the apartment," I tell her. "I'm moving to Beijing!"

The phone slips from my fingers as Brett wraps his arms around me, pulling me into his lap and kissing me all over. He reaches for the cooler, pulls out two plastic flutes, and a bottle of champagne. The Dom. Of course. Such a Brett move. Typically, I would avoid plastic stemware for a splurge bottle of champs, but I make an exception.

"This calls for the good stuff," he says, smiling and pours two glasses. "Cheers, love," he toasts, holding up his glass, "To us. Forever."

"Cheers!" I toast, and we kiss.

Like always.

Chapter 25

THE SET BACK

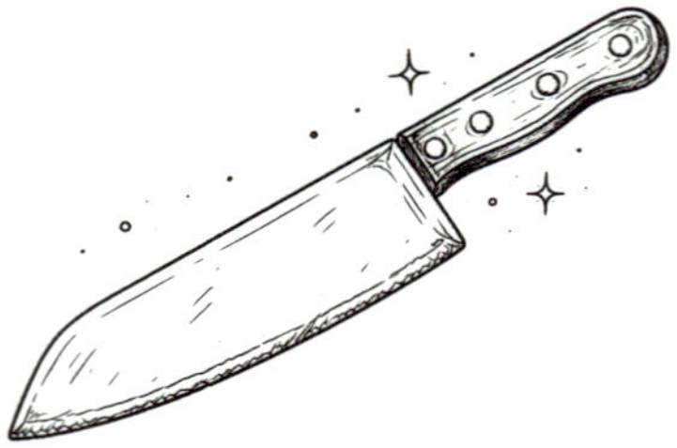

FALL 2009
New York City

It's human nature to want a villain. When something goes wrong, especially something as unsettling as mental illness and suicide attempts, we look for the "cause." If we pinpoint the "cause," then we can remove it and move on. Problem solved.

I think those closest to me, and some small part of me, too, want to believe that Richard was the root of it all. As if mental illness works like a bad roommate you can politely ask to leave.

But that's not how it works.

Richard may not have made things easier. He may not have had the bandwidth or desire to be my support system, but he didn't create my illness. Removing him from my life has not removed the diagnosis. Bipolar disorder doesn't pack up its bags because your marriage does, nor does it go away when you find a new, wonderful love. It would have been comforting if it were that simple. Clean. Cause and effect. But the truth is less convenient and far more nuanced.

November and December are blurring past at warp speed. My darling little nook in New York, the jewel box that felt, just three months ago, like such a declaration of independence suddenly reveals itself to be far more temporary than I'd imagined. After chatting for hours about our decision, I set my move date for Beijing just after Christmas. December 27. A clean break. A new year, in every sense.

There is a lot to do, in a short amount of time, but the biggest of all, are the goodbyes to make. Not to mention another trip to Beijing. This one is far less romantic, more logistical. Not to imply it won't be fun, just challenging. Brett is worried about me coming back to an empty apartment, cold and so far away from family and friends. The isolation is not lost on me, or him.

A visit back to select furniture and start the design process for our new apartment seems like the right thing to do. To have touches of me already in place when I arrive. More of a home, less of a sterile space where I don't know a soul outside of Brett. It feels strangely grown-up to be choosing sofas and dining tables for a life I haven't fully stepped into yet. And it feels undeniably strange to be spending Brett's money.

At one point, I let myself shift the narrative. I tell myself I'm his interior designer. A role that isn't much of a stretch given my background and college major. Suddenly, it becomes a project. A vision to execute.

I sift through markets, buying gorgeous silks and ordering custom curtains at insanely lower prices than back in the States. I pick out lamps and rugs, some from IKEA, some from beautiful home stores and some from the Chinese version of a swap meet, right on the streets of Beijing. I find art and have it framed in creative and over-the-top ways for pennies on the U.S. dollar. It is exhilarating to design with these resources. But it's also slightly terrifying to design a home in such a foreign place.This trip back to China is shorter than my first two trips. A quick in and out.

It's important that I get back to my goodbyes in the States. To tie up loose ends. Not because I won't return often. I know I will. It's one of the key subjects of conversation with Brett. The importance of coming back, of staying connected to the people I love. Reassuring them that I'm okay. This move isn't just geography; it's a signal that my life is moving on, changing.

It also means stepping away from Jet Set Lingerie. And that is harder than I expect. I hadn't realized how much of my identity is woven into the brand. The late nights, the risks, the inside jokes, the way it feels like ours in a way nothing else ever has. I'm also slightly caught off guard by the Twins. I mistakenly think the babies on the way, combined with the slow unraveling of our three major opportunities, might make them want to pause, too.

Instead, they ask to buy me out. And none of us is prepared for the letter. Drafted by Pornkiat's lawyer. Cold. Formal. Final.

It demands we end our partnership immediately, and with it, our ability to produce both the shapewear and intimacies collections. In an instant, the factory is no longer ours to rely on. A forced buyout. The loss of our production home. Years of infrastructure pulled out from beneath us with the clean detachment of legal language.

It's devastating to the brand. But the grief that follows isn't just about business. What unsettles me more is the strain it places on the longest and most important friendships of my life.

Stress has a way of distorting things. Of taking what is true and sharpening it just enough to cut. Conversations that would have once felt easy start to carry edges. At one point, one of the Twins says it, carefully, but still:

"Well . . . it's easier for you to walk away."

A pause.

"The money you put in . . . it's from your ex-husband, so what does it matter?"

And then, softer but heavier, "Ours came from our dad."

I know what they mean.

Their inheritance wasn't just money. It represented him. The father they loved unequivocally. The father who would do anything for his girls. The man who gave 110% to those he cared about, even from his deathbed. It was a piece of him, carried forward into something we built together. Of course, it feels heavier to them. But hearing it, in that moment, stung. Like my stake in our company was somehow less real. Less earned. Less mine.

Something in me pulls taut. They're not wrong. But they're also not right. And I know, somewhere underneath it, that this is what stress does. It pulls the hardest truths to the surface, but without gentleness. Without the correct context.

Their stress makes it come out harsher than they mean. And mine, my stress of staying with Richard, of trying to hold together something already fractured, makes my decision to pause the business sound lighter than it actually feels. Like I'm walking away easily. But I'm not. I'm choosing between two things that both matter to me. And somehow, in the pressure of it all, that nuance gets lost.

The fear of losing Greer and Addy, of something altering permanently between us, hurts more than anything. More than the brand. More than my marriage.

It's strange how you can be so sure about a decision, so genuinely excited for a fresh start, and still grieve what you're leaving behind.

In the middle of all of it, I am doing what I am supposed to do. I am taking my medication. Responsibly. Diligently. No shortcuts. No skipped doses.

Still, my sleep slips. Just a little. The rhythm gets off-balance, and with it, so do I. I pull out every cognitive therapy trick up my sleeve. I reread crayon scribbled journal entries from East Pines, underlining the parts where I'd promised myself that I'd recognize the warning signs. I try to stay ahead of it.

Brett is working nonstop, preparing to take the week of Christmas off to come back and help me move. Christmas isn't a work holiday in China, and the investors aren't thrilled about him stepping away, mostly from an optics standpoint. He needs to get ahead. To prove himself. To show that he isn't distracted. I can see he feels he has to earn the right to leave. So, he works longer days. Later nights. I try not to need him too much. But I am not going to make myself small.

This move to Beijing is as much an adventure for me as it is a way to be near Brett. Our love is so new. He jokes about me being "his," but never as a possession. It was sharing me with another man that he didn't want. He loves my gusto for life. My courage to go out, to do, to explore, without asking him to always be by my side.

Even with the existing disractions, I can feel something coming. I fear it. Brett is deep into reading multiple books about bipolar and is now starting to understand the signs and triggers. I'm not trying to, nor do I want to, hide anything from him, but our time apart makes it easy to do. From the very beginning, I've been an open book. And he has always been receptive, interested, never judgmental. But I mistakenly think that I can handle what I know is happening inside me on my own.

November 29, 2009, 5 a.m.—Brett's Apartment, Beijing

It's is getting colder by the day. The city sits at a similar latitude to Denver, which equates to highs of 40 and lows in the teens come fall. The blustery winds from the Mongolian Plateau add another layer of cold, which I discover upon googling, "Why is it so cold in Beijing?" Naturally, I stock up on fun puffer jackets and gorgeous furs from the Russian markets, far too many of them.

Brett isn't mad, but he is concerned. Impulsive purchases like these are a major indicator of mania on the horizon. Sensing something might be off, we do what we can to reduce my alone time during the last few days of my visit. The driver brings me out to Brett's office every day to have lunch with him, and I start meeting him at restaurants for dinner, rather than waiting for him to get home. It shaves hours off as the traffic can be unbearable at that time of day.

But there is only so much you can do. Sometimes, the disease takes over. Even in happy times, it creeps in. I had been unhappy so long before this, I never dreamed I could slip now.

A few days before my return flight to the States, my last trip before my official move, I wake up before dawn. On a typical day, Brett would pull my body to his and roll me on top. We would make love. Sometimes soft and sweet. Sometimes so passionate, I thought I might explode. A fantastic way to wake up. In all my years of marriage, morning sex was never a part of the equation.

From a disease point of view, the endorphins from physical touch have the potential to curb the depressive lows. But with mania on the horizon, it becomes a trigger. New territory for me indeed.

I get out of bed. Make coffee, something I only recently learned to do well, and try to read my journals. My eyes bounce all over the page. I desperately want to go for a walk, but it's dark and freezing. I go to the spare bedroom and do a few sets of jumping jacks. Trying to expell the extra energy. My skin, crawling from the inside out, feels like it is full of ants just under the surface.

When Brett wakes up, he finds me on my knees, beside the guest bed, praying. Not to say it's a last resort, but I often try the more medical options before this one, even though I know how much it helps.

Praying is not something that would ever alarm Brett. The jumping jacks, on the other hand, would have been a tell-tale sign.

We shower together and get ready side by side. When he leaves for the office, I feel like I should ask him to stay, but I shove the desire deep inside.

"Can't wait to see you tonight," he says, walking out the door, "Da Dong in Sanlitun at 7, right?"

"Yes, of course, see you then, love," I say and close the door behind him.

As soon as it warms up a bit, I get outside. I spend all day distracting myself. Meandering. I even find my way inside the commercial signage shop just across the street and order a giant, custom Lucite sign, a clear back with *Nĭ Hao* in bold neon pink. The perfect welcome art for our entryway. A bright "HELLO" as soon as you walk in. I start to feel a bit less buzzy, so I feel safe to go home. Even though I will be alone.

Around 4 p.m., the stirring inside my body is back, almost too much to bear. Brett has texted a few times, but I can't focus long enough to type a response.

I scratch. Conitnuously. Eventually, tearing through my tights. The spot on my thigh is already red. Then, the skin finally breaks.

By 6 p.m., I am in a full tailspin. Overwhelmed by my own existence. I need out. Out of my body. Out of this place. I'm trapped. I can hear myself mumbling, "Get me out, get me out."

It's as if I'm watching myself from above, hovering over this mess of a human. I walk, almost mechanically to the kitchen and take a large chef's knife from the magnetic strip mounted to the sleek backsplash, all white and shiny—the most modern kitchen I've ever seen in real life.

I walk to the far-left window, one of the few that opens wide. I place my right hand, holding the butcher knife against the screen and pull down with all my force. Puncturing right through it. The metal mesh tears back toward me, and I punch it forward, creating a full opening.

In my bare feet, wearing only a lightweight sweater dress, I step onto the cold metal ledge. Only concrete and the massive lily pad pond are beneath me, 11 floors below. I stand there with the knife, still in my hand. Ready to step off . . .

Time passes.

I don't hear the front door open.

But suddenly, Brett is there.

His arms reaching through the window, beyond the broken screen. His hands wrap around my waist, tighter than I've ever felt them. It hurts, startling me. The knife falls from my hands, dropping onto the ledge and sliding to the far end of the window sill, teetering on the edge.

He pulls me inside, my heels hitting the bottom of the window frame. I can't feel it. I hear it, though. My feet are numb from the cold. I don't have a concept of time. Everything seems to happen at once.

"Baby, are you okay?" Brett gasps. "What were you doing out there? Why would you . . . ? When you didn't text me back, I got so worried, so I rushed home. God, what would I do without you. What would any of us do? Please, please talk to me. What can I do?"

My mind slips back to another moment like this.

Fall 2008, Dallas

The bathroom light is too bright. It flattens everything; the tile, the mirror, the water climbing too high along the edge of the tub. I'm already in. Under the weight of it. It's warm. Welcoming.

The water laps just below the rim, threatening to spill. The room is quiet except for the dull, underwater sound filling my ears. Everything feels distant, muted, like I'm on the ceiling, looking down at another version of my body, slightly removed, slightly delayed.

The water wraps around me. I close my eyes. I'm tired. Not just physically. A deeper kind of tired. I can't keep up with the constant noise in my head, the churn of it, the effort. It's the kind of tired quietly suggesting the world might run more smoothly without me in it.

The water feels calm. Still. Like a place I can settle into. A place that doesn't ask anything of me. A place to rest. To disappear. No questions asked. And then, I hear it. Muffled at first, through the warmth surrounding me.

Richard's voice.

Sharp. Immediate. Breaking through everything. Closing in fast. Hands are on me before I can react, pulling my arms, abrupt, unceremonious. The water surges over the edge, spilling hard onto the ceramic tile. The air hits my skin cold and sudden, shocking me back into my body. My cotton wrapdress clings, heavy, dripping, pooling at my feet as he drags me up and out.

I cough. Blink. Desperately trying to orient myself. The room feels louder now. Even brighter than before. Mostly wrong.

And there's Richard, standing in front of me, pushing a monogrammed towel at me. My instinct isn't to wrap myself. It's to bend quickly drying my dripping mess before he comments.

"I knew you'd do something stupid like this," he says as I kneel to clean up the mess I've made. Disgust fills the air.

No pause. No softness. No asking if I'm okay. Just anger. Exasperation. I'm not fully back in my body, but I do understand that I interrupted his Saturday. I created a problem he now has to deal with.

In this fragile space, somewhere between disappearing and being pulled back, Richard doesn't meet me with concern. He meets me with contempt. Not because he found me. Though I wish he hadn't. But because of how he did.

It's painfully clear that my illness is too much for him. It probably is for anyone. And I get it now. I will have to leave. For good.

I just don't know how to do it yet.

November 29, 2009, Around 7 p.m.—Brett's Apartment, Beijing

Brett wraps me in a quilted blanket and carries me to the couch. When my body warms, my trance subsides along with the shivers. His forehead is touching mine. Tears in his eyes. Fear all over his face. His Italian skin, white as a ghost.

"Oh God, I'm so sorry, Brett," I cry. "I don't know . . . it just happened. Like I was watching myself do it. I really thought . . . " I paused. "I really tricked myself into believing I might be cured." The tears rolled down my face. "But I'm not. This darkness is a part of me. I don't think it's going anywhere. I don't think it ever will. It's something I will always have to manage."

"No, my love," he said, "it's something we will always have to manage. I'm in this with you. But you have to talk to me. I knew something was wrong this morning. I should have said something. I should have stayed. But like you, I wanted to believe that, maybe, by a miracle . . ." He doesn't want to say it, but it has to be said. "That being together might change things."

"Oh, Brett," I assure him, "It has, in so many ways. But just because I'm happy and safe with you, doesn't mean I'm healed. But it does mean that I have even more of a reason to keep going, to keep learning how to treat and live with the imbalances my body throws at me. Thank you for being kind, for not making me feel like a burden."

"You are never a burden. Ever," he says.

He goes to the kitchen. Fixes me a bowl of soup, with a big stack of saltines. The brand name ones. A splurge here in Beijing at $12 USD for a box at the international market, but it's something he has stocked in the pantry or in the hotel room for every one of my visits.

We crawl into bed before 9 p.m. Exhausted, nestled in his arms, I fall into a deep sleep.

Chapter 26

THE BLONDE IN BEIJING

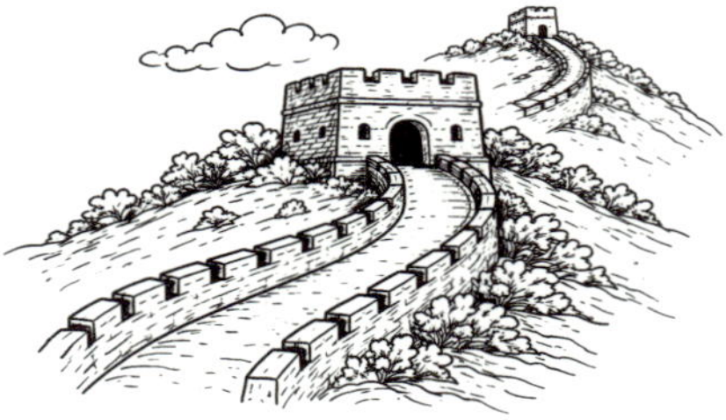

DECEMBER 9, 2009
New York City

Back in the States for less than three weeks before my move, and after my setback in Beijing, I schedule biweekly calls with my doctor. We're trying to figure out what medicinal shifts we need to explore, but also, he's worried that any major change during the move, one he doesn't fully support, could cause more problems. His biggest concern is that I find a permanent doctor in Beijing as soon as I arrive. Brett is already on the case.

Surprisingly, it turns out that international mental health care is much easier than it is in the States. No insurance hoops to jump through. No wait times. Brett produces a list of doctors for me to choose from within a week. This would have taken months in the US.

I decide to go with an expat, from Georgia actually. And blonde. We are able to have a call ahead of my move, and we scheduled my first in-person appointment for the second week of January.

Not surprising, my mom, similar to my psychiatrist, is also not on board with my move. She also doesn't love that my dad encourages it so freely. He doesn't approve of long-distance love; he's notorious for his opposition of it. He strongly believes you need to understand the ins and outs of everyday life to know if a relationship will work out long-term. He told me I was living in a "layover." Quite a fitting reference seeing as

I've been dressing as a fake flight attendant for the last four years.

For better or worse, I decide to tell Mom and Dad about the setback. In the name of my newly embraced transparency, it was, without question, for the worse.

Naturally, it scares everyone. It's one thing to suspect instability; it's another to have it confirmed out loud. Like Brett, and, if I'm honest, like a small hopeful part of myself, they wanted to believe that Richard was the primary catalyst. If you removed him, the volatility would disappear. Now, it's painfully clear he was never the cause.

And yet, oddly, there is also peace.

They listen closely as I share the difference between the two instances—how Brett handled it versus Richard. The way Brett reacted. His steadiness. The fact that he stayed grounded when things wobbled. And I think that gives them something solid to hold onto.

Because if I'm not moving back home, which, at this point, is absolutely not an option, then they can at least see that I'm not alone in this.

The last few weeks in New York are filled with packing, shedding things I don't need or want, and visiting with friends all over the city. Uptown, Downtown, East Side, West Side.

Brett arrived back in New York a few days ahead of our planned trips. First to Knoxville, Tennessee, to meet Addy's baby girl. Then to Kentucky to see my family, and finally, to Ohio to see his.

But sadly, a surprise blizzard hits the city. Dumping 15 inches of snow in record time. Thousands of flights are cancelled, including ours. We can't fly out for at least two days. In fact, we can't get out of New York fast enough to not encroach into time with both of our families, a non-negotiable for either side. Brett makes calls and finds a flight leaving from Philly to Nashville the next day and books a car service to take us first thing in the morning. I find a special comfort in his take-charge attitude. It provides a peace inside that I didn't even know I needed. But I do.

Addy and I sob on the phone together when I share the news. I'm devastated that I'll have to wait to meet her precious new addition. Our future foursome. Made harder by the fact that I don't know exactly when I'll even be back to the States.

As I talk with her on the phone, crying between my words, Brett chimes in, "How about we book you a ticket to Dallas after Greer's baby is born. Addy, you'll be there for that, right? Then, you can meet them both?"

Though it didn't go exactly how I wanted it to, this was a nice consolation prize.

After I hang up with her, Brett and I decide to shake off the sad mood. We get dressed in our warmest clothes and venture out to see what restaurants might be open. Luckily, Pearl Oyster Bar, one of our mutual faves, has two seats left at the counter. We order the largest seafood tower on the menu and toast with La Chouffe. Even with puffy eyes, red from the tears, it's one of those nights that I oddly know I will never forget. The warmth of the restaurant. The snow falling outside. A glistening city looking so fresh and clean entirely covered in snow.

We talk about our families, practicing names, connecting all the dots between which uncle belongs to which aunt. The cousins' names, where they live and what they do. We prepare for our visits and talk about family Christmas traditions.

Buzzy on beer, we walk back to my apartment for the last time, Brett's arm wrapped around my shoulders. Me bundled in a fur coat and hat with snow boots. Him in a camel overcoat and suede Ferragamo shoes, being ruined by the unexpected snow.

The next morning, the town car picks us up bright and early, and we hustle to Philadelphia to make our flight. First stop, Nashville. My mom and dad will pick us up together. We will celebrate with my dad's side of the family in my hometown, a two-hour drive from the

Nashville airport, the closest option.

Christmas at my dad's house is, first and foremost, about the food. Becky outdoes herself every year. An extravagant spread appears as if conjured, rack of lamb cooked perfectly pink, a bubbling lasagna that could feed a small army, and no fewer than three salads to convince us we're exercising restraint.

And then there's dessert. Becky's mother is the family's secret weapon. She's an expert baker. The dessert lineup is impressive: pies, bars, layered creations that require both engineering and patience. But the Italian cream cake reigns supreme. It is, without question, the crown jewel and forever at the top of my list.

Somewhere between second helpings and a nip of bourbon-infused eggnog, Brett makes his rounds.

He meets my dad's only sister, the one with bipolar, and her two boys. He listens, and he asks thoughtful questions (in between all the questions they're asking him). He laughs at the right moments. He spends real time with Mama Jean, the matriarch of the family and the unofficial gatekeeper of her only granddaughter. She grills him the hardest, naturally. Direct questions. Long pauses. Evaluating eyes.

He doesn't flinch.

By the end of the night, after the plates are cleared and the stories get louder, the consensus is unanimous: Grandy Mac, my dad's dad—a treasured man, gone to soon—would have loved Brett. The jokes. The easy charm. The ability to spin a little nonsense with total confidence. The big, steady energy.

Somehow, that feels like the highest approval of all.

The next day, we drive four hours to northern Kentucky, just outside of Cincinnati to my Aunt Lorna's. This is the portion of our tour where Brett meets my mother's entire side of the family—both of her sisters, their husbands, their only-child daughters, and my grandparents, Nannie and Bubba.

I'm not as close to this set of grandparents, but they are

loving, kind, and funny. Bubba is the best joke-teller this side of the Mason-Dixon. The kind who leans back in his chair, clears his throat dramatically, and absolutely commits to the punch line. Sometimes a little dirty, sometimes with the cleanness of a joke off the back of a Laffy Taffy wrapper.

Lorna, my mom's middle sister, will be the hardest on Brett. She's a tough crowd. Sharp. Observant. Not easily impressed. But she'll soften eventually, probably somewhere between offering her tenth casserole and the best mashed potatoes you've ever had. Her love language is starch. Her husband, Greg's, is bacon.

Mom brings her homemade fudge, her signature dish and Bubba's favorite, wrapped neatly in wax paper, inside a Christmas tin, like it's currency. It disappears faster than anything else on the table.

By the time dinner winds down, we gather in the living room for the annual Chinese Gift Auction. Dirty Santa. White Elephant. It has a thousand names, but the rules are sacred, and competitiveness is real. Alliances form. Betrayals happen. Someone inevitably fights over a Christopher Radko ornament.

The gifts Brett and I packed are actually from China, which feels poetic in a way no one else quite understands. Little pieces of the life we're building, folded into this loud, crowded, full of creamed corn room.

I watch Brett hold his own, laughing, swapping gifts, letting Bubba finish long stories without interrupting. I realize he doesn't need to try that hard. He fits.

Suddenly, I'm nervous about how I'll fit at his parent's house.

Mom and Lorna drive us to Columbus the next day. Mom is buzzing with curiosity. She wants to know all the details. Who Brett's parents are. What their house looks like. Where it sits, what kind of neighborhood. She's mentally cataloging everything before we even arrive.

Lorna, on the other hand, is mostly focused on confirming that they're not serial killers. A very Lorna concern.

We get there early. It's a quick drive from Cincinnati, and before long, the seven of us are seated at their country club for lunch. Cory, Brett's brother, is in town, too.

Somehow, it's . . . easy.

The conversation flows in that cautious but genuine way these things sometimes do. Of course, there are a few pauses, small pockets of silence where everyone recalibrates. But Donna, Brett's mom, handles them effortlessly. One of 14 children, she has clearly spent a lifetime navigating noise, filling gaps, and smoothing edges. She knows exactly what to say and when to say it. She's kind. A little dry but deeply loving.

Brett's dad, Tom, is funny. Every other sentence has a tinge of sarcasm. He's the kind of man who shows affection by lightly picking on you. But deep down, you know he's a softy, a teddy bear in a jokester body. Mom and Lorna, having been raised by Bubba, immediately recognize this dialect of love.

And Cory, he's exactly what a little brother (who is no longer little) should be. Supportive without hovering. Warm without trying too hard. He makes the whole table feel relaxed. Me especially.

At some point, I realize I've unclenched. The worlds aren't colliding. They're blending. What a relief.

When Mom and Lorna go to leave, Tom walks them to the car.

"Thanks for driving them up here," he says. "So glad we got to meet and spend some time together before these two head 6,000 miles away. And hey, at least you know now that we aren't serial killers."

Mom and Lorna keel over in laughter. What are the odds that he would say the exact thing Lorna had been thinking since we planned the visit? She filled him in on why they were laughing so hard, and everyone got the giggles.

Brett and I follow Mom all the way to the car. Lorna gets in the driver's seat this time. Knowing her sister all too well. Driving through the tears would be too dangerous.

Mom hugs Brett first.

"I know she can take care of herself, but you take care of her, too. Take care of each other," she says, holding back the tears for as long as she can.

"Mona, you come anytime you want," Brett says. "Just pick a date. And yes, I will always take care of her. I love her more than I've ever loved anything."

My turn.

Neither of us have the words to fit the moment. Everything and nothing to say at the same time. How do you move across the world from the one person who loves you unconditionally?

"Morgie, call anytime. Don't let the 14-hour time change stop you. And I'm just a 24-hour flight away," she says, mustering up a laugh. "You'll have to give me a little extra warning if you need me."

"I'll always need you, Mom," I say. "But I've got this. Don't make me cry too hard. I've got to look cute to meet all their friends tonight at their Christmas party!" I tease.

We both laugh a little, and she takes her place in the passenger side. Life will be different now. This is the farthest I've ever lived from home. Even farther than London, and far more foreign. But I know deep down, she's excited for me. Even if she can't say it out loud. Brett and I stand at the end of his parents' driveway, waving one last time before their car fades out of sight.

That night, 50 or 60 of Tom and Donna's closest friends pour into the house for their annual Christmas party. The kitchen counters disappear under trays of food, salty, savory, sweet. Bowls of dip, platters of cheese, and all kinds of things wrapped in bacon. Towering above it all are piles of Tom's famous garbage cookies with every conceivable ingredient packed into one chaotic, glorious bite. They are exactly what they sound like and somehow completely perfect. Tom is deep in his Food Network phase, post his recent retirement.

The living room is filled with men ranging in age from Cory's to older than Tom. It's loud and animated. Lots of talk about the Detroit Lions. The formal dining room, however, is a different ecosystem entirely. It's Donna's lioness den. She sits at the head of it, surrounded by her closest friends. About an hour into the party, she invites me in.

Brett is stunned. He leans toward his mom and reminds her, intentionally loud enough for the entire room to hear, that he has never once been invited into that circle. Not him. Nor any girl he has ever brought home.

Nervous as all get out, I smooth down my red fit-and-flare dress. It's vintage, a remake of a timeless 1950s silhouette, but made in the '80s by Victor Costa. There's just enough swing in the skirt to feel festive but still tasteful. I hope she approves. I hope all of them do.

Of course, Brett has brought home girls before. Beautiful ones. Smart ones. Interesting ones. None of them were previously married. None of them were openly living with mental illness. (Or at least none who admitted it . . .)

After 38 years of waiting for him to "find the one," I can't help but wonder if I look like what they'd imagined.

I step into the lioness den.

And it is . . . lovely.

They are warm. Curious in the best way. Supportive. Genuinely approving. They remind me so much of my mom's friend group, the women who helped raise me, who showed up in enormous ways when I returned to Murray in August.

For over an hour, we talk about families, about travel, about marriage, about life. They ask real questions. They listen to the answers. I ask them questions back, curious who belongs to whom outside the walls of this room.

When Brett finally hovers at the doorway, half-grinning, asking if they are ever going to let him have me back, I stand up right in front of Donna.

"I know you've waited a long time for him to find the one, and I'm sure that you weren't expecting or hoping for a bipolar divorcée—"

She stops me right there. She won't allow whatever is coming. "Morgan, you're exactly what we've been waiting for," she interrupts, stepping in for a hug. She wraps her arms around me, deeply, like I already belong here as a part of the family.

The next day, they drove us to the Columbus airport. We spend one last night in my tiny, New York City apartment. And then, in the morning, as the sun rises over the city, we hop in a long black suburban, stuffed to the top with everything I'm bringing to Beijing.

I look up at the building, snow still resting on almost every windowsill. I look to the left, at the giant arch standing at the front of Washington Square Park and to my right, all the way Uptown on Fifth. Oh, what a difference six months can make. After a decade of hiding myself, my symptoms, and my disease, here I am, taking a chance on a fresh start. I know it will be hard. But I can do hard things.

I thought I might cry a little on the drive, but I'm too excited. Too happy to be with Brett. His smile is too contagious. It puts me at ease—always.

We drop off six suitcases and four moving boxes with the lovely people at the Continental desk, and head straight through security to begin our 14-hour journey east. The significance that this is our first time to make the flight together, moving me there for good, isn't lost on me.

On the plane, we toast the move with welcome champagne from the flight attendants. My favorite flight attendant is on board. This is now my third leg with her. Between all the back and forth, it seems we are flying in parallel schedules. She's not supposed to, but I encourage her to pour a glass and toast with us. She discreetly obliges. Brett and I celebrate for the first few hours, making plans of what we will do for our first weekend of my permanent residence in old Peking.

And then, we pop on our noise-cancelling earphones, matching gifts to each other that made us laugh when we opened them simultaneously. Perfectly in sync, we push the buttons on the screen to turn on a movie to watch in unison—*When Harry Met Sally*.

At some point, we both drift off to sleep and wake up to omelettes for breakfast and the notice that we are landing soon. We kiss as the wheels touch down on the runway.

As I step off the plane, the stub of a one-way ticket, layered with baggage claim stickers, in my left hand, and Brett's hand tightly gripped in my right, I see mountains in the distance. The tiniest glimpse of the Great Wall. It's a rare bluebird sky kind of day. The kind Beijing only sees a dozen times a year.

I might always be a Bipolar Blonde, but for the next little while, I'm going to focus on being a Blonde in Beijing.

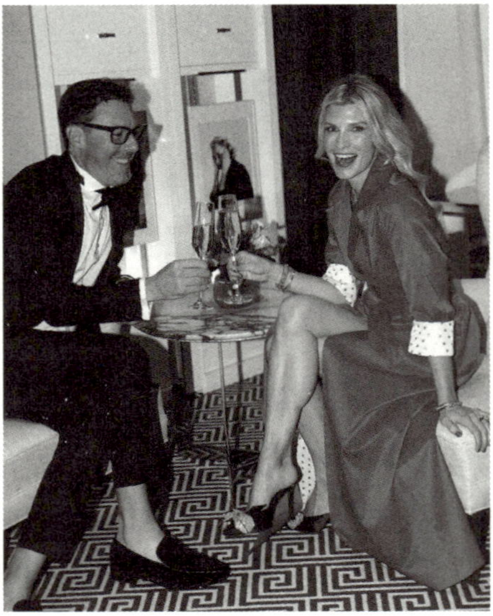

WHERE IS SHE NOW?

Nearly 20 years after her bipolar diagnosis, Morgan lives in California with her husband, Brett, her favorite plot twist, whom she's rarely been apart from since that fateful night at The Carlyle 17 years ago. Married for 15 years, Morgan and Brett spend their days running Buru, the women's clothing brand they cofounded in 2013, and raising their three children—Olive Bee, Schafer, and Carlyle—who keep them equal parts grounded and on their toes.

Morgan continues to navigate a full, vibrant life, while managing bipolar disorder with an openness about her experience, the right mix of medicines, thoughtful mental health care, and a support system of people who show up, again and again.

She chooses life every day—even when it's hard.

What once felt like a life sentence has, in time, revealed itself to be something else entirely—something powerful, even a superpower at times, if met head-on.

MADISON AV
E 76TH ST
Diet
Coke
M+B
25¢